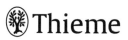

Reconstructive Facial Plastic Surgery

A Problem-Solving Manual

2nd Revised and Expanded Edition

Hilko Weerda, MD, DMD

Professor Emeritus
Department of Otorhinolaryngology—Head, Neck, and Plastic Surgery,
University Hospital Schleswig-Holstein, Campus Lübeck
Lübeck, Germany

1390 illustrations

In 2001, the first edition of this book was awarded the
George Davey Howells Memorial Prize in Otolaryngology
by the University of London and the Otology Section of the
Royal Society of Medicine, London, UK.

Thieme
Stuttgart · New York · Delhi · Rio

Library of Congress Cataloging-in-Publication Data is available from the publisher.

Illustrator: Original illustrations by Katharina Schumacher, Munich
Fig. 5.54: Illustration by Joachim Quetz, MD, originally published in Facial Plastic Surgery 2014; 30: 300–305
Additional illustrations by Thomson, India

Correspondence:
Prof. Hilko Weerda, MD, DMD
Freiburg, Germany
hubweerda@yahoo.de

1st English edition 2001
Reprint of 1st English edition 2007

© 2015 Georg Thieme Verlag KG
Thieme Publishers Stuttgart
Rüdigerstrasse 14, 70469 Stuttgart, Germany
+49 [0]711 8931 421
customerservice@thieme.de

Thieme Publishers New York
333 Seventh Avenue, New York, NY 10001 USA
1-800-782-3488 customerservice@thieme.com

Thieme Publishers Delhi
A-12, second floor, Sector-2, NOIDA-201301
Uttar Pradesh, India,
+91 120 45 566 00 customerservice@thieme.in

Thieme Publishers Rio Thieme Publicações Ltda.
Argentina Building, 16th floor, Ala A, 228 Praia do Botafogo,
Rio de Janeiro 22250-040 Brazil,
+55 21 3736-3631

Cover design: Thieme Publishing Group
Typesetting by primustype Robert Hurler GmbH,
Notzingen, Germany
Printed in Germany by Aprinta Druck, Wemding

ISBN 978-3-13-129642-9

Also available as an e-book:
eISBN 978-3-13-69632-8

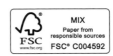

Contents

I   Anatomy, Principles of Facial Surgery, and Coverage of Defects

Special Part

II Coverage of Defects in Specific Facial Regions

III Rib Cartilage, Myocutaneous and Free Flaps, and Microvascular Surgery

Foreword to the 2nd Edition

The eagerly awaited second edition of Professor Hilko Weerda's beautifully concise, and influential guide to reconstructive facial plastic surgery combines a clarity of vision that results from years of analytical thought, with exemplary text. Almost 1,400 illustrations portray the approach and surgical planning for a myriad of surgical defects. While students of facial plastic surgery will find his instructions clearly described in a stepwise manner, more senior colleagues will also benefit from his insight into more complex problems. While there are numerous books on similar topics, those that can in any way rival this text in its scope and wisdom are few and far between. In my capacity as President of the European Academy of Facial Plastic Surgery, I would urge all surgeons interested in this field to have this book close at hand, on their work desks, and in the operating room's library, where it can act as a timely reminder of the best techniques available and a valuable teaching aid.

From a practical point of view, the surgeon is initially guided through the most important principles of facial reconstructive surgery, before being introduced to specialized sections that deal systematically with each of the major subunits of the face. Professor Weerda's pioneering work in auricular reconstruction is also clearly reflected in the appropriate sections in the book.

The specialty of facial plastic surgery has been growing exponentially over the past few years. This remarkable book will certainly act as a major leading light for our trainees and mentors. I would like to congratulate Professor Weerda and his team for this impressive achievement. It has already found permanent residence on my desk.

Professor Pietro Palma
President
European Academy of Facial Plastic Surgery
University of Insubria Varese
Milano, Italy

Foreword to the First Edition

Balancing the twin needs of functional and aesthetic facial defect reconstruction has challenged surgeons over the centuries to develop practical and utilitarian repair solutions. Professor Hilko Weerda, in typical meticulous fashion, presents in this text atlas a virtual encyclopaedia of reconstructive options for the thoughtful repair of a wide-ranging group of facial, head, and neck defects. The multiple options and alternatives available for defect repair and reconstruction presented in this volume have met the test of time world-wide.

Reconstruction in the head and neck region requires a dedication to meticulous planning. Facial plastic and reconstructive surgery is, in it's finest sense, a craft best developed over time and seasoned with experience. The thought process required in the planning of facial repair probably supercedes the technical skill involved in the surgical event itself. Techniques highly useful and indicated in one region of the face may not serve well for adjacent regions. Skin thickness, skin mobility, the presence of hair-bearing structures, and the junctions of facial landmarks must all be considered when the *most appropriate surgical option* is chosen. A tissue price is paid (by the patient) whenever regional tissues are advanced, rotated, transposed, or interposed to reconstruct defects–scarring, distortion, and asymmetries of the donor as well as the recipient site are everpresent possibilities. The surgeon's critical responsibility is to diminish the amount of that price to be paid by employing the correct reconstructive option. Given our present state of knowledge, the majority of challenging facial repairs should produce a *functionally useful* and *aesthetically admirable* outcome. As the brilliant reconstructive surgeon Gary Burget states: "the eye does not perceive cover, lining or support. It sees a pattern of graduated light and shadow ... color, texture and most importantly contour create the visual image ...".

Professor Weerda has succeeded admirably in authoring a comprehensive compendium designed to aid the reconstructive surgeon in assessing the various options and alternatives for facial repair.

M. Eugene Tardy, M.D., F.A.C.S.
Professor Emeritus of Clinical Otolaryngology–
Head and Neck Surgery
Director of Facial Plastic Surgery
Department of Otolaryngology–
Head and Neck Surgery
University of Illinois Medical Center
Chicago, Illinois, USA

Preface to the 2nd Edition

Particularly in this age of mass media, the face plays a pivotal role in human self-identification. Malformations, defects, and bony or soft-tissue changes caused by trauma or neoplasms can drastically alter the patient's appearance, frequently impacting on his or her feeling of self-worth. Drawing on our experience in the operating room and our many years of planning and conducting courses in plastic and reconstructive surgery, we have created an easy-to-use, step-by-step surgical textbook for the face and neck, based on informative illustrations and concise text. Sequences of drawings provide both the novice and the experienced facial surgeon with simple, reproducible solutions to many of the most commonly encountered problems and questions in facial plastic surgery.

In the 2nd expanded edition we were able to add color photographs, partly taken from slides, to show the situation before and after reconstruction. Along with the most commonly practiced reconstructive procedures, a number of other proposed technical solutions are presented, largely without commentary.

I express thanks to my colleagues Stephan Remmert, Konrad Sommer, Ralf Siegert, and Joachim Quetz for their excellent contributions. I thank Dr. S. Storz, Tuttlingen, for letting me use the illustrations of the basic instrument set and Mrs. Schumacher for providing most of the drawings that consistently conformed to the author's wishes. I also thank Mr. Konnry, Ms. Hengst, Ms. Hollins, and Ms. Kuhn-Giovannini of Thieme Publishers for their outstanding work in the production of this book.

Hilko Weerda

Contributors

Joachim Quetz, MD
Supervising Physician
Department of Otorhinolaryngology, Head and Neck Surgery
University Clinic Schleswig-Holstein, Campus Kiel, Germany

Stephan Remmert, MD
Professor
ENT Clinic
Department of
Otorhinolaryngology—Head and Neck Surgery
Malteser Hospital St. Anne
Duisburg, Germany

Ralf Siegert, MD, DMD
Professor
Head of ENT Clinic, Plastic Surgery
Prosper Hospital
Recklinghausen, Germany

Konrad Sommer, MD
Professor
Head of the ENT Clinic
Marien Hospital
Osnabrück, Germany

I Anatomy, Principles of Facial Surgery, and Coverage of Defects

1 Anatomy of the Skin and Skin Flaps

The Skin
(Fig. 1.1)

The skin is composed of epithelial layers (epidermis) and the dermis. Below the skin are the subcutaneous tissue, fascia, and muscle (**Fig. 1.1**).

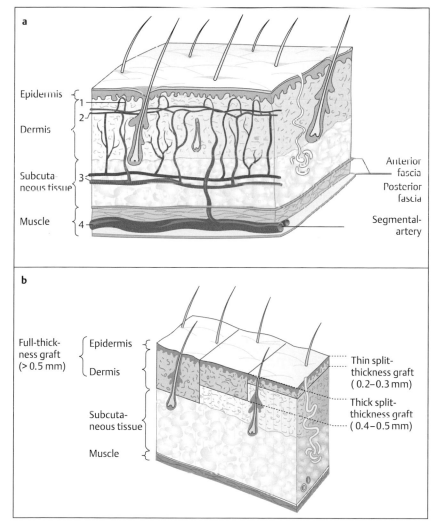

a

Epidermis
Dermis
Subcuta-
neous tissue
Muscle

Anterior
fascia
Posterior
fascia
Segmental-
artery

b

Full-thick-
ness graft
(> 0.5 mm)

Epidermis

Dermis

Subcuta-
neous tissue

Muscle

Thin split-
thickness graft
(0.2–0.3 mm)

Thick split-
thickness graft
(0.4–0.5 mm)

Fig. 1.1a, b
a Structure of the skin:
   1. Subpapillary vascular plexus
   2. Dermal vascular plexus
   3. Subdermal vascular plexus
   4. Segmental vascular plexus.
b **Composition of free skin grafts.**

Types of Skin Flaps

Random Pattern Flaps

(**Fig. 1.2**)

Random pattern flaps derive their blood supply from the dermal and subdermal plexus (**Fig. 1.2**). The **ratio of flap length to flap width** in the face is approximately **2:1**.

Axial Pattern Flaps

(**Fig. 1.3**)

An axial pattern flap is designed to be supplied by a specific arterial vessel. For example, a forehead flap can be mobilized on the frontal branch of the superficial temporal artery, and the median forehead flap can be based on the supratrochlear artery (see **Fig. 5.15**). A **3:1 or 4:1 length-to-width ratio** can be achieved with these flaps.

Island Flaps

(**Fig. 1.4**)

In an island flap, the skin is transposed into the defect on a pedicle composed of only the nutrient vessels (**Fig. 1.4**; see also **Fig. 5.9**; **Fig. 10.5a**).

Myocutaneous Island Flaps

(**Fig. 1.5**; see also **Fig. 12.1**)

The myocutaneous island flap is an axial pattern flap that generally includes skin, subcutaneous fat, muscle fascia, and muscle tissue. Familiar examples are the myocutaneous pectoralis major island flap and the myocutaneous latissimus dorsi island flap (see **Fig. 12.2**).

Neurovascular Island Flaps

With some flaps, sensory or motor nerves can be mobilized in addition to nutrient vessels. For example, authors have transferred neurovascular island flaps from around the mouth for use in lip reconstruction (Karapandzic 1974; Weerda 1983a, b; Remmert et al. 1994; see **Figs. 6.19, 6.28, 12.3**).

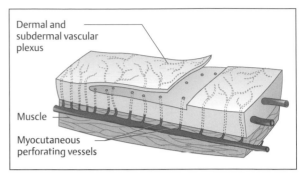

Fig. 1.2 **Random pattern skin flap** for facial use has an approximately 2:1 ratio of length to width. A special type is the subcutaneous pedicle flap (Barron et al. 1965; Lejour 1972; see **Figs. 5.44** and **5.45**).

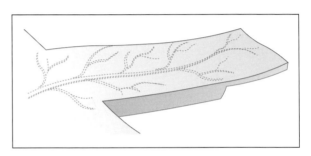

Fig. 1.3 **The axial pattern flap** is based on a specific artery. Examples are the forehead flap, Esser's cheek rotation, and the median forehead flap (see **Figs. 5.51b, 6.17, 8.1**).

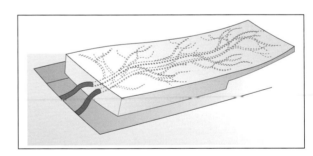

Fig. 1.4 **Island flap.** A variant of this flap is the neurovascular island flap, which includes a nerve supply (Karapandzic 1974; Weerda 1980c; Weerda and Siegert 1991; see **Fig. 6.19**).

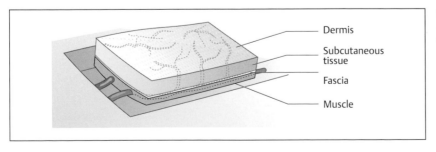

Fig. 1.5 **Axial-pattern myocutaneous island flap** (see **Figs. 12.1** and **12.2**).

2 Basic Principles of Facial Surgery

Suture Materials and Techniques

We use atraumatic cutting needles for the skin, and we generally use round needles for the mucosa. Our suture material of choice for the face is 6-0 or 7-0 monofilament on a very fine needle. Occasionally, we use 5-0 monofilament for areas that are not visible (Prolene, PDS, P 1 and P 6 5-0 needle with P 3 or PS 3 needle).

Our subcutaneous sutures are composed of absorbable or fast-dissolving braided or monofilament material (Vicryl or PDS, P 1, P 3 needle Ethicon, Norderstedt, Germany).

A suture or suture line must remain in place only until the wound has healed to an adequate tensile strength. Leaving sutures in for too long results in ugly scarring of the needle tracks.

Sutures are removed as early as possible. Sutures in the eyelid area or near the border of the lip should be removed on the fifth postoperative day, and sutures in other facial areas on day five or six. If sutures have been placed under tension, we remove them on day seven or eight. Sutures in the posterior auricular surface are removed on day eight.

The simple interrupted suture (**Fig. 2.1**) is most commonly used. Each surgical knot should be tied with at least two, or preferably three, throws tied in opposite directions.

We generally use continuous sutures (**Fig. 2.2**) for the lid area, for long traumatic wounds, and behind the ear in auricular reconstructions. After every three or four stitches, we usually tie an intermediate knot to obtain a secure coaptation.

The tightened suture should raise the wound edges slightly, so that the scar will be at skin level following scar contraction. With deep wounds, a subcutaneous approximating suture is placed initially with a buried knot (**Fig. 2.1a, b**).

In areas where two skin incisions meet at an angle, we generally use a Donati or Allgöwer type of vertical mattress suture to coapt the wound edges (**Fig. 2.3**).

Wounds under tension are additionally reinforced with mattress sutures tied over ointment-impregnated gauze or silicone button (**Fig. 2.4**). These sutures are removed in 7 to 10 days.

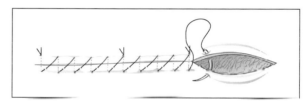

Fig. 2.2 Over-and-over continuous suture, intermediate knot after four stitches.

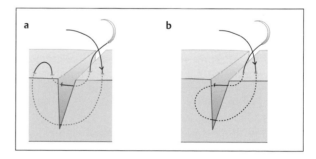

Fig. 2.3a, b
a Vertical mattress suture (Donati type).
b Vertical mattress suture (Allgöwer type).

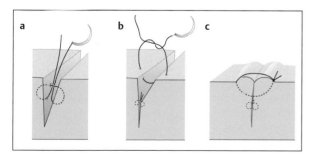

Fig. 2.1a–c Simple interrupted suture.
a Subcutaneous approximating suture of absorbable material, with a buried knot.
b The entrance and exit points are placed symmetrically.
c The suture is tightened, slightly pursing the wound margins, and is tied on one side.

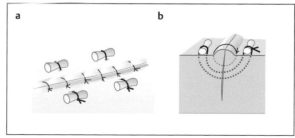

Fig. 2.4a, b
a **Mattress sutures** can be used to reinforce a suture line that is under tension. The monofilament threads are tied over bolsters consisting of swabs, silicone tubing, etc.
b Schematic view in cross-section.

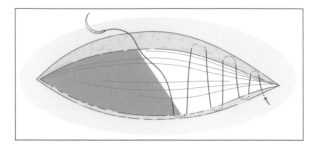

Fig. 2.5   Continuous intracutaneous suture.

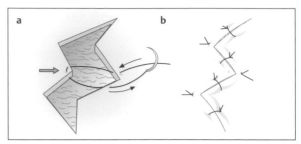

Fig. 2.6a, b   Gillies corner suture.

The continuous intracutaneous suture can yield a more favorable cosmetic result in many surgical procedures (**Fig. 2.5**). We use 4-0 or 5-0 monofilament material for this type of suture.

Adhesive strips can be added to the sutures, to further relieve tension on the wound edges and ensure a cosmetically acceptable scar.

The Gillies corner suture is used in angled suture lines and for the dispersion of scars (**Fig. 2.6a**). The needle is passed subcutaneously through the wound angle and brought out on the opposite side (**Fig. 2.6b**).

Basic Instrument Set for Reconstructive Facial Plastic Surgery
(Weerda 2006; Weerda and Siegert 2012)
(**Fig. 2.7**)

We generally use a 2× to 2.5× binocular loupe when operating and suturing. A high-quality instrument set (**Fig. 2.7a, d, e**) is needed that includes no. 11, no. 15, and no. 19 knife blades ① and one small and one slightly larger needle holder for atraumatic needles ②. The set should include fine surgical forceps (e.g., Adson forceps), dissecting forceps ③, fine, angled bipolar forceps for vascular electrocautery, two or three fine hemostatic clamps, mucosal clamps, and assorted sharp-pointed scissors and dissecting scissors ④. Fine, single-prong and double-prong hooks ⑤ are useful for holding and manipulating flaps. The Weerda hook forceps (**Fig. 2.7b**) is a good alternative, but care must be taken not to crush the flap margins with the forceps. Important accessories are a millimeter rule, a caliper (**Fig. 2.7a**, ⑥), and sterile color markers or methylene-blue marking pencils. Suture materials consists of 5-0, 6-0, and 7-0 monofilament, along with 4-0 and 5-0 absorbable braided and monofilament sutures. For cutting the auricular cartilage and other cartilaginous structures, we use assorted carving tools available from KARL STORZ—ENDOSKOPE, Tuttlingen, Germany (**Fig. 2.7a**, ⑦ and **2.7f**; see also **Figs. 11.1** and **11.3**).

We also use various lengths of adhesive tape for dressings, and emollient ointments that often contain petroleum jelly. We routinely use suction drains and mini-suction drains to aspirate wound secretions and help contour the skin to the wound bed.

The Binocular Loupe
(**Fig. 2.7c**)

We have become accustomed to using a binocular loupe (2.0 to 2.5× magnification), both when performing operations and when placing sutures.

Here we will describe only the basic instrument set. The tray setups that we recommend for reconstructive facial plastic surgery are illustrated on p. 8.

The high-quality basic instrument set consists of the following items (**Fig. 2.7d**): ① scalpels with no. 11, no. 15, and no. 19 blades; ②needle holders—one small and one slightly larger, for atraumatic needles; ③ fine tissue forceps (e.g., Adson forceps); ④ fine, angled bipolar forceps for vascular electrocautery; ⑤ two or three small hemostatic clamps; ⑥ mucosa clamps; ⑦ assorted pointed scissors; and ⑧ dissecting scissors.

We additionally use ⑨ fine, single- and double-prong hooks for holding and manipulating the flaps. A good alternative is the Weerda hook forceps ⑩ (**Fig. 2.7e**). Ordinary forceps should not be used, as they are liable to crush the flap margins. Other important accessories are a millimeter rule ⑪ and a caliper ⑫ (**Fig. 2.7f**) and sterile skin markers or methylene blue marking pencils. We use an assortment of craft knives for carving and sculpturing cartilaginous frameworks (e.g., for an auricular reconstruction; see **Fig. 2.7a** ⑦ and **g**).

Additional instruments:
• Dermatome
• Mucotome
• Assorted needle holders
• Special clamp (or needle holder) for twisting the suture ends
• Wire cutters
• A Luniatschek gauze packer for burying wire sutures

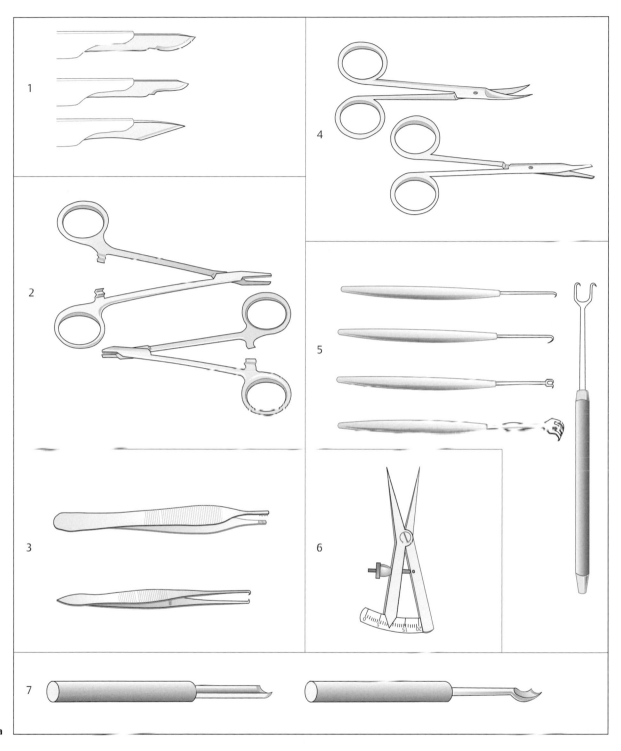

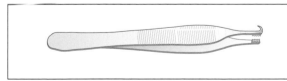

Fig. 2.7a–g

a Instruments for facial surgery (see text; from KARL STORZ—ENDOSKOPE, Tuttlingen, Germany).

b Weerda hook forceps (KARL STORZ—ENDOSKOPE, Tuttlingen, Germany) see **Fig. 2.7e.**

(Continued on next page) ▶

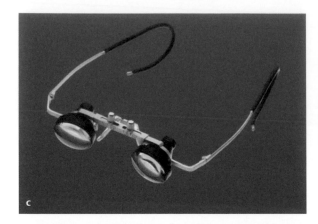

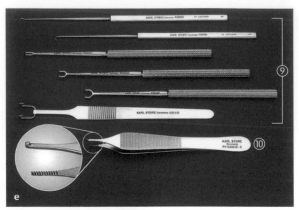

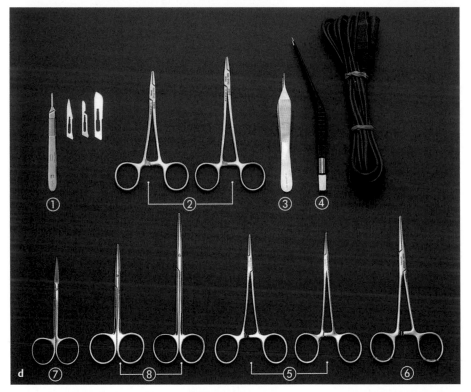

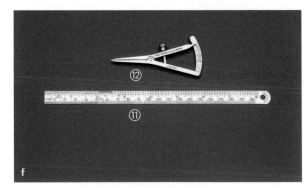

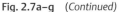

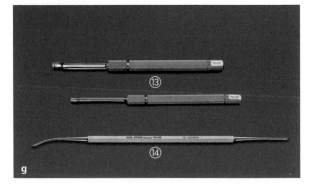

Fig. 2.7a–g *(Continued)*

c   **Binocular loupe** (from Weerda 2007, K. Storz Endo-Press).

d   **Basic instrument set for reconstructive facial plastic surgery** (from Weerda 2007).

e–g **Basic instrument set for reconstructive facial plastic surgery** (from Weerda 2007). A summary of instruments will be found in the appendix; see text, p. 6.

With kind premission of Karl Storz-Endoskope, Tuttlingen, Germany (Weerda 2006, Weerda and Siegert 2012).

Wound Management, Repair of Small Defects, and Scar Revision

Surgical procedures of up to 2.5 hours can be conducted under local anesthesia. More extensive operations and scar revisions call for general anesthesia. Care should be taken that the tape-secured endotracheal tube does not distort the face. The face should not be taped over during operations in the facial nerve area. We use a transparent film drape for this purpose (to allow facial nerve monitoring).

Relaxed Skin Tension Lines, Vascular Supply (Fig. 2.8i), and "Esthetic Units" (Fig. 2.20)

The facial surgeon must be familiar with the location and distribution of the relaxed skin tension lines (RSTLs) in the face, the facial "esthetic units" (see **Fig. 2.20a–d**), and the vascular supply of the face (**Fig. 2.8i**). Besides the RSTLs, attention should also be given to **wrinkle lines** in the aging face.

Incisions or small excisions and sutures placed in the RSTLs will heal with fine, unobtrusive scars. Incisions and excisions made at right angles to these lines will often lead to broad, unsightly scars. Thus, the plastic surgeon should always try to place the cuts used for incisions, excisions, and scar revisions in these lines, to achieve good cosmetic results.

The term **"esthetic units"** (see **Fig. 2.20a–d**) refers to circumscribed facial regions that should each be reconstructed as a separate unit whenever possible. The radical excision of tumors takes precedence over esthetic units, however. We shall return to this reconstructive concept in the sections that deal with specific facial regions.

Wound Management and Scar Revision

It is a general rule in facial plastic surgery to sacrifice as little skin as possible. Small wounds that extend obliquely into the tissue should be straightened whenever the surrounding tissue can be mobilized and the wound edges coapted without tension. A subcutaneous suture with a buried knot should always be placed to allow tension-free approximation of the wound margins (see **Fig. 2.1**). Because the subcutaneous tissue, epidermis, and dermis take different lengths of time to achieve adequate wound strength, early removal of the skin sutures from a wound without subcutaneous sutures would result in a broad, unsightly scar.

Management of Wounds with Traumatic Tattooing

If a wound contains embedded grit and dirt, it should first be scrubbed with a sterile toothbrush or hand brush and antiseptic soap, until all dirt residues have been removed. It can be extremely tedious to remove these particles after the wound has healed.

Scar Revision by W-Plasty and the Broken-Line Technique of Webster (1969)
(Fig. 2.8a–j)

If time permits in trauma cases, the wound should be dispersed with a **W-plasty**, broken-line excision, or Z-plasty that conforms to the RSTLs. If this is not possible, scar revision should be postponed for at least 6 months to 1 year. Long scars are very conspicuous, especially when they cross RSTLs at right angles. Scar revision therefore has two goals:

- **Dispersing a long scar into smaller individual scars**
- **Positioning the smaller scars in RSTLs.**

Revision techniques involve excising the scar and dispersing the wound line into multiple segments. The **W-plasty** consists of segments 4 to 5 mm long arranged in a zigzag pattern (**Fig. 2.8a2, c, e–j**). The new scars run in alternating directions and are barely perceptible after the wound has healed. In the **broken-line technique**, the segments are placed in an irregular pattern (**Fig. 2.8a3, c**). In both the W-plasty and broken-line techniques, the margins of the excision are fashioned so that they will fit together precisely like a lock and key. Generally, this is done with a no. 11 blade that is held perpendicular to the skin surface when the cuts are made. The wound edges are then undermined with a no. 15 blade or pointed scissors (Webster 1969; Borges 1973; Haas 1991). Fine scars can also be managed by dermabrasion (see Chapter 17). The suture material of choice is 6-0 or 7-0 monofilament, and subcutaneous sutures should be placed whenever possible. Corners and triangles are secured with Gillies corner sutures (**Fig. 2.6**).

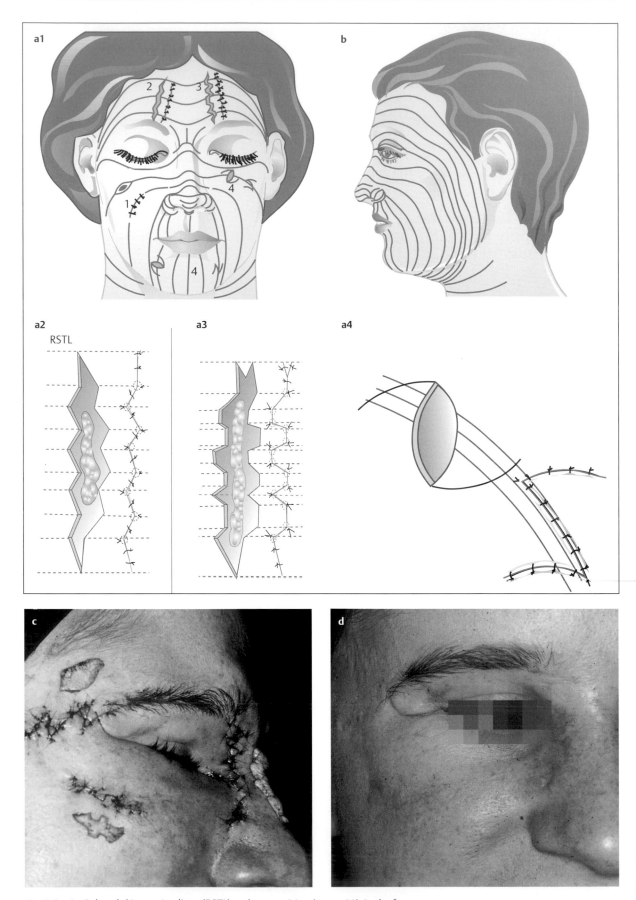

Fig. 2.8a–j   Relaxed skin tension lines (RSTL) and scar revision (see p. 11) in the face.

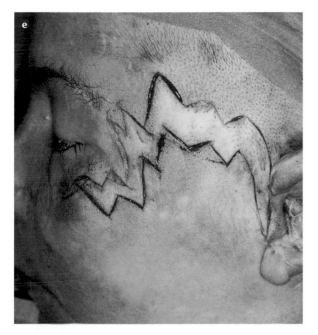

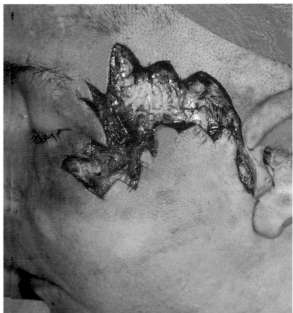

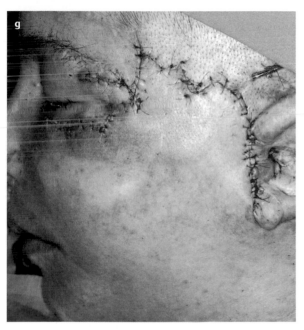

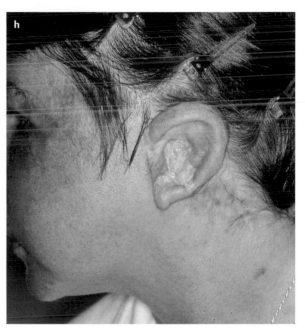

Fig. 2.8a–j   *(Continued)* Relaxed skin tension lines (RSTl) and scar revision in the faces

a1 **Elliptical excision** in the RSTLs, front view.

a2 Scar excision by W-plasty. The **W-plasty** is an interdigitating, zig-zag-shaped excision with segment lengths of 3 to 4 mm.

a3 Scar excision by the **broken-line technique** creates skin tags of varying shape with an edge length of 3 to 5 mm. The edges interdigitate and should follow the RSTLs as closely as possible.

a4 **Z-plasty** following scar excision in the face. The new scar is orientated along the RSTLs (see **Fig. 2.15, 2.16**).

b Side view.

c Scar revision with w-plasty and broken-line technique.

d Result.

e Large temporal scar and auricular loss with additional facial palsy. Scar revision with W-techniques and with broken-line technique. The ear was reconstructed 2 years previously: scar incision.

f Scar excision following the RSTL (see **a2, a3**).

g Closure of the wounds and face lift.

h 5 months after revision.

(Continued on next page)   ▶

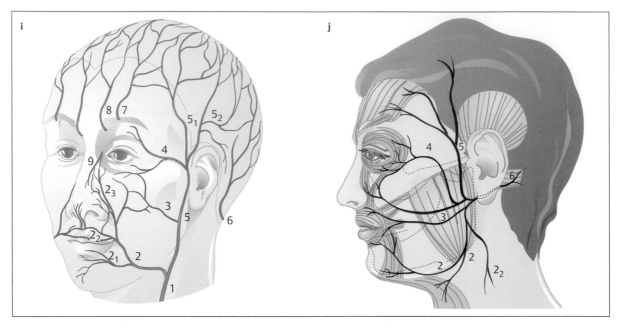

Fig. 2.8a–j   *(Continued)* Relaxed skin tension lines (RSTL) and scar revision in the face.

i The face derives its **arterial blood supply** from the external carotid artery and anastomotic areas:

  1 External carotid artery
  2 Facial artery
  2₁ Inferior labial artery
  2₂ Superior labial artery
  2₃ Angular artery
  3 Transverse facial artery (from 5)
  4 Zygomatico-orbital artery (from 5)
  5 Superficial temporal artery
  5₁ Frontal branch
  5₂ Parietal branch
  6 Occipital artery
  7 Supraorbital artery (see **Figs. 5.51b; 5.52b, d, e; 5.53**, and **5.54o**)
  8 Supratrochlear artery (see **Figs. 5.51b, 5.53**, and **5.54o**)
  9 Dorsal nasal artery (see **Fig. 5.8a**).

j The **facial nerve** and its distribution in the face:

  1 Trunk from the stylomastoid foramen
  2 Marginal mandibular branch
  2₂ Cervical branch   **2+3:** cervicofacial branch
  3 Buccal branches
  4 Zygomatic branches
  5 Temporal branches   **4+5:** temporofacial branch
  6 Posterior auricular branch.

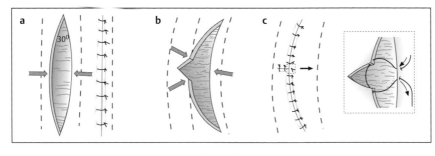

Fig. 2.9a–c
a **Elliptical excision** in the RSTLs. The excision angle is ~30°.
b Crescent-shaped excision.
c Suture.

Small Excisions

When an **elliptical excision** is made in the RSTLs, the wound angle should not exceed 30° (**Figs. 2.8a** and **2.9**). Various excision techniques can be used (**Figs. 2.10–2.14**).

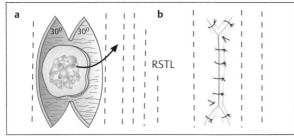

Fig. 2.10a, b
a **Double M-plasty.** Each excision angle is 30°.
b Closure.

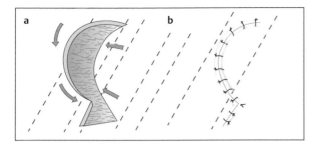

Fig. 2.11a, b
a Crescent-shaped **advancement flap** of Jackson (1985).
b Closure of the defects.

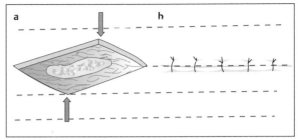

Fig. 2.12a, b
a **Rhomboid excision**.
b Closure.

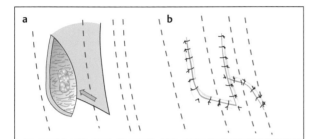

Fig. 2.13a, b
a **Small flap advancement** for an elliptical excision.
b Closure.

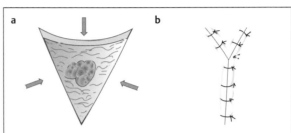

Fig. 2.14a, b
a **Triangular excision**.
b Closure.

Z-Plasty
(Figs. 2.15 and 2.16)

The Z-plasty is used to relieve tension on tissues that have been distorted by a contracted scar (**Fig. 2.15**). This technique can also disperse and redirect wounds that cross RSTLs at right angles, in which case a multiple Z-plasty can also be used (**Fig. 2.16**) (Jackson 1985a).

Numerous variations of the Z-plasty are available for repairing defects of varying size (**Fig. 2.8d** and **Figs. 2.17** and **2.18**). These techniques require a high degree of flap mobility (Cummings et al. 1986).

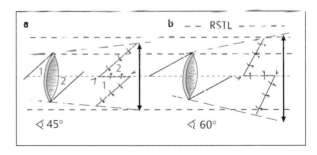

Fig. 2.15a, b **Simple Z-plasty**.
a The scar, which crosses the RSTLs (– –) almost at right angles, is excised and dispersed with a 45° Z-plasty. Flaps 1 and 2 are transposed, causing a slight lengthening of the tissue in the direction of the arrow.
b Transposing flaps 1 and 2 in a 60° Z-plasty produces even greater tissue lengthening (arrow).

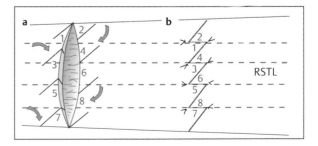

Fig. 2.16a, b **Multiple Z-plasty**.
a The scar is excised, and the long scar is dispersed into multiple Zs that more closely follow the RSTLs.
b Transposing the flaps lengthens the tissue in the direction of the scar and disperses the scar into multiple smaller flaps (see Wound Management and Scar Revision, p. 9).

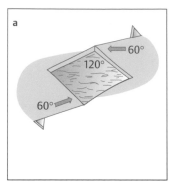

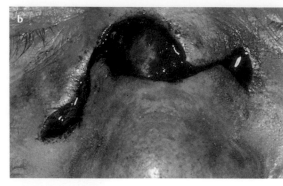

Fig. 2.17a–d
a Rhomboid defect repaired by a **Z-plasty**, using the technique of Pate and Wilkinson (1991).
b Defect, a **Z-plasty** is incised, with a Burow's triangle at the end of the incision.
c, d Closure of the defect.

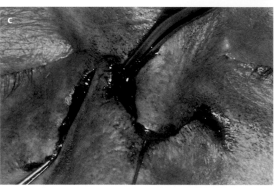

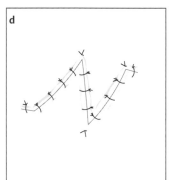

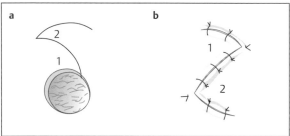

Fig. 2.18a, b   **Z-plasty** for the closure of small circular defects.

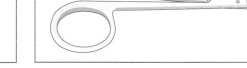

Fig. 2.19   Weerda **suture microscissors** with micro-cutting edge (KARL STORZ—ENDOSKOPE, Tuttlingen, Germany).

Postoperative Treatment of Scars

We use microscissors (**Fig. 2.19**) for cutting and removing the sutures on postoperative day five, six, or seven. A cortisone ointment is massaged into the scar for 15 minutes in the morning and evening, for 2 weeks. If the patient is prone to hypertrophic scarring, we inject a 1:2 dilution of Volon A crystal suspension (10 mg Volon A diluted with 2 mL of physiologic saline).

Esthetic Units of the Face
(**Fig. 2.20**)

If portions of the face need to be reconstructed, better cosmetic results are achieved by reconstructing areas as complete units (see **Fig. 5.54**). This is not always possible, however, especially in tumor resections.

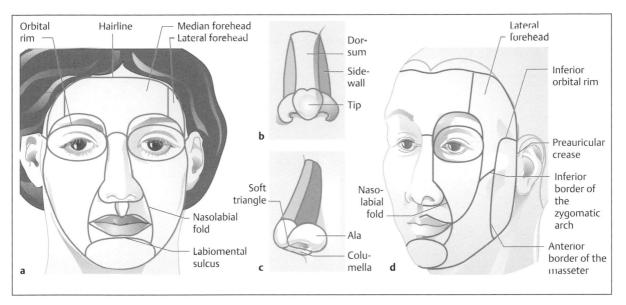

Fig. 2.20a–d **Esthetic units** of the face.
a In the face.
b Nasal subunits, anterior view.
c nasal subunits, lateral view.
d Esthetic subunits of the cheek (Sherris and Larrabee 2009).

Tumor Resection with Histologic Control
(Fig. 2.21)

Complete tumor removal takes precedence over all cosmetic and reconstructive concerns. Regardless of whether the tumor is a basal cell carcinoma, squamous carcinoma, or melanoma, it must be certain that adequate marginal and deep clearance has been achieved in accordance with oncologic principles. Wherever possible, we practice a modified form of histologically controlled tumor resection. This means that the tumor is first excised with a margin of healthy tissue, marked with threads to indicate its position in the face or neck, and outlined on paper (**Fig. 2.21a**). The specimen is sent to pathology, and additional samples are taken from the margins and base of the tumor bed (**Fig. 2.21b**), marked on a sheet of paper (e.g., glove paper), and sent to pathology for separate evaluation. The defect is not reconstructed until the histologic results are known (secondary or delayed coverage). This can minimize the recurrence rate, and the cosmetic results are as good as with a primary reconstruction. This procedure is followed even if re-excision is necessary, owing to positive margins.

Small tumors are elliptically excised in the RSTLs, and the wound margins are sparingly undermined and closed in two layers (see **Figs. 2.8a** and **2.9a**). Various skin flaps can be used to cover larger defects.

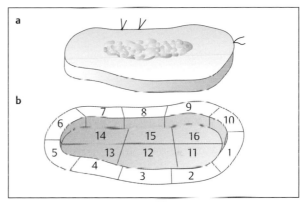

Fig. 2.21a, b **Tumor resection with histologic control**.
a The skin tumor is removed with a margin of healthy tissue, and the edges of the specimen are marked with threads.
b The margins and base of the tumor bed are resected in a clockwise direction and checked histologically to verify complete **tumor clearance**.

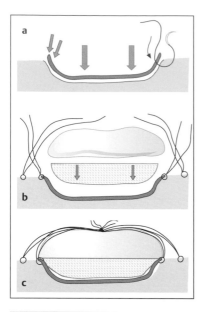
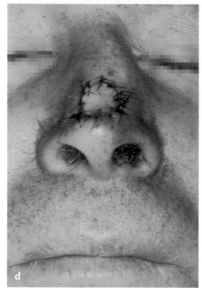
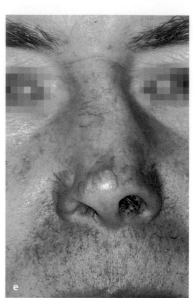
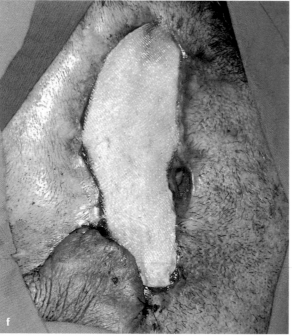
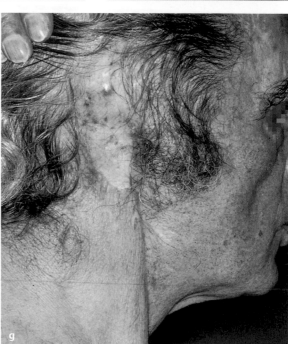

Fig. 2.22a–g Free skin grafts.

a Following meticulous hemostasis, the split-thickness or full-thickness skin graft (see **Fig. 1.1b**) is sutured to the wound margin on one side. A thin film of fibrin glue (Tissucol, Baxter Germany, Heidelberg) is applied to the base of the wound, and the graft is pressed firmly against the wound bed for 30 seconds.

b A light pressure dressing is particularly recommended in more mobile facial areas. The graft-fixation sutures are left long, and additional 4-0 sutures may be placed 1 cm from the wound margin. We cover the graft with a 1- to 2-mm

thickness of petrolatum foam, followed by a foam or gauze bolster over which the suture tails are tied, exerting gentle pressure on the grafted site.

c The tie-over dressing remains in place for at least 6 to 8 days.

d Full-thickness skin graft from retroauricular.

e Colors match after healing.

f Split-thickness skin graft after tumor resection (see **Fig. 10.86**). The skin is glued and sutured, the sutures are left long (**b, c**).

g Result 1 year after covering the defect.

Free Skin Grafts

(Fig. 2.22)

Although our tendency is to cover facial defects with local skin flaps, sometimes it is better to use a full-thickness or split-thickness skin graft to repair a tumor resection site, especially in older patients. This is especially true if the tumor cannot be excised with the requisite safety margin, or if it is uncertain that the tumor has been fully encompassed. We use skin from the postauricular or retroauricular area to cover facial defects, as it most closely matches the color and texture of the facial skin. Other acceptable donor sites are the supraclavicular area and the medial surface of the upper arm. Groin skin can be used in less conspicuous areas. We have found the scalp above the ear to be a good donor region. When this skin is used for split-thickness grafts that are no more than 0.3 mm thick, the hair is cut very short and the skin is harvested above the level of the hair bulbs with a dermatome or mucotome. The regrowth of hair will conceal the donor scars.

Large split-thickness grafts can be obtained from the buttock, from the abdominal skin, or, as a last resort, from the thigh. They are harvested using various types of dermatomes, which are set to the desired thickness of the graft. Thin split-thickness skin grafts are harvested with a thickness of 0.2 to 0.3 mm; thick split-thickness skin grafts are in the range of 0.35 to 0.50 mm, and full-thickness skin grafts are over 0.5 mm thick (see **Fig. 1.1b**).

The wound bed to be grafted must be free of bleeding sites and clotted blood, otherwise the graft will not adhere to the wound bed and will be lost to necrosis. Harvesting the graft from the groin area leaves an unobtrusive, streaklike scar. The free graft should be slightly larger than the primary defect. We use a pattern made from aluminum foil (suture wrapping material) or glove paper to outline a graft of sufficient size.

Generally, the graft is sutured into the wound bed with 5-0 or 6-0 monofilament (**Fig. 2.22a**). Fibrin glue (Baxter Germany, Heidelberg) is additionally used to support hemostasis and ensure adequate fixation of the graft in the recipient bed. The grafted site is covered with a layer of foam coated with a mixture of Betadine and petrolatum. This is covered with a petrolatum gauze bolster, over which the suture tails are tied to create a light pressure dressing (**Fig. 2.22b**). The tie-over dressing remains in place for 6 to 8 days (**Fig. 2.22c**). The dressing can also be covered with adhesive strips.

A successful graft requires a well-perfused recipient bed. A graft placed on bare bone, for example, will not survive. If bone is exposed, or if the level of the graft does not match that of the surrounding skin, special measures must be taken. When cortical bone has been exposed, drilling multiple holes down to cancellous bone will promote the formation of granulation tissue. The soft granulations are periodically removed and light pressure dressings applied to condition the graft bed. When the level of the bed has reached that of the surrounding skin, graft inset can be performed (see **Figs. 5.52j, l** and **10.100**).

Composite Grafts

(Fig. 2.23)

Grafts from the auricle can be harvested from the posterior (**Fig. 2.23c–f**) or anterior region (**Fig. 2.23g–l**) as particularly, two-layer chondrocutaneous grafts (**Fig. 2.23g–l**) and full-thickness (three-layer) grafts composed of anterior skin, cartilage, and posterior skin. They are most commonly used for nasal reconstruction (**Fig. 2.24**) and (**Fig. 5.54**) but can be used in the auricle as well (**Fig. 2.23m–o**). Because the skin of the graft contracts slightly, it should be cut slightly larger than the defect and thus larger than the cartilage layer. Again, we use a pattern made from aluminum foil (**Fig. 2.23c**) (suture material wrapper) or glove paper as a guide. The skin on the anterior side is more firmly adherent to the perichondrium and cartilage than the posterior skin. If the retroauricular skin is included in the graft, it should be tacked to the cartilage with a few simple interrupted sutures, to prevent separation.

The donor defect may be closed by direct suture or covered with a retroauricular island flap (see **Figs. 10.2–10.5**). When the composite graft is handled, care must be taken not to crush its edges with the forceps, and the fixation sutures should not be placed too close together. Dark discoloration of the graft during the first few days is no cause for alarm, but more than 20% of these grafts do not survive (**Fig. 2.23b–d**) (Walter 1997). The dressing over the composite graft should keep it immobile for 6 to 7 days if possible, to avoid tearing the capillary buds that revascularize the graft (Weerda 2007, p. 42, Table 3.11; **Fig. 2.23b–d**).

Cartilagenous and Composite Grafts for Auricular and Nasal Reconstruction

(Figs. 2.23 and 2.24; rib cartilage see pp. 207–211 and see also **Fig. 5.54**)

For partial (**Fig. 5.48d, e**) or total reconstruction (**Fig. 5.54**), we need cartilaginous grafts of different sizes, commonly harvested from the cavum conchae and cymba (**Fig. 2.24**). These grafts can be taken from the posterior (**Fig. 2.24a–d**) or from the anterior aspect of the auricle (**Fig. 2.24e–g**). For the nasal dorsum, we use a compound septal rotation flap (see **Fig. 5.54a–h**) and usually a rib cartilage strut (see **Fig. 11.1**).

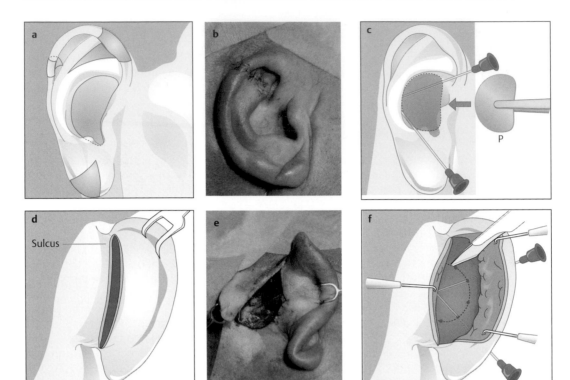

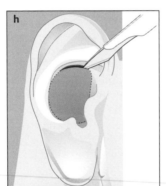

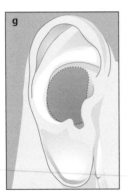

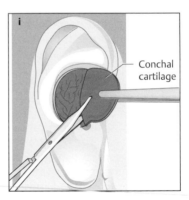

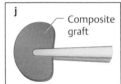

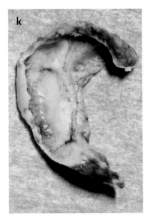

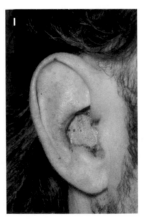

Fig. 2.23a–o

a Donor sites where two-layer and three-layer **composite grafts** or conchal cartilage can be obtained with primary closure of the defects. A fat–dermis graft can be harvested from the earlobe.

b Situation after harvesting a three-layered wedge-shaped composite graft and closure of the wound in the upper part of the auricle (see **Fig. 5.41**).

c Harvesting conchal cartilage from postauricular region, using a pattern (P) of aluminum foil, the graft is outlined with needles from the anterior aspect.

d, e Incision in the sulcus, preparation of the skin.

f Outline of the cartilage.

g, h Harvesting a conchal two-layered composite graft from the anterior aspect.

g The composite graft is outlined with a pattern (see **c**).

h Incision through skin and cartilage with a no. 11 or 15 blade.

i–l Preparation of the graft and excision of the composite graft (**j, k**).

l A full-thickness or split-thickness skin graft is sutured and glued into the defect. The free graft has taken (see **Fig. 10.3**).

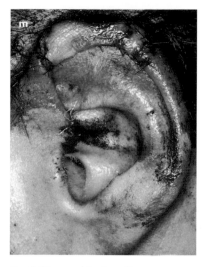
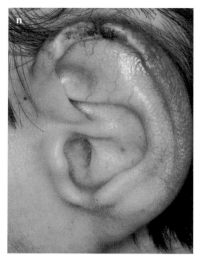
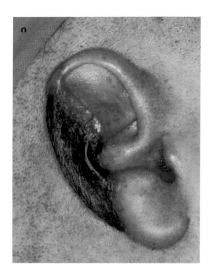

Fig. 2.23a–o *(Continued)*
m Replantation of a small part of the helical rim after a dog-bite.

n Healing with a small central defect after 3 months (Weerda 2007, p. 36).

o Replantation of a medium-sized composite graft, a necrosis resulted.

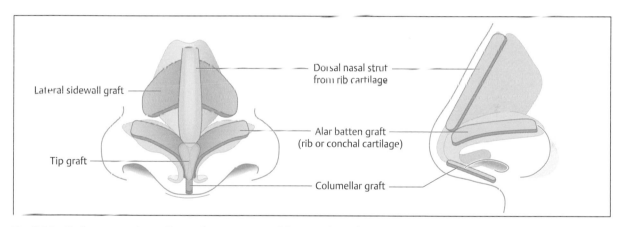

Lateral sidewall graft

Dorsal nasal strut from rib cartilage

Alar batten graft (rib or conchal cartilage)

Tip graft

Columellar graft

Fig. 2.24   Grafts commonly used in nasal reconstruction (Sherris and Larrabee 2009). For nasal reconstruction we use rib cartilage (see **Fig. 5.54**, p. 68) and cartilage from one or both conchae (see **Fig. 5.54w–y**).

Graft Nomenclature

Autologous:
The donor and recipient are the same (*autograft*).

Isogeneic:
The donor and recipient are genetically identical (e.g., monozygotic twins, animals of a single inbred strain; *isograft* or *syngraft*).

Allogeneic:
The donor and recipient are of the same species (human–human, dog–dog; *allograft*).

Xenogeneic:
The donor and recipient are of different species (e.g., bovine cartilage; *xenograft* or *heterograft*).

Prosthetic:
Lost tissues are replaced with synthetic materials such as metal, plastic, or ceramic (*prosthetic implants*).

3 Coverage of Defects

Local Flaps

Local flaps are flaps that are raised from tissues in the immediate vicinity of the defect.

Advancement Flaps

Advancement Flap of Burow (1855)
(Fig. 3.1)

Simple triangular defects can be covered by advancing the adjacent skin. A small Burow's triangle is excised at the opposite end of the flap (**Fig. 3.1a**) to prevent formation of a **dog ear**.

Burow's U-Advancement
(Figs. 3.2–3.7)

The U-shaped skin advancement requires the excision of two Burow's triangles (**Fig. 3.2a**). The length-to-width ratio of the standard U-flap should not exceed 2:1, and a 3:1 ratio is allowed only in exceptional cases.

In the Stark modification of the U-advancement (quoted in Jost et al. 1977), the flap is widened toward its base. Cut-backs can be added to increase the flap length (**Fig. 3.3a**). The extra small defects created by the flap are closed by mobilizing the surrounding skin (**Fig. 3.3b**). Other modifications are shown in **Figs. 3.4–3.7**.

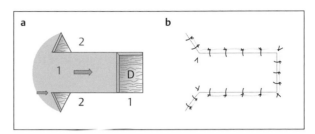

Fig. 3.2a, b   U-advancement of Burow.
a The ratio of defect (D) length to flap length is ~1:2, and the base-to-length ratio of the flap should not exceed 1:2. The flap is advanced by excising two small Burow's triangles and mobilizing the surrounding skin.
b Closure of all defects (see **Figs. 5.14, 5.26, 10.17**).

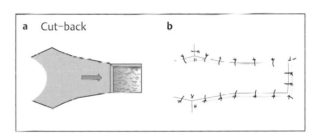

Fig. 3.3a, b   Modifications of defect closure using Burow's triangles.

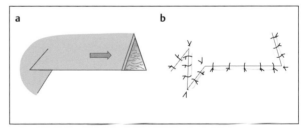

Fig. 3.4a, b   Modifications of defect closure using Burow's triangles.

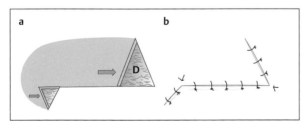

Fig. 3.1a, b   **Advancement flap** of Burow (1855).
a The flap is incised along the base of the wedge-shaped defect, and a small Burow's triangle (arrow) is excised on the opposite side. The skin is mobilized and shifted in the direction of the arrow to close the defect. Excising the small Burow's triangle eliminates a dog ear at the base of the flap.
b Appearance after coverage of the defect (see **Figs. 5.1** and **5.24**).

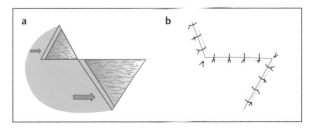

Fig. 3.5a, b   Modifications of defect closure using Burow's triangles.

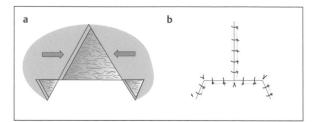

Fig. 3.6a, b   Modifications of defect closure using Burow's triangles.

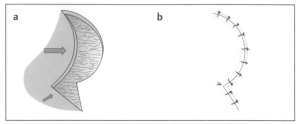

Fig. 3.7a, b   Modifications of defect closure using Burow's triangles.

V-Y and V-Y-S Advancement of Argamaso (1974) (Figs. 3.8–3.10)

The V-Y advancement and double V-Y-S advancement of Argamaso (1974) are special designs used for releasing contracted scars, for columellar reconstruction from the upper lip, and for lengthening the frenulum (**Fig. 3.8**).

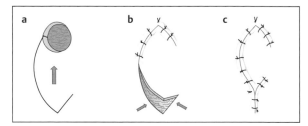

Fig. 3.9a–c   Modification of the V-Y plasty (see **Figs. 5.2** and 5.10).

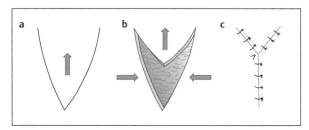

Fig. 3.8a–c   V-Y advancement (see **Fig. 5.4**).
a A contracted scar or the frenulum can be lengthened by making a V-shaped incision, mobilizing the flap, and advancing it in the direction of the arrow.
b The skin is mobilized.
c Closure of the defects.

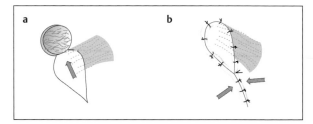

Fig. 3.10a, b   V-Y-S advancement of Argamaso (1974).

Flaps without Continuous Epithelial Coverage (Rettinger 1996a, b)

Sliding Flap
(**Figs. 3.11–3.14**)
Another interesting type of advancement flap is the sliding flap, which is based entirely on subcutaneous tissue. Barron and Emmett (1965) devised a flap with a lateral subcutaneous pedicle (**Fig. 3.11**; see also **Figs. 5.33, 5.44, 6.16**). The skin flap is outlined, and the pedicle is mobilized on one side. The flap is slid into the defect on the subcutaneous pedicle. Lejour (1975) described a similar flap based on subcutaneous tissue (**Figs. 3.12–3.14**; see also **Fig. 5.7**). We have used this type of flap to repair defects in the tongue (Weerda 1985; **Fig. 3.14**).

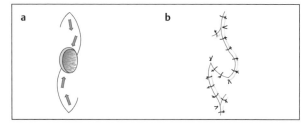

Fig. 3.11a, b   Sliding flap of Barron and Emmett (1965, see **Fig. 5.7**, p. 37).
a Flap with a lateral subcutaneous pedicle.
b Closure of the defects.

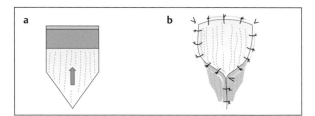

Fig. 3.12a, b   Sliding flap of Lejour (1975), based on the subcutaneous tissue below the flap. (see **Fig. 3.13**; see also **Fig. 5.7**).

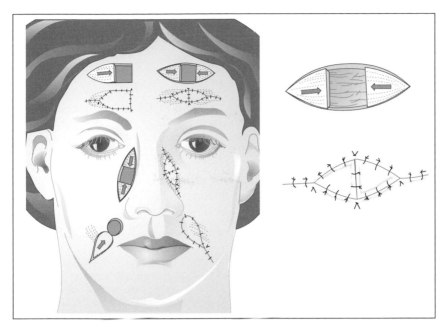

Fig. 3.13 Examples and modifications of sliding flaps for facial plastic surgery (see Figs. 5.33, 5.44, 5.45, 6.16).

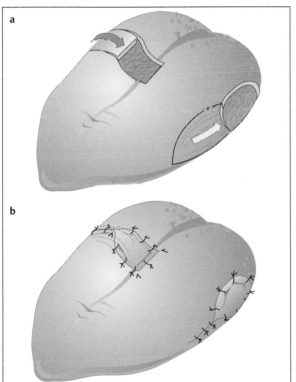

Fig. 3.14a, b   **Myomucosal sliding flap** of Weerda (1985b).
a The sliding flaps have been outlined.
b The flaps are slid into the defects on a lateral muscle pedicle, and the defects are closed.

Pedicled Flaps

Transposition Flap
(Fig. 3.15)

This flap must be large enough for transfer into a local defect (D). The surrounding skin can be mobilized for primary coverage of the secondary defect (S) (**Fig. 3.15b, c**; **Figs. 3.16** and **3.17**). The flap may be swung through an acute angle (**Fig. 3.17**), a 90° angle, or even more than 90°, depending on the mobility of the surrounding skin. If the transposition flap is too short but has a broad enough base, the flap can be lengthened by adding a back-cut (**Fig. 3.18**). Care is taken that the residual base is still adequate for flap nutrition (Weerda 1978b; Haas 1991); see **Figs. 5.12, 10.16, 10.64**.

Rotation Flap
(Fig. 3.19)

This is a semicircular skin flap that is rotated into the defect on a pivot point. Again, the flap must be sufficiently broad, and a broad base is necessary if a backcut is needed to lengthen the flap (**Fig. 3.20**; see also **Figs. 6.25, 8.1, 8.17**). If the rotation flap is too small (**Fig. 3.21a**), the residual defect can be covered by mobilizing the surrounding skin (**Fig. 3.21b, c**; see also **Fig. 6.14**).

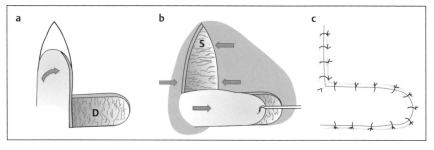

Fig. 3.15a–c   Transposition flap (see **Figs. 5.6; 5.29b, c; 10.16**).
a The transposition flap is outlined at a 90° angle to the defect (D).
b The flap is swung into the defect, and the secondary defect (S) is closed by advancing the surrounding skin.
c Appearance after closure of all defects.

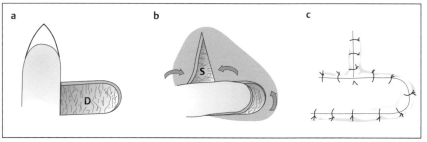

Fig. 3.16a–c   Other options for **closing the secondary defect** (S). D = defect.

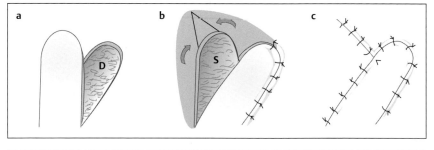

Fig. 3.17a–c   Other options for **transposition and mobilization** (see **Fig. 5.19**).
a Transposition flap. D = defect.
b Additional skin is excised to allow closure of the secondary defect (S).
c Closure.

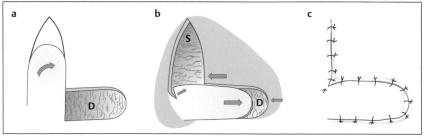

Fig. 3.18a–c   The surrounding skin is mobilized and advanced in the direction of the arrow.
a The transposition flap is too short. D = defect.
b A back cut is made to lengthen the flap (while **preserving an adequate base**). S = secondary defect.
c Closure of all defects.

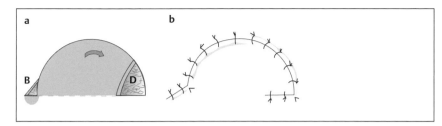

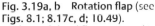
Fig. 3.19a, b Rotation flap (see Figs. 8.1; 8.17c, d; 10.49).
a The mobilized flap is rotated into the defect (D) after excision of a Burow's triangle (B).
b Appearance after closure of the defects.

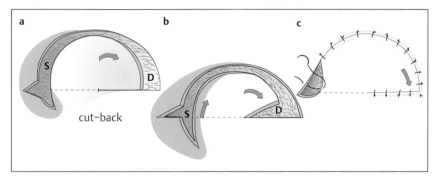

Fig. 3.20a–c Transfer of a too-small rotation flap aided by a **cut-back** (see Fig. 3.18).
a The flap is lengthened by making a cut-back.
b The defect (D) is closed, and the secondary defect (S) is mobilized in the area of the cut-back.
c Closure of all defects.

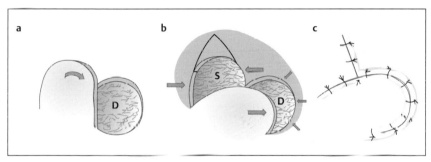

Fig. 3.21a–c Transfer of a too-small rotation flap aided by **mobilizing the surrounding skin** (see Fig. 8.17c–g).
a Flap.
b The flap is rotated, and the surrounding skin is mobilized to close the residual defect (D) and secondary defect (S). If necessary, a skin triangle is excised over the secondary defect (←).
c Closure of all defects.

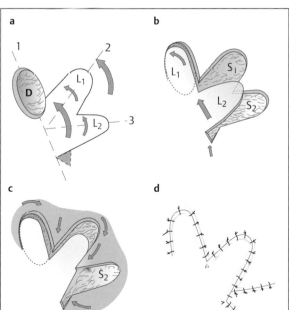

Fig. 3.22a–d Bilobed flap (Esser 1918) (see Figs. 5.6, 5.8, 5.13, 5.29, 5.46, 6.15, 8.8, 8.19, 10.65, 10.87).
a The angle between the defect (D) and the first lobe L_1 equals the angle between L_1 and lobe L_2. If the skin is mobile, **lobe 1 is approximately two thirds of the size of the defect**, and **lobe 2 is approximately two thirds** of the size of lobe 1.
b The flaps and surrounding skin are mobilized, and lobe L_1 is swung into the defect. Lobe L_2 is swung into the secondary defect S_1.
c The surrounding skin is mobilized, and all secondary defects are closed.
d Appearance after closure of all defects.

Bilobed Flap
(Fig. 3.22)

An interesting flap design is the "bilobed flap," described by Esser (1918). The two flaps have a common base and form an angle between 45° and 180°. Smaller angles make it easier to rotate the two attached transposition flaps (Fig. 3.23), while larger angles require longer flaps and cause greater skin bunching. Other combinations of such flaps are possible (see Fig. 5.29).

These flaps are used in areas where the surrounding skin is not mobile enough to close the secondary defect, such as the **nasal flank**, the junction of the

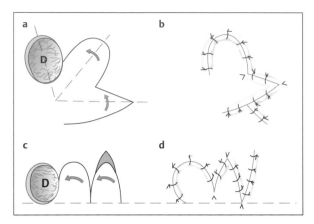

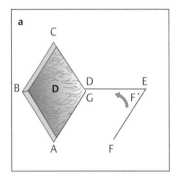

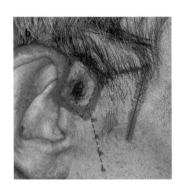

scalp and neck, the cheek, and the nasal tip area (Zimany 1953; Elliot 1969; Weerda 1978c, d, 1980d, e) (see **Figs. 5.6, 5.8, 5.13, 5.28, 5.46, 8.19, 9.5, 10.87**).

Fig. 3.23a–c Modifications of the bilobed flap. D = defect.

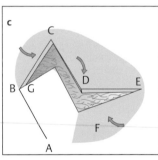

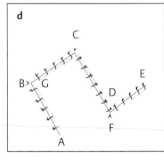

Fig. 3.24a–f Rhomboid flap of Limberg (1967).
a The first flap incision is an extension of the axis B–D, and the second incision (E–F) is made parallel to G–A.
b Outline of tumor excision and rhomboid flap.
c The flap is mobilized.
d, e Appearance after closure of all defects.
f Result (see **Fig. 10.42**).

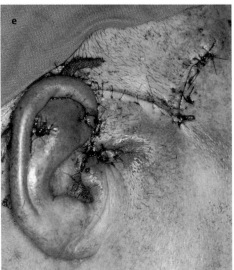

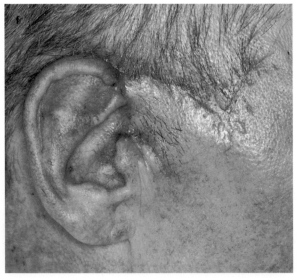

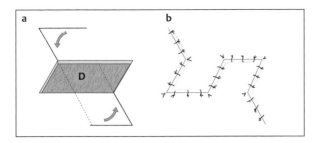

Fig. 3.25a, b Two opposing Limberg flaps are mobilized (arrows) (**a**), and all the defects (D) are closed (**b**).

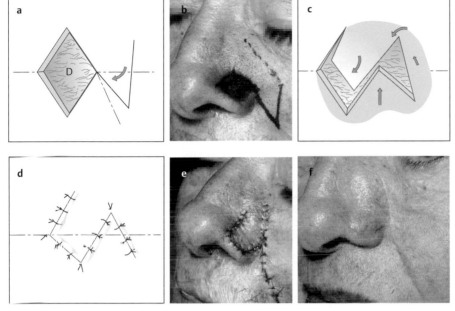

Fig. 3.26a–f Rhomboid flap of Dufourmentel (1962).
a, b Pattern of the flap incision. The tumor is incised, the flap outlined.
c Mobilization and flap transfer.
d, e Closure of all defects.
f Result.

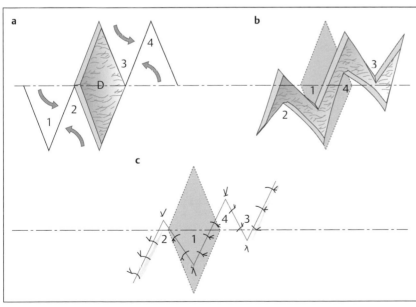

Fig. 3.27a–c Defect covered with two modified rhomboid flaps corresponding to a Z-plasty. D = defect.

Rhomboid Flap
(**Figs. 3.24–3.27**)

The rhomboid flap described by Limberg (1967) is useful for reconstructing temporal or cheek defects (**Fig. 3.24b, c** and **Fig. 3.25**; see also **Fig. 8.13**). A simi-

lar flap was described by Dufourmentel (1962) (**Figs. 3.26** and **3.27**).

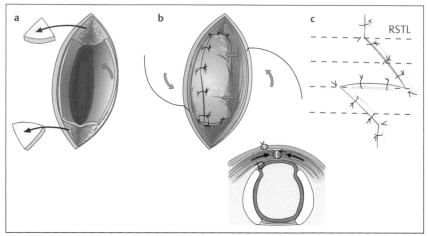

Fig. 3.28a–c   Turnover flaps are used for tracheostoma closure, closing a tracheal groove, or reconstructing alar defects (see **Fig. 5.39**).

a   A flap of appropriate size is outlined lateral to the tracheostoma and dissected to its margin. Skin triangles are excised above and below the defect and are discarded. The tracheostoma margin on the opposite side is freshened.

b   The flap is hinged over and sutured to the freshened epithelial border. The long laryngeal muscles are mobilized to cover the turnover flap (middle layer →).

c   A Z-plasty is performed to close the wound and place the scar in the RSTLs (dashed red line).

Turnover Flap
(**Fig. 3.28**)

Turnover flaps can be used for nasal reconstruction, especially in the alar area (see **Figs. 5.37, 5.39, 5.46**). They can also be designed as island flaps (see **Fig. 5.45**) and are useful for closing a tracheostoma (**Fig. 3.28**).

Tubed Pedicle Flap (Bipedicle Flap)
(**Fig. 3.29**)

The tubed flap or tubed pedicle flap is generally designed as a delayed bipedicle flap (**Fig. 3.29a**). Transfer is delayed for ~3 to 4 weeks, to promote the development of a central vascular supply. First the flap is cut with a 5:1 or 6:1 length-to-width ratio (**Fig. 3.29a**) and tubed, preferably by sewing epithelium to epithelium. The proximal end of the flap is preserved as a nutrient pedicle for the "long flap." The defect below the tube can be mobilized and closed by direct suture (**Fig. 3.29b**). After 3 to 4 weeks, the distal end of the bridge segment is clamped off with a thin rubber tube (Nelaton catheter). If livid discoloration occurs, the catheter is applied only briefly as a tourniquet (**Fig. 3.29c**). The tourniquet times are then gradually lengthened each day until the entire flap receives its blood supply from the proximal end. Finally, the other end is detached (**Fig. 3.29d**) and sutured into the defect. This process is repeated, and in about 3 weeks the residual tube flap is removed and insetting is completed (see **Figs. 5.17, 5.18, 10.37, 38**).

Distant Flaps

Distant Tubed Pedicle Flap

As noted above, tubed pedicle flaps can be transferred to the face from the upper arm or abdominal skin, if necessary by using a jump-flap technique. With the development of myocutaneous flaps and free tissue transfers, however, this technique is rarely used today.

Myocutaneous and Myofascial Flaps
(see **Figs. 12.1–12.3**)

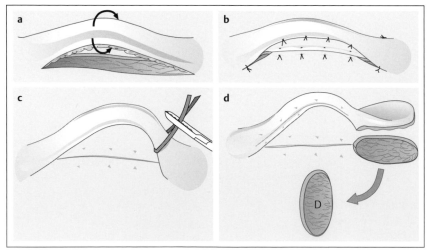

Fig. 3.29a–d   Delayed transfer of a **tubed bipedicle flap** (see text).

a   The bipedicle flap is raised and its bridge segment is tubed. The donor defect is closed.

b   Appearance after closure of the defects.

c   About 3 weeks later, the distal end of the bridge segment is clamped off with a Nelaton catheter and clamp.

d   The distal end of the flap is detached and inset into the defect. In a second operation 3 weeks later, the residual tube is divided, insetting at the recipient site is completed, and the unused portion of the flap is returned or discarded (see **Fig. 10.37**).

Special Part

II Coverage of Defects in Specific Facial Regions

For smaller facial defects, an attempt is made to achieve coverage by means of flap advancement or local flaps (**Plate 1**). Keep in mind that these flaps should be placed in RSTLs whenever possible (see p. 9).

If flaps cannot be obtained from the immediate vicinity of the primary defect, regional flaps are used. These are larger flaps involving the movement of tissue somewhat more distant from the recipient site.

The classic "regional flaps" from the neck and chest are no longer in common use. For the most part they have been replaced by myocutaneous island flaps (see p. 213) and free flaps. Even the classic "distant flaps," transferred as tubed flaps from the chest or abdomen over a period of weeks or months, are very rarely used today and have been replaced by myocutaneous flaps and free tissue transfers with microvascular anastomosis (see pp. 221 and 227).

Small facial defects can be excised and reconstructed with small flaps using a technique that will place the scars as close to the RSTLs as possible (see **Fig. 2.8a** and **Plate 1**).

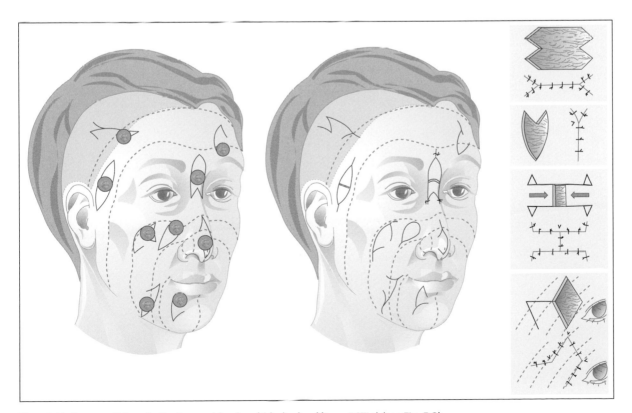

Plate 1 Various small flaps in the face and forehead (dashed red lines: RSTLs) (see Fig. 5.2).

4 Forehead Region

Median Forehead Region

The RSTLs run along the forehead and are perpendicular to the frown lines in the glabellar area (see **Fig. 2.8a**). Forehead defects up to 3.5 cm in size, especially when near the midline, can be closed by mobilizing the surrounding tissue. Primary closure can be facilitated by making parallel or perpendicular incisions in the galea. Small defects can be managed with various advancement, rotation, and transposition flaps (see **Figs. 3.1–3.27**) and Z-plasties (see **Figs. 2.15–2.18**).

Wedge-Shaped Defects
(**Fig. 4.1**)

Wedge-shaped midline defects that are based on the glabella (**Fig. 4.1a**) or frontal hairline (**Fig. 4.1b**) can be closed primarily by making an incision above the eyebrow or along the hairline and mobilizing the forehead skin.

H-Flap
(**Fig. 4.2**)

The H-flap is suitable for defects ~4 cm wide. Incisions are made along the eyebrow and hairline, extending through all layers in their lateral portions. The inferior Burow's triangles are placed near the eyebrow to preserve the frontal branch of the superficial temporal artery. The brow portion of the flap should be anchored to the periosteum, to avoid eyebrow distortion. As a rule, scars are no longer visible by 6 months to 1 year after surgery. A visible midline scar can be revised with the broken-line technique, or dispersed

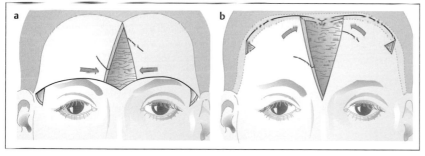

Fig. 4.1a, b
a Wedge-shaped defect in the forehead with an inferior base. An incision is made above the browline, and Burow's triangles are excised just lateral to the brow (see **Fig. 4.2**). The forehead skin is mobilized in the direction of the arrows. A Z-plasty (red line) can be used to disperse the scar.
b For a superiorly based defect, an incision is made ~1 to 1.5 cm behind the hairline. Lateral Burow's triangles are excised.

Fig. 4.2a, b H-flap (bilateral U-advancement flaps).
a For a midline forehead defect over 4 cm wide, an incision is made above the eyebrow and below the hairline. Lateral Burow's triangles are excised on the hairline and just behind the eyebrow, to avoid cutting the frontal branch of the superficial temporal artery. The midline scar can be dispersed with a Z-plasty (red line).
b All defects are closed.

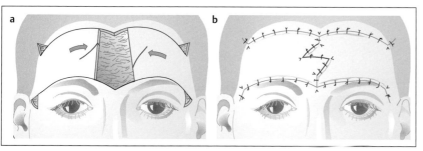

Fig. 4.3a, b Double rotation flap. An elliptical forehead defect is covered by incising and rotating the forehead skin and closing all defects. Again, a Z-plasty can be used to disperse the scar.

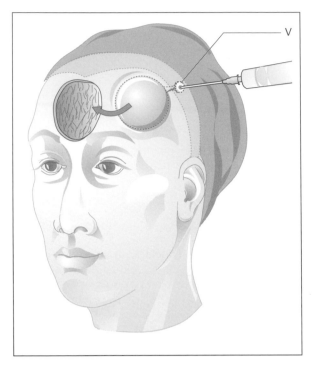
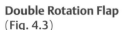

Fig. 4.4   Use of a **tissue expander** with a volume of ~100 cm³. V = valve for injecting sterile saline solution into the expander.

with a primary Z-plasty (**Fig. 4.2b**; see also **Figs. 2.8a4** and **2.15**). Smaller defects can be managed with a Burow's U-advancement on one side (**Fig. 4.2a**).

Double Rotation Flap
(**Fig. 4.3**)

A double rotation flap can be used to close larger midline and paramedian defects in the forehead. Again, the scars are located principally along the eyebrow and hairline (**Fig. 4.3b**).

Soft-tissue expansion can also be used for the primary closure of large midline defects (**Fig. 4.4**).

Lateral Forehead Defects
Forehead Rotation
(**Fig. 4.5**)

A wedge-shaped lateral forehead defect can be closed by making a long incision behind the frontal hairline, widely mobilizing the forehead skin, and rotating the skin into the defect. A dog ear is excised at the pivot point in the central forehead, and the wound is closed (**Fig. 4.5b**).

Similarly, wedge-shaped defects in the lateral forehead can be covered by a modification of the Esser cheek rotation flap (**Fig. 4.6**). Burow's triangles are excised below the earlobe and on the neck, to close the secondary defect. In the area of the zygomatic arch, the flap should be carefully dissected on the subcutaneous plane, to avoid damaging the temporal branch of the facial nerve, which is very superficial in that area.

Other options for covering lateral forehead defects are described in the section on reconstructing cheek defects (Chapter 8, see **Figs. 8.10, 8.16, 8.19, 8.22, 8.24**).

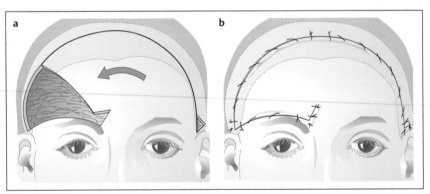

Fig. 4.5a, b   Lateral forehead defect closed with a **rotation flap**.
a The flap incision is placed ~3 to 4 cm behind the hairline (see **Fig. 5.48a, b**).
b The primary defect is closed. A Burow's triangle is excised at the pivot point (this may be postponed, owing to risk of flap necrosis).

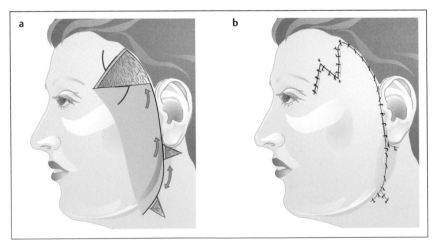

Fig. 4.6a, b   Lateral forehead defect closed with an **Esser cheek rotation flap**.
a Cheek rotation with Burow's triangles.
b Closure of all defects. Z-plasty (red line) can be added to disperse the scar (see **Fig. 2.8, Fig. 8.1**).

5 Nasal Region

The reader is advised at this point to review the esthetic units of the nose (see p. 15 and **Fig. 2.20b, c**).

Glabella and Nasal Root
(**Figs. 5.1–5.9**)

U-Advancement Flap of Burow
(**Fig. 5.1**)

A simple U-shaped advancement flap can be used to cover smaller defects in the area of the glabella and upper nasal dorsum (see p. 21). Burow's triangles are excised just above the eyebrow, resulting in unobtrusive scars.

V-Y Advancement
(**Fig. 5.2**; see also **Figs. 3.8–3.10**)

Trapezoidal rotation flaps are useful for reconstructing defects of the upper nasal dorsum (**Fig. 5.2a, b**) and canthal area (**Figs. 5.3–5.6**). The flap geometry corresponds to a V-Y advancement, and the secondary defect is closed by mobilizing the surrounding skin (**Figs. 5.2b, 5.3, 5.4**). Because these flaps receive a good blood supply from the supratrochlear artery on one side, the pedicle can be kept relatively thin, allowing for good mobilization and downward rotation of the flap.

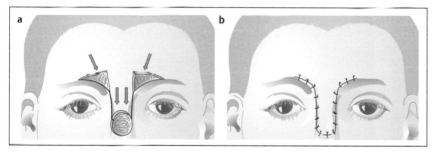

Fig. 5.1a, b U-advancement flap from the glabella, used to reconstruct a defect in the superior nasal dorsum.
a Burow's triangles are located just above the eyebrows.
b Appearance after closure of all defects (see **Fig. 3.2**).

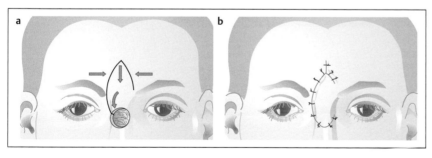

Fig. 5.2a, b Trapezoidal V-Y advancement (see **Figs. 3.9** and **5.4**).

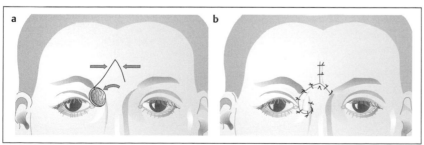

Figs. 5.3a, b Modification of the V-Y advancement (see **Fig. 5.4**).

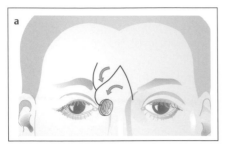

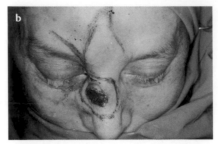

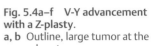

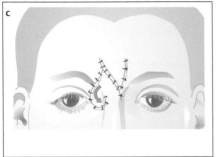

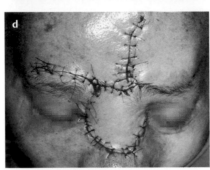

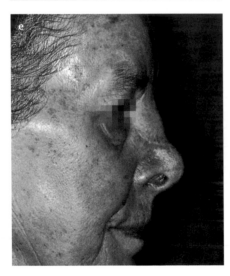

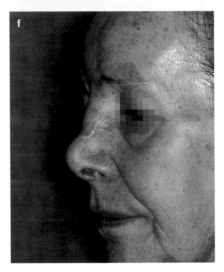

Fig. 5.4a–f   V-Y advancement with a Z-plasty.
a, b Outline, large tumor at the nasal root.
c, d Closure of the defect after tumor excision. An incision near the eyebrow and mobilization of the skin of the forehead allows primary closure.
e, f Result 1 year after reconstruction.

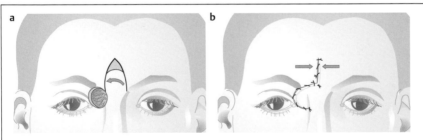

Fig. 5.5a, b   Closure with a **small transposition flap**.

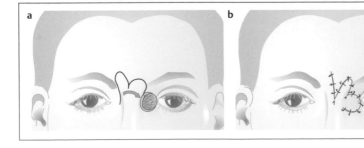

Fig. 5.6a, b   Closure with a **bilobed flap** (see **Fig. 5.8**).

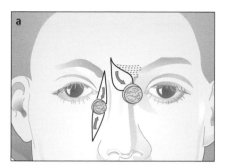

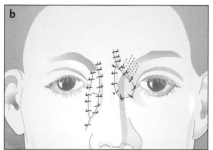

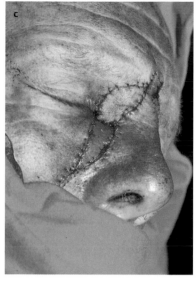

Fig. 5.7a–f **Sliding flap** with a lateral subcutaneous pedicle (see p. 22).
a Outline of the flap on the left side.
b Closure of all defects.
c Superiorly and inferiorly merged sliding flap to close the defect at the right lateral nasal root.
d Upper sliding flap on the left side.
e Results after reconstruction.
f One year after reconstruction.

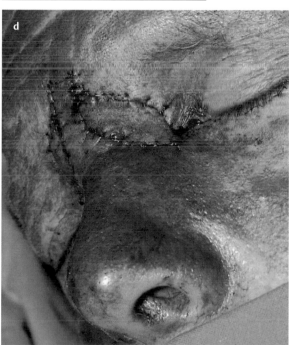

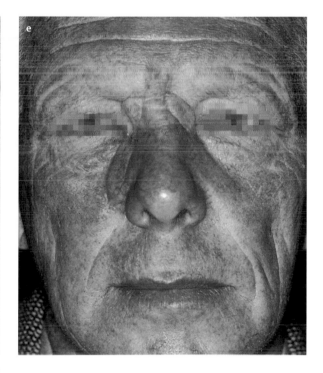

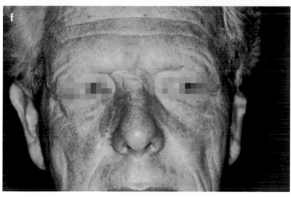

Sliding Flap
(**Fig. 5.7**)

The sliding flap of Barron and Emmet (1965), which has a lateral subcutaneous pedicle (see p. 22 and **Figs. 3.11–3.14**), has proven useful for reconstructing defects located more in the upper lateral portion of the nasal bridge. Besides a simple transposition flap (**Fig. 5.5**), a specially designed V-Y advancement flap (**Fig. 5.3**) or V-Y advancement with a Z-plasty (**Fig. 5.4**) can be used.

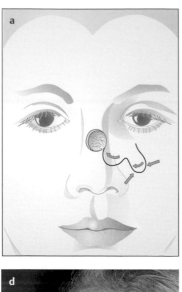

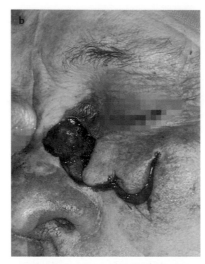

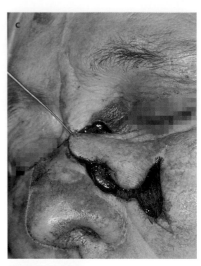

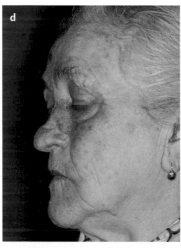

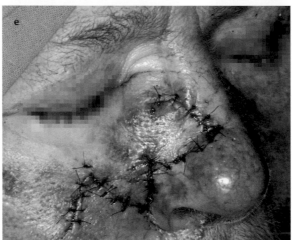

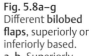

Fig. 5.8a–g
Different **bilobed flaps**, superiorly or inferiorly based.
a, b Superiorly based bilobed flaps for the reconstruction of the dorsum and the lateral nose.
c The flaps are rotated into the defect.
d Result after 1 year.
e Superiorly based bilobed flaps on the right side. The defect is closed.
f Result.
g Inferiorly based bilobed flap to recover a defect on the dorsum (distortion of the lower eyelid should be avoided!).

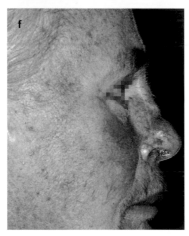

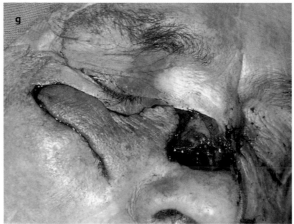

Nasal Dorsum
(Figs. 5.8–5.12)

Because the skin of the nasal dorsum is very tight, only relatively small defects extending across the dorsum can be closed by mobilizing the surrounding skin. A great many defects in this area can be closed with local tissue transferred from above or from the side. It should be noted, however, that the skin of the cheek and forehead is considerably thicker than the dorsal nasal skin.

Bilobed Flap
(Fig. 5.8)

Superiorly or inferiorly based bilobed flaps have proven excellent for the reconstruction of defects in the nasal dorsum and sidewall (**Fig. 5.8**; see pp. 25,

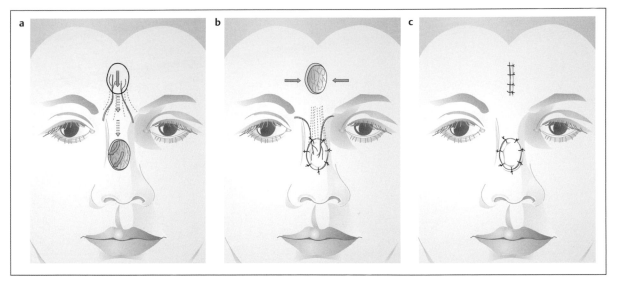

Fig. 5.9a–c **Island flap** based on the supratrochlear artery (Converse 1977).
a The flap is outlined, and subcutaneous dissection is performed without vascular injury.
b The bridge of skin between the flap and defect is undermined, and the island flap is pulled through.
c Closure of all defects.

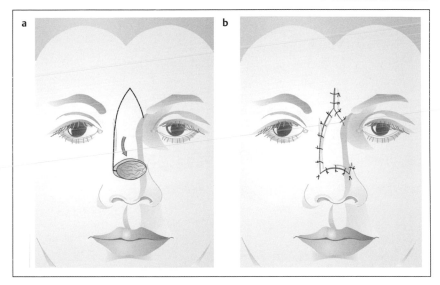

Fig. 5.10 **Trapezoidal V-Y advancement** of Rieger (can also reach the nasal tip; see **Fig. 5.14**).

26 and **Fig. 3.23**). Both small and larger defects can be managed in this way. The first lobe of the flap is moved into the primary defect, the second lobe is moved into the defect created by the first lobe, and the other secondary defect is closed by cheek mobilization (**Fig. 5.8a, b**). The angle between the primary defect and first lobe should approximately equal the angle between the first and second lobes, and all the angles should be 90° or less if possible. Larger angles lead to greater torsion and a bulkier dog ear at the pivot point of the flap (see pp. 25, 26 and **Figs. 3.22** and **3.23**). If the transfer creates a relatively large cheek defect, care should be taken that **the closure does not distort the lower eyelid**. For this reason, the subcutaneous tissue of the lower wound margin is usually attached to the periosteum of the upper wound margin after the cheek has been mobilized.

Island Flap
(**Fig. 5.9**)

The island flap described by Converse (1977), based on **one or both** trochlear arteries, is also useful for reconstructing defects in the nasal dorsum (**Fig. 5.9**). The bridge of skin between the island flap and the primary defect can be partially or completely divided if the flap shows livid discoloration because of excessive pressure on the pedicle. This flap can also been taken more laterally based on one supratrochlear artery.

Rieger Flap
(**Fig. 5.10**)

The trapezoidal Rieger flap (**Fig. 5.10**) is another option for reconstructing dorsal nasal defects (see also **Figs. 5.2, 5.3**).

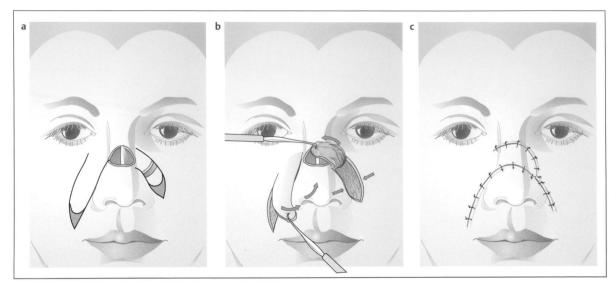

Fig. 5.11a–c **Nasolabial flaps** (Cameron 1975) used to reconstruct a full-thickness defect.
a One nasolabial flap (left side) is de-epithelialized in the septal   **b** A second nasolabial flap (right) is used for cover.
area to reconstruct the lining.   **c** Closure of all defects.

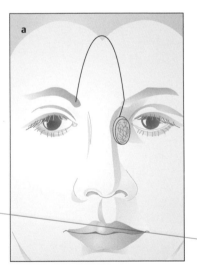
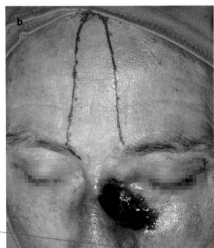
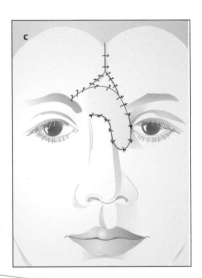
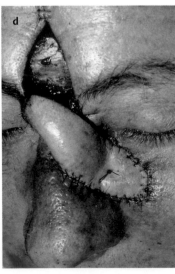
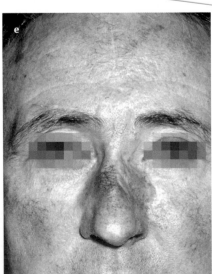

Fig. 5.12a–e   Reconstruction of a defect of the lateral nose and dorsum with a median forehead flap inner lining (with a full-thickness free skin graft).
a, b Outline.
c, d Closure of the defects.
e Results after 2 years.

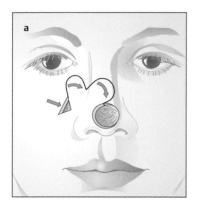

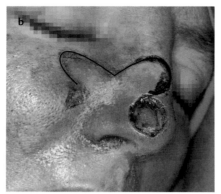

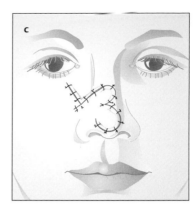

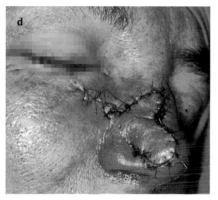

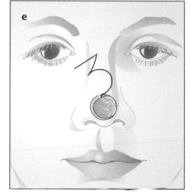

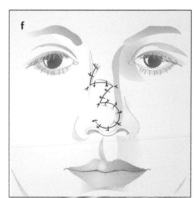

Fig. 5.13a–h Various designs of the bilobed flap.
a, b Inferiorly based bilobed flaps.
c, d Closure.
e–h Various designs of the bilobed flap (see **Figs. 3.22** and **3.23**).

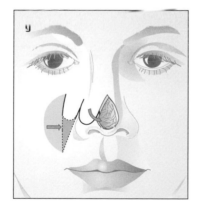

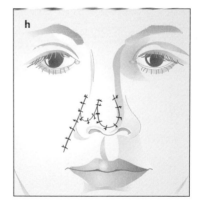

Nasolabial Flap
(**Fig. 5.11**)

Cameron (1975) suggested using two nasolabial flaps to reconstruct full-thickness nasal defects. The first flap (**Fig. 5.11a, b**) is swung into the defect with the epithelial side inward, after first removing the epithelium from the area that will overlie the septum. The second flap is then used for cover (**Fig. 5.11c**). One nasolabial flap is sufficient for reconstructing a two-layer defect.

Median Forehead Flap
(**Fig. 5.12**)

If a large defect of the nasal flank cannot be adequately covered with a bilobed flap (see **Fig. 5.8**), the median forehead flap is useful for this type of reconstruction (**Fig. 5.12**; see also **Fig. 5.15**).

Nasal Tip
(**Figs. 5.13–5.17**)

While small defects in the nasal tip area can be reconstructed with local flap transfers, larger defects that extend to the ala and columella require the use of median forehead flaps or the relatively difficult frontotemporal flap described by Schmid and Meyer (1962) (see **Figs. 5.17** and **5.18**).

Bilobed Flap
(**Fig. 5.13**)

The nasal tip area can be reconstructed using bilobed flaps that are based inferiorly (**Fig. 5.13a**), laterally (**Fig. 5.13e**), or superiorly (**Fig. 5.13g**). The scars should be placed approximately in the RSTLs. If the flaps are sufficiently large and mobile, a defect in the

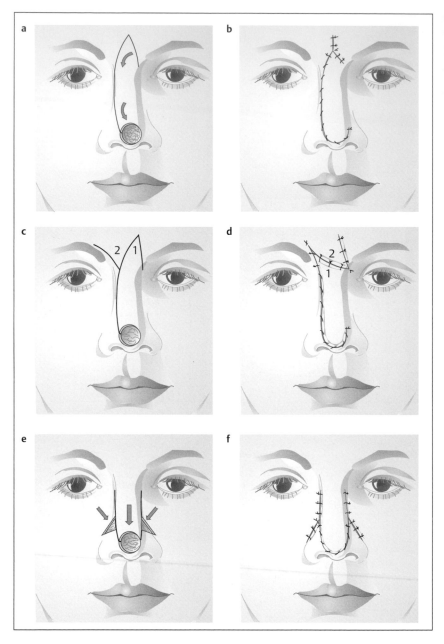

Fig. 5.14a–f **Various designs of advancement flaps** used to reconstruct the dorsal nasal skin (see **Figs. 3.9, 5.10**).
a–d Long Rieger flap
   (see **Fig. 5.10**).
e, f U-shaped advancement.

upper columella can be repaired concurrently with the tip defect (see **Figs. 3.22, 5.6, 5.8, 5.28, 5.29, 5.46**).

V-Y Advancement Flap of Rieger (1957)
(**Fig. 5.14**)

Larger nasal tip defects can be covered with a Rieger advancement flap based on the side of the nose (**Fig. 5.14a**). The glabellar portion of the flap has a trapezoidal design. The flap is mobilized along the opposite nasal flank, and a V-Y advancement is performed (**Fig. 5.14b**). A small Z-plasty may be necessary with larger defects (**Fig. 5.14c, d**). The U-advancement is another option (**Fig. 5.14e, f**).

Median and Paramedian Forehead Flap
(**Fig. 5.15**)

The median and paramedian forehead flaps are used to reconstruct larger defects of the nasal dorsum, sidewall, and tip, as well as partial and total nasal reconstruction (see **Figs. 5.47, 5.51a and 5.54**). The flap receives its blood supply from the supratrochlear artery on **one or both sides** (**Fig. 5.15a, b**). These vessels can be identified with a Doppler probe. The forehead should be high enough to permit the end of the flap to reach the nasal tip (using a pattern as a guide). The width of the flap should not exceed 3 to 3.5 cm, so that the donor defect in the forehead can be closed primarily without special preparations. The flap can

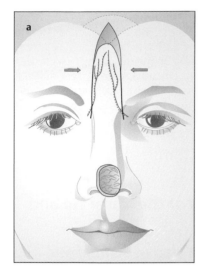
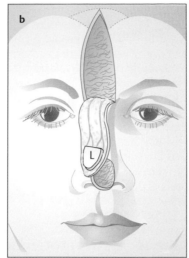
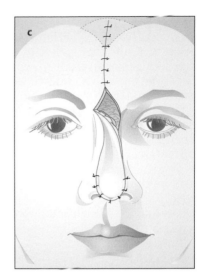
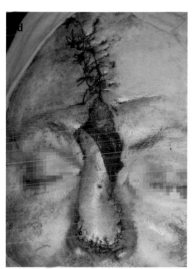
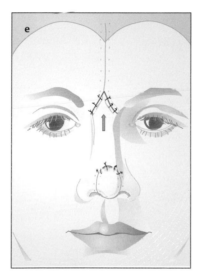
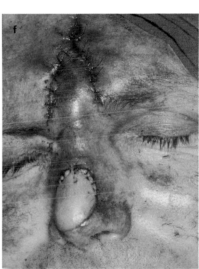
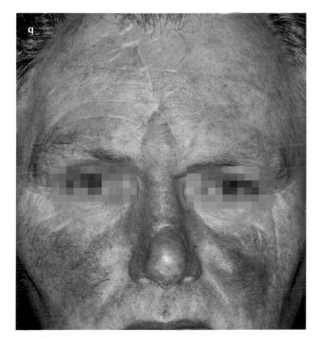

Fig. 5.15a–g   The median and paramedian forehead flap.

a   Outline of the forehead flap, which is based on the supraorbital and supratrochlear arteries. The maximum flap width is 3.5 cm, to close the primary defect (see **Figs. 5.49–5.54**).

b   The flap is dissected, leaving the galea and periosteum on the bone. If necessary, a split-thickness or full-thickness skin graft or composite graft (L) can be attached to the distal end of the flap (L).

c, d   The flap is sutured into the tip defect and the forehead wound is closed, leaving a wedge-shaped defect between the eyebrows.

e, f   The flap has been detached and its inset completed. The pedicle is reimplanted in the interbrow area 3 to 4 weeks later (see **Fig. 5.16c**).

g   Result one year after reconstruction (see **Figs. 5.51, 5.52, 5.55**).

be used immediately, owing to its excellent blood supply. The medial vertical scar in the forehead can be dispersed with a primary Z-plasty or W-plasty (see pp. 10 and 33). If the flap is broad, resulting in a tense suture line, we prefer secondary revision of scars that are still conspicuous 1 year after the operation (**Figs. 5.53** and **5.54**; see also **Figs. 4.1–4.4**).

The flap incision can be made through all layers down to the level of the eyebrow (**Fig. 5.15a**). In the glabellar area, the flap is bluntly dissected with a sponge stick or curved clamp to expose and preserve the artery on one or both sides (if we use the median forehead flap) (**Fig. 5.15c, d**). The skin incision can then be continued down below the brow level. If one artery is lost, the second artery ensures adequate flap perfusion. The residual triangular defect in the interbrow area (**Fig. 5.15d, e**) is covered with meshed tulle or a similar dressing. About 17 to 20 days are needed for the forehead flap to take at the recipient site (**Fig. 5.15d, f**). At that time, its pedicle is divided and inset into the triangular interbrow defect, which is first cleared of granulation tissue (**Fig. 5.15e**). The interbrow wound should not be reapproximated at the time of flap transfer, as this would distort the eyebrows by drawing them toward the midline. The wound edges should be freshened prior to inset of the flap pedicle (**Fig. 5.15f**).

As in all operations, meticulous hemostasis is required.

The flap takes from 6 months to 1 year to heal completely (**Fig. 5.15g**). If it is too thick, or if unsightly scars have formed, the flap may be thinned (defatted) and/or the scars revised by means of small Z-plasties or W-plasties (see pp. 10 and 11). For larger defects, we recommend using 50- to 100-mL tissue expanders on one or both sides (see **Fig. 4.4**) before raising the median or oblique forehead flap.

Modifications are asymmetric, paramedian forehead flaps (**Fig. 5.16a–c**) and oblique forehead flaps (**Fig. 5.16d; s. Fig. 5.54**).

Larger Defects of the Nasal Tip and Ala

Frontotemporal Flap of Schmid and Meyer
(**Figs. 5.17** and **5.18**)

If the median or oblique forehead flap cannot adequately cover a defect, or if larger, full-thickness

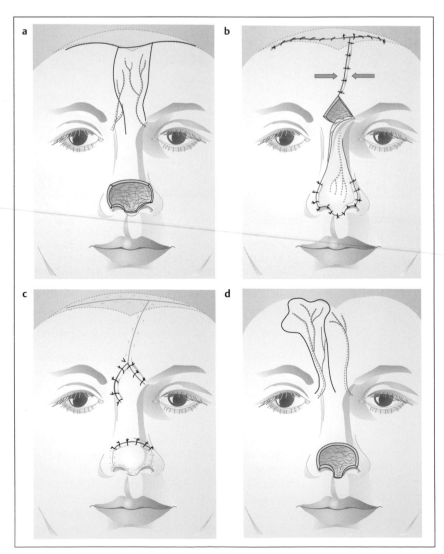

Fig. 5.16a–d   Straight and oblique median and paramedian forehead flaps of varying sizes (see Fig. 5.49).
a   Paramedian forehead flap based on one supratrochlear artery.
b   Closure of the defects.
c   About 20 days later, the flap is detached and the pedicle returned (see Fig. 5.15d).
d   Oblique forehead flap. The flap width may exceed 3.5 cm, but this precludes a simple direct closure of the secondary defect (see Figs. 4.1–4.4; Fig. 5.54q ff.).

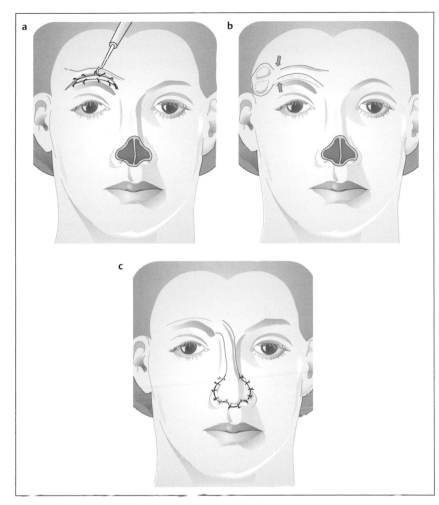

Fig. 5.17a–c Frontotemporal flap of Schmid and Meyer (1964) (see **Fig. 5.50**).
a A narrow bipedicle flap is raised above the eyebrow, to function as a **"transport flap."** The cut is widened slightly toward the bone. The defect is closed primarily, tacking the upper wound edge to the frontal periosteum, to avoid drawing the eyebrow upward. The bipedicle flap is sheathed with split-thickness skin. The reconstructive flap is outlined in the temporal area, using a pattern.
b A small bridge of skin (arrows) is left between the temporal flap and the bipedicle flap.
c About 6–7 weeks after creating the bipedicle flap, and 3 weeks after dividing the small bridge between the two flaps, the temporal flap is transferred and inset into the nasal defect. About 3–4 weeks later, the nutrient pedicle is detached at the nasal tip. If the tubed flap will be used to reconstruct the columella, the pedicle is divided at the eyebrow.

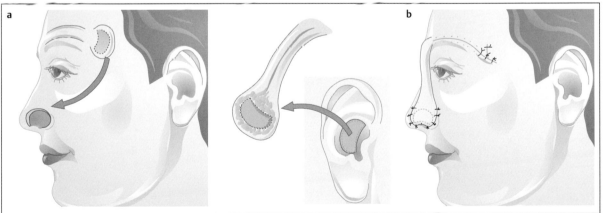

Fig. 5.18a, b
a The frontotemporal flap is precut, and its temporal end is lined with a composite graft.

b The flap is inset into the alar defect.

defects are present, excellent results can be achieved with the somewhat difficult frontotemporal flap of Schmid (1952) as modified by Meyer (1964, 1988) (**Fig. 5.17**). Because of its technical complexities, however, this flap is no longer widely used.

The flap is mobilized in stages ~16 to 20 days apart. In ~8 weeks, the surgeon can swing the flap downward, freshen the wound edges, and inset the flap into the defect.

Stage I:
First, a narrow, superciliary bipedicle flap is created. The flap incisions above the eyebrow should be spaced at a width of no more than 8 mm, but the lateral ends can be angled superiorly and inferiorly in a trapezoidal design. The superciliary defect below the bipedicle flap is closed by mobilizing the forehead skin (**Fig. 5.17a**). The upper edge of the wound is tacked subcutaneously to the periosteum of the frontal bone, to prevent eyebrow distortion. The superciliary segment of the flap is then sheathed with a split-thickness skin graft. The bipedicle flap serves merely as a transport flap; the reconstructive flap is outlined in the temporal area, to conform to the nasal defect (**Fig. 5.17b**). Split-thickness skin, cartilage, or composite grafts can be added to the temporal flap during the initial sitting (**Fig. 5.18**).

Stage II:
About 15 to 20 days later, the bridge between the prelined temporal flap and the transport flap is incised (**Fig. 5.17b**).

Stage III:
After a total of 3 to 4 weeks, the entire flap can be raised on its median pedicle, and the temporal flap is inset into the nasal defect (**Fig. 5.17c**).

Stage IV:
About 3 to 4 weeks later, the pedicle can be divided or opened up, inset to reconstruct the columella (Meyer 1988), or discarded.

Additional stages:
Further steps may be needed to complete the insetting of the temporal flap in the nose, or scar revisions may be necessary to improve the outcome. This technique can also be used for alar reconstruction using a composite graft from the auricular concha (**Fig. 5.18**). Other flap options for partial nasal reconstruction are described on the next pages.

Nasal Flank

We use small **transposition or rotation flaps** from the cheek to reconstruct defects of the nasal flank (**Figs. 5.19–5.21**).

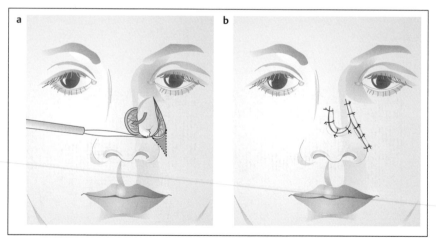

Fig. 5.19a, b   Superiorly based **lateral transposition flap (see Fig. 3.17 and Fig. 5.23d, e).**

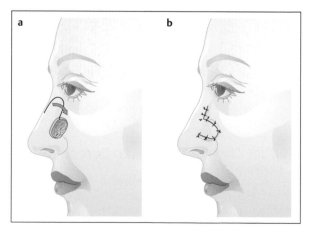

Fig. 5.20a, b   **Small transposition flap** based inferomedially.

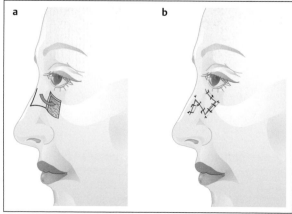

Fig. 5.21a, b   **Small Limberg flap.**

Fig. 5.22a, b Burow's advancement flap.
a Wedge-shaped defect on the nasal flank. Burow's triangle is in the nasolabial fold.
b Closure of all defects (see **Fig. 3.1**).

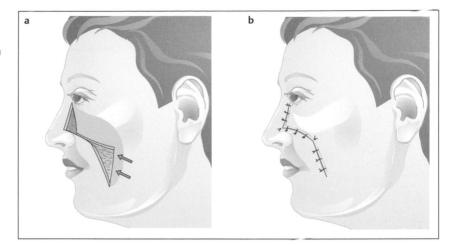

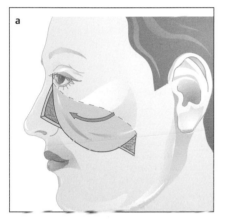

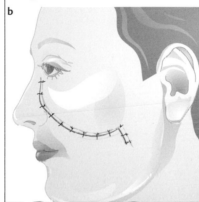

Fig. 5.23a–e Superiorly based **cheek rotation** of Sercer and Mündnich (1962).
a The cheek rotation flap is outlined, Burow's triangle is excised.
b Closure of all the defects.
c Nasal tumor, the superiorly pedicled transposition flap is outlined (see **Fig. 5.19**).
d Situation after reconstruction of a nasal defect; a cheek rotation flap is incised and mobilized to close the secondary defect.
e The defects are closed.

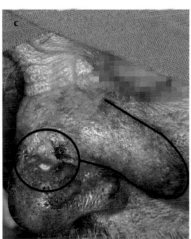

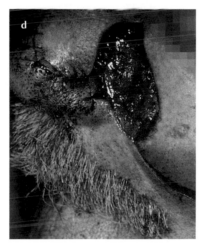

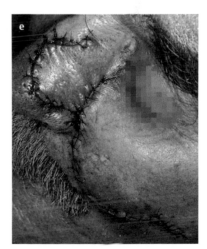

Below we shall illustrate some special flap designs that can be used when the flaps described above are inadequate for reconstruction.

Flap Advancement of Burow (1855)
(Fig. 5.22).

Wedge-shaped defects in the nasal sidewall can be closed using a simple Burow's advancement flap. The scars run along the nose at the boundary of the esthetic unit (see **Fig. 2.19**) and in the nasolabial fold.

Median Cheek Rotation of Sercer and Mündich (1962)
(Fig. 5.23)

Rotating the cheek medially on a superiorly based flap results in scars at the boundary of the esthetic units.

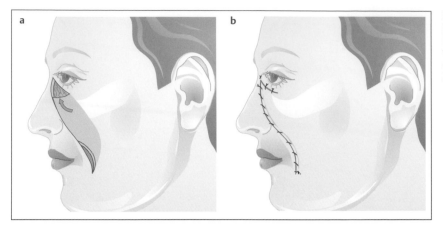

Fig. 5.24a, b   Burow's laterally based **cheek advancement** is a hook-shaped flap for repairing nasal flank defects (also suitable for lower eyelid reconstruction) (see **Fig. 3.1**).

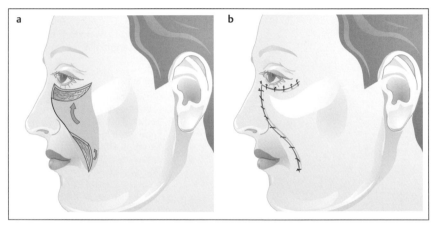

Fig. 5.25a, b   **Cheek rotation** of Imre (1928) with a banana-shaped skin excision.
a Flaps outlined for reconstructing the lower eyelid.
b Closure of all defects (subcutaneous tissue is fixed to the orbital periosteum) (see Fig. 2a in Weerda, 1980).

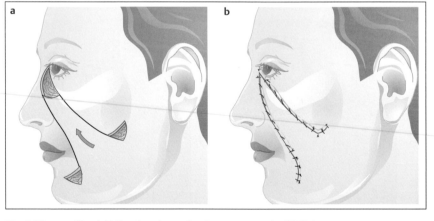

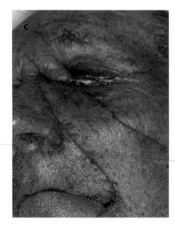

Fig. 5.26a–c   Cheek U-flap (rarely used as it runs across the RSTLs).
a Paranasal defect and outline of the U-flap.
b Closure of all defects.
c Result one month later, the upper defect was reconstructed by a supra-eyebrow flap.

Burow's Laterally Based Cheek Advancement Flap
(**Fig. 5.24**; see also **Fig. 3.1**)

Imre's Cheek Rotation (1928)
(**Fig. 5.25**)

Imre developed a laterally based, wedge-shaped cheek rotation flap for reconstructing nasal flank defects that extend into the lower eyelid. Instead of a Burow's triangle, a banana-shaped incision is made in the nasola-bial fold. The subcutaneous tissue of this flap should be fixed to the periosteum of the orbital margin, to prevent eversion of the lower eyelid. For the same reason, the flap should not be sutured under tension.

Cheek U-Flap
(**Fig. 5.26**)

This flap is rarely used because it conforms poorly to the RSTLs, especially in its superior portion. It can be used in cases of tumor recurrence involving the nasal

Fig. 5.27a–d   Double Dufourmentel flaps (see Fig. 3.26).

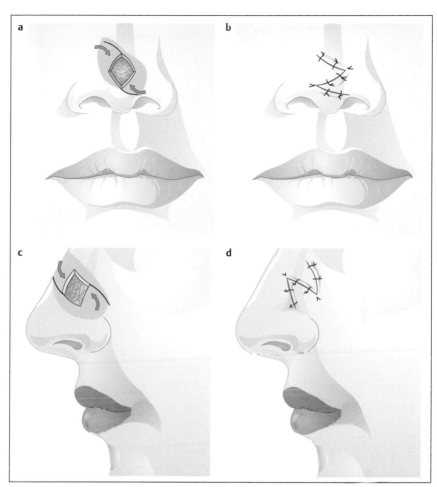

Fig. 5.28a–c   Bilobed flap.

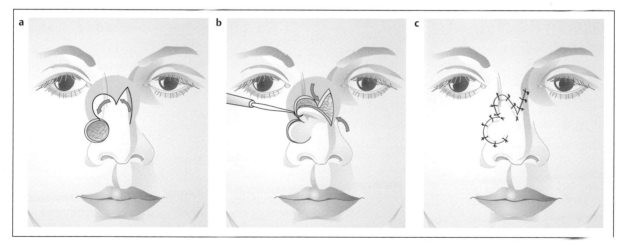

flank and medial canthal area, especially if median forehead flaps have already been used. Banana-shaped excisions can be made at the end of the flap instead of Burow's triangles. One alternative to the U-flap is the Esser–Imre cheek advancement (see **Fig. 8.2**).

Figs. 5.27–5.31 illustrate several practical flap techniques that can be used to reconstruct smaller defects throughout the nasal region:

- The double Dufourmentel flap (**Fig. 5.27**), well suited for reconstructing smaller defects
- The bilobed flap (**Figs. 5.28** and **5.29**)
- Transposition flaps (see **Fig. 5.19**)
- Advancement flaps (**Fig. 5.30**)
- Double transposition flaps (**Fig. 5.31**).

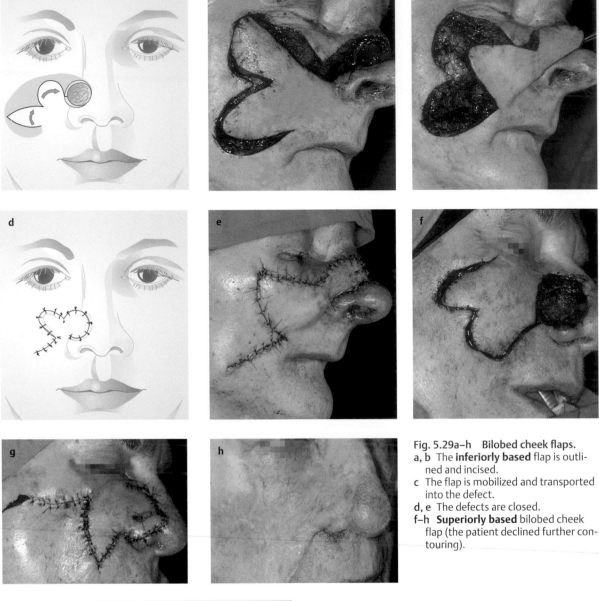

Fig. 5.29a–h Bilobed cheek flaps.
a, b The **inferiorly based** flap is outlined and incised.
c The flap is mobilized and transported into the defect.
d, e The defects are closed.
f–h Superiorly based bilobed cheek flap (the patient declined further contouring).

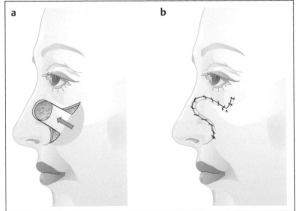

Fig. 5.30a, b U-advancement flap. Burow's triangles are excised from the nasolabial fold and nasal flank (see **Fig. 3.2**).

Island Flap
(**Fig. 5.32**)

An island flap from the cheek is also useful for reconstructing small defects in the nasal flank area. The flap may be based on the facial artery or may be designed with a subcutaneous pedicle that has an inferolateral or superolateral position in relation to the flap. The skin between the flap and the defect is undermined, and the pedicle is pulled through. Care is taken not to place excessive torsion or pressure on the flap pedicle. Because the subcutaneous pedicle often creates fullness at the pull-through site, this is not one of our favorite flaps. The cheek must be mobilized somewhat more widely than with other flaps, to avoid distorting the upper lip.

Fig. 5.31a–c   Double transposition flap with V-Y advancement (see Figs. 5.23c–e).

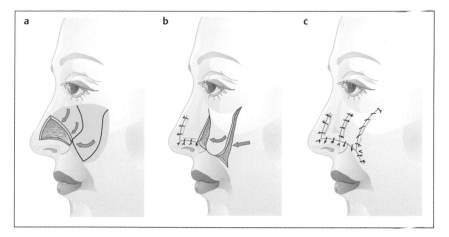

Sliding Flap
(Fig. 5.33)

A better choice is the sliding flap (**Fig. 5.33**). A sliding flap from the nasolabial fold is well suited for reconstructing the area where the lower or middle third of the nose meets the cheek. Like the island flap described above, the sliding flap is generally slid into the defect on a lateral pedicle (see **Figs. 3.11–3.13**) (Barron et al. 1965). Other examples are shown in the chapters on the cheek region (p. 115) and eyelid region (p. 129).

Nasal Ala

Smaller alar defects, especially when they are less than full thickness, can be covered using small rotation and transposition flaps or an island flap (**Fig. 5.32**; see also **Figs. 5.28–5.31**).

Full-Thickness Reconstructions

Z-Plasty of Denonvilliers and Joseph (1931)
(Fig. 5.34)

A defect in the alar rim can be corrected by mobilizing the ala as a full-thickness flap based on the alar groove, and performing a Z-plasty to bring down the superior nasal soft tissues.

Anteriorly Based Alar Rotation (Weerda 1984)
(Fig. 5.35)

Our technique differs from Denonvilliers', in that we use a flap based anteriorly on the nasal tip to bring down the alar rim. This allows us to place the Z-plasty more in the area of the nasolabial fold and cheek, where the skin is generally more mobile. The somewhat thicker cheek skin must be adequately thinned, and secondary refinement of the alar rim may be necessary at a later time.

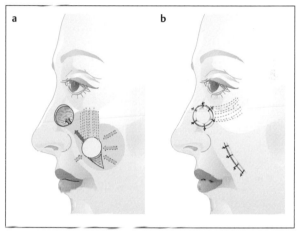

Fig. 5.32a, b   Island flap on a subcutaneous pedicle.
a The pedicle is undermined (red arrow) to create a tunnel.
b The flap is inset into the defect, and the donor site is closed primarily. (The flap can also be designed as an axial pattern flap based on the facial artery.)

Modification of the Anteriorly Based Alar Rotation
The defect formed by downward rotation of the ala can also be closed with a small, superiorly based transposition flap from the adjacent region (**Fig. 5.36a–c**).

Coverage with a Transposition Flap
A turnover flap is outlined in the skin above the alar rim defect and turned down to reconstruct the nostril lining (**Fig. 5.37a**). A laterally based transposition flap is then raised from the cheek and nasolabial fold, to cover the partial-thickness defect (**Fig. 5.37b, c**).

Lowering the Alar Rim as a Full-Thickness Bipedicle Flap and with a Composite Graft
(Fig. 5.38)

The alar rim can also be lowered by making a full-thickness incision ~7 to 8 mm above and parallel to the alar rim (**Fig. 5.38a**). After the ala has been brought down, the secondary defect is repaired with a three-layer composite graft from the auricle (see also p. 55 and **Fig. 2.23a**).

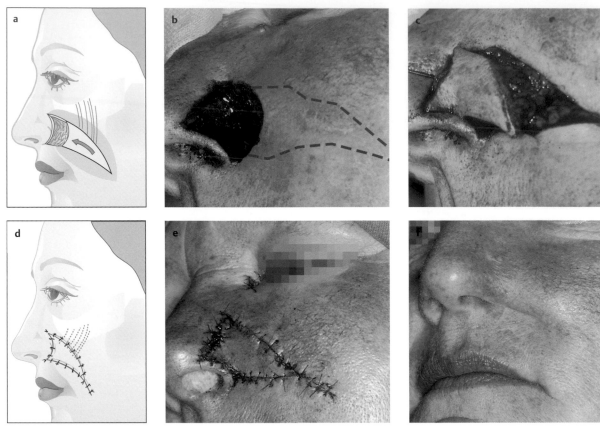

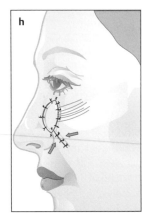

Fig. 5.33a–f   Sliding flaps for reconstructing defects behind the ala (**a–f**) or lateral nasal wall (**g, h**). These flaps are of variable size and may be transferred on a subcutaneous pedicle (see **Figs. 3.11** and **3.12**).

a, b Outline of the superiorly based sliding flap (see **Fig. 3.11**).
c The flap is transported into the defect.
d, e The defects are closed.
f Result after 5 years (the patient did not want contouring of the alar groove).
g, h Sliding flaps with a lateral subcutaneous pedicle.

Fig. 5.34a, b   Z-plasty of Denonvilliers and Joseph (1931) (see **Fig. 5.35**).

a Laterally and medially based flaps (1, 2) are transposed to bring down the alar rim.
b Closure of all defects.

Fig. 5.35a–f   Anteriorly based alar rotation of Weerda (1984) and Z-plasty.

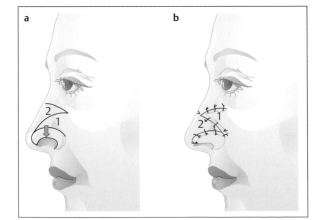

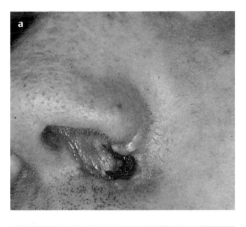

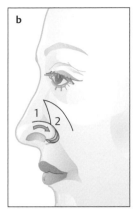

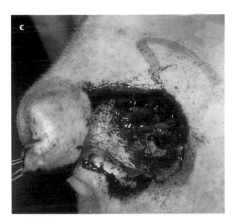

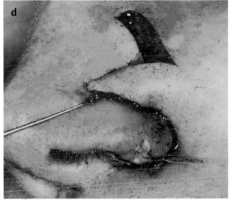

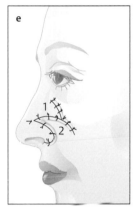

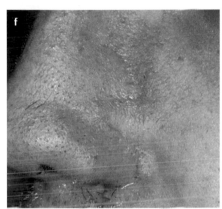

a Defect, the alar rim is too high.
b Outline.
c Incision and mobilization of the alar flaps.
d Z-plasty.

e Closure of all defects.
f Result.
Fig. 5.36a–c   Modification of the anteriorly based **alar rotation**.

a An incision is made around the ala, and two adjacent flaps are outlined.
b The ala is brought down to the desired position, and the flaps are transposed.
c Appearance after the reconstruction.
Fig. 5.37a–c   Reconstruction of the ala using a **turnover flap** and a

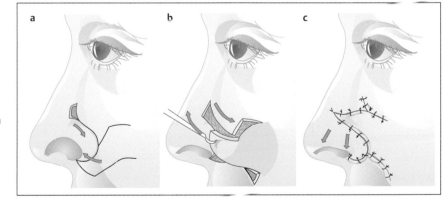

Turnover Flap and Composite Graft
(Lexer 1931, modified by Kastenbauer 1977)

A bipedicle turnover flap is used for intranasal lining (**Fig. 5.39a, b**), similar to the technique just described. Then a two-layer composite graft is used to reconstruct the alar rim. The skin of the composite graft is infolded to create a natural-appearing rim (**Fig. 5.39c**).

Converting a Peripheral to a Central Defect (Haas 1991) and Reconstructing the Alar Rim with a Transposition Flap
(**Fig. 5.40**)

In this technique, a two-layer or three-layer composite graft is inserted to repair the central defect (**Fig. 5.40a**).

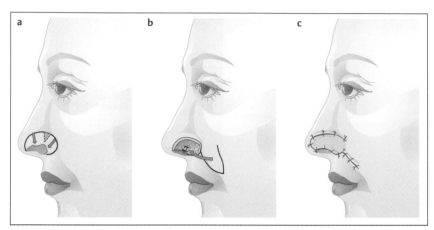

transposition flap from the nasolabial fold.

a The turnover flap for lining the defect is outlined, excising a small triangular skin flap as needed.

b Lining of the defect is completed, and the transposition flap is raised.

c Appearance after the reconstruction. (Additional inset of the pedicle may be necessary.)

Fig. 5.38a, b   Lowering the alar rim with a full-thickness bipedicle

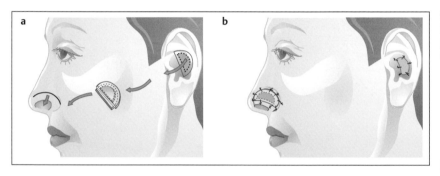

flap, and closing the defect with a full-thickness auricular composite graft (see **Fig. 2.23**).

a A full-thickness incision is made around the ala, the rim is lowered, and a full-thickness composite graft is harvested from the auricle (making the skin component slightly larger than the cartilage component). The auricular defect is covered with a retroauricular island flap.

b The defects are closed. The retroauricular surface of the composite graft faces outward.

Fig. 5.39a–c   Turnover flap and composite graft (see **Fig. 5.37**).

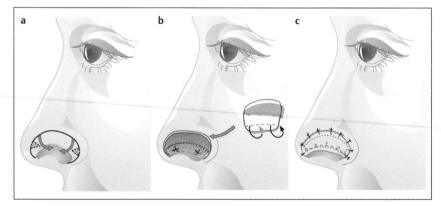

a An incision is made around the alar rim.

b The flap is hinged over, its edges are freshened, and the turnover flap is sutured in place. A two-layer composite graft is harvested with a slightly larger skin island, and its distal edge is folded over to create an alar rim.

c The composite graft is inset into the defect.

Fig. 5.40a–c   Reconstruction of the alar rim with an **inferiorly based transposition flap**.

a The lining is reconstructed with a turnover flap.

b The ala is reconstructed with an inferiorly based transposition flap (1).

c The central defect is repaired with a composite graft (2).

Fig. 5.41a–f   Wedge-shaped alar defect reconstructed with a **composite graft**.

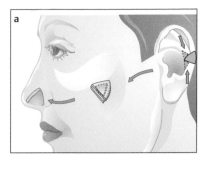
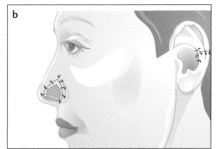
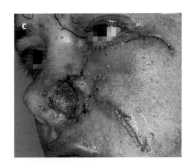
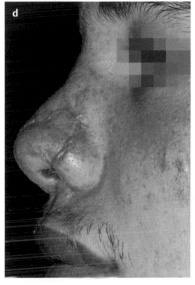
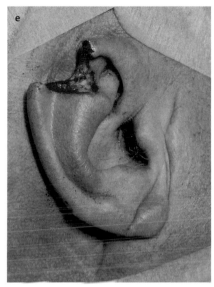
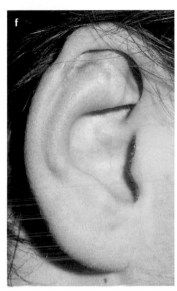

a A full-thickness composite graft is taken from the auricular border, which is closed with the excision of small Burow's triangles, slightly shortening the overall length of the auricle (see also **Fig. 5.28**).

b Reconstruction of the ala.

c Poor color match after 9 days.

d Results after 2 months, slight edema of the composite flap.

e Defect of the auricle after excision of the composite graft.

f Result some weeks after primary closure (see **Fig. 10.21**).

Fig. 5.42a–c **Larger alar defects** can be reconstructed with a Nelaton transposition flap from the alar groove.

Wedge-Shaped Defect in the Alar Rim
(**Fig. 5.41**)

Wedge-shaped defects in the alar rim that are no larger than 1 cm can be covered with a full-thickness composite graft from the auricle (**Fig. 5.41**). These composite grafts have a success rate of 80%, and livid discoloration during the initial days after graft inset should not cause concern (**Fig. 5.41c**). The skin component should be cut slightly larger than the cartilage, and the fine monofilament sutures should not be spaced too close together. The reconstructed ala should be immobilized for 8 to 10 days. Above all, the dressing should not be changed for the first 6 days, as this would jeopardize capillary ingrowth. Harvesting of the composite graft is guided by a pattern matched to the size and shape of the defect (**Fig. 5.41e, f**). We generally use the aluminum foil wrapper from suture materials to make the pattern.

Nelaton Flap (Nasolabial Flap)
(**Fig. 5.42**)

The Nelaton flap has proved useful for reconstructing larger partial-thickness and full-thickness defects of the ala. The defect should be carefully measured and the flap designed so it is slightly larger and longer. The flap is less satisfactory for bearded patients. The Nelaton flap is a superiorly based flap that is swung into the defect from the nasolabial fold. It can be infolded to reconstruct the alar rim. In men with heavy facial hair, the end of the flap should be thinned; the hair bulbs will be resected. Generally, there is no need to add cartilage for structural support. If the entire ala has been resected, the alar groove must be reconstructed in a second procedure. The donor defect in the nasolabial fold is easily closed by mobilizing the surrounding skin (**Fig. 5.42b**), which gives a barely perceptible scar. The alar rim can also be reconstructed with a nasolabial flap (**Fig. 5.43**).

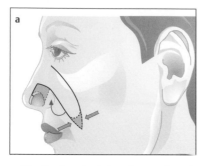

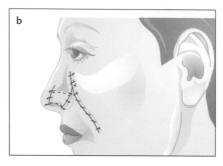

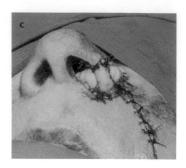

a The flap is cut ~1.5 cm longer than the measured length, as the end is used for lining (that portion is thinned). Flaps for bearded patients are cut above the hair bulbs.

b, c Appearance after closure of all defects (some revision of the flap base may be required) (see **Fig. 5.49**).

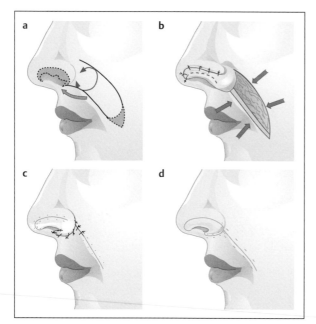

Fig. 5.43a–d   Reconstruction of the alar rim in two stages.
a, b Stage I.
c Stage II: the end of the flap is inset ~3 weeks later.
d Result.

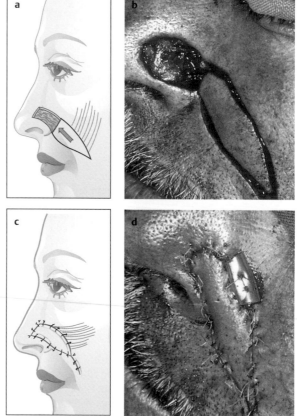

Fig. 5.44a–d   Reconstruction of an alar defect with a sliding flap from the nasolabial fold (after Barron and Emmett 1965; see **Fig. 5.33**).
a, b The flap is based superiorly on a subcutaneous pedicle.
c, d Closure of all defects (see **Figs. 3.11** and **5.33**).

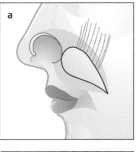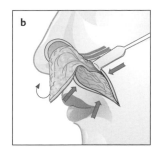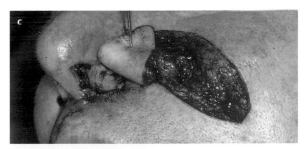
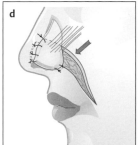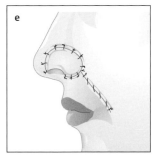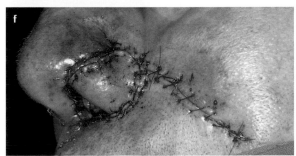

Fig. 5.45a–f   The **"in-and-out flap"** of Peers (1967), used to reconstruct a full-thickness alar defect.

a A large sliding flap is cut from the nasolabial fold and based on an anterosuperior subcutaneous pedicle. (Do not incise too deeply; dissect on a superficial subcutaneous plane in the cheek.)

b The upper portion of the flap is used for intranasal lining.

c, d The lower portion of the flap is thinned and inset into the external defect.

e, f Appearance following the full-thickness reconstruction. (see **Fig. 3.11**).

Sliding Flap of Barron and Emmett (1965) and Lejour (1972) from the Nasolabial Fold
(**Fig. 5.44**)

To slide a nasolabial flap to an alar defect with an adequate blood supply, the flap should have a subcutaneous pedicle that is placed laterally above the flap (**Fig. 5.44**; Barron and Emmett 1965) or directly below it (Lejour 1972) (**Fig. 5.44b**). The end of the flap is tapered to create a V-Y type of advancement in the nasolabial groove (see **Figs. 3.11–3.13** and **3.29**).

In-and-Out Flap of Peers (1967)
(**Fig. 5.45**)

This flap has an anterior superior subcutaneous pedicle (**Fig. 5.45a, b**) similar to the sliding flap above. The anterior portion of the flap is used for lining (**Fig. 5.45b, c**). The lower portion of the nasolabial flap is partially cleared of fat and inset into the alar defect for cover (**Fig. 5.45c–f**).

Median Forehead Flap
(see **Figs. 5.15** and **5.51**)

Besides providing nasal tip coverage, a median or oblique forehead flap is useful for reconstructing large defects in the nasal ala (**Fig. 5.15**). The technical details are the same as described on pages 40, 43 and 44.

Bilobed Flap from the Cheek (Weerda 1983c)
(**Fig. 5.46**)

In elderly patients with a large excess of cheek skin, an anterosuperiorly based bilobed flap can be taken from the cheek to reconstruct a large alar defect. With older defects, a turnover flap above the nostril can be used for lining (**Fig. 5.46a**; see also **Fig. 5.42a, b**), and an alar rim is fashioned by hinging over the lateral part of the first bilobed flap (**Fig. 5.46a**). The secondary defect is closed by mobilizing the surrounding skin. The cheek just below the eyelid should not be mobilized, and the lower portion of the cheek that has been mobilized upward should be fixed to the periosteum of the orbital rim (**Fig. 5.46b**). If the secondary defect cannot be closed by primary mobilization of the cheek, it should be closed by means of an Esser cheek rotation like that used with large nasolabial flaps (see **Fig. 8.1**) or by applying other flap techniques (see **Figs. 8.18** and **8.19**).

Large Defects of the Lateral Nose
(**Figs. 5.47** and **5.48**)

If a nasolabial flap (Nelaton flap, see **Figs. 5.42** and **5.43**) or bilobed flap (see **Fig. 5.46**) are not large enough to cover large lateral defect of the nose, we use a median (see **Fig. 5.12**) or paramedian forehead flap (see **Fig. 5.16**). Sometimes a lateral frontal flap can be used (**Fig. 5.48**).

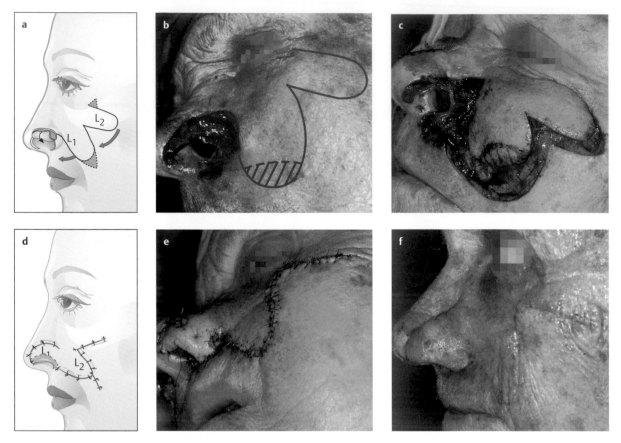

Fig. 5.46a–f   Bilobed flap from the cheek to reconstruct a large alar defect (Weerda 1983c).

a, b Outline of the bilobed flap. A turnover flap from the upper nasal defect is used for lining. A small flap is turned over at the lateral edge of the first flap (L_1).

c The bilobed flap is incised.

d, e The bilobed flap is rotated into place, and all defects are individually closed. The alar rim is in a good shape (**e**).

f Result after 6 weeks.

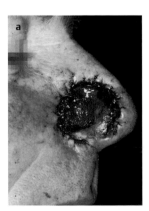
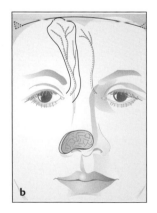
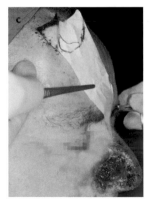

Fig. 5.47a–j   Oblique forehead flap for reconstruction of the alar and lateral nose.

a Large defect of the lateral nose and ala.

b Outline of the forehead flap.

c Template.

Fig. 5.47d–j   ▶

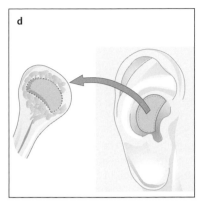

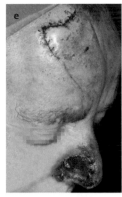

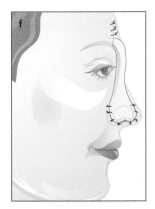

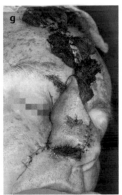

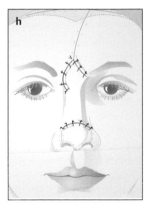

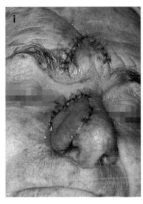

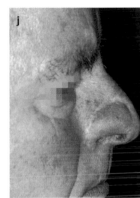

Fig. 5.47a–j *(Continued)*

d, e A composite graft of the concha is situated to the flap (see **Fig. 10.2**) as inner lining and as support.

f, g Insertion of the flap into the defect after 10 days; the frontal defect is closed primarily.

h, i Dissection of the flap after 4 weeks, the flap is modeled and inset, and the pedicle stump replanted to prevent a distortion of the eyebrows (see **Figs. 5.15** and **5.16**).

j Result months later.

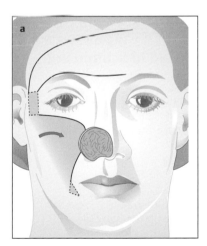

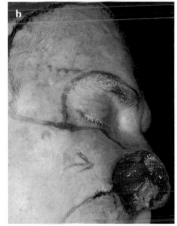

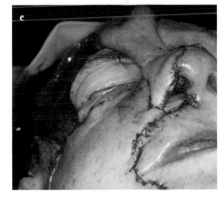

Fig. 5.48a–e   Lateral frontal flap (the patient did not want a median forehead flap).

a, b Defect of the lateral nose and cheek. The lateral frontal flap is preauricular extended and a cheek advancement flap is outlined.

c The lateral frontal flap is incised and sutured into the nasal defect with a good inner lining. The cheek defect is closed. The preauricular defect will be covered with a retroauricular full-thickness skin flap (see **Fig. 5.53b**).

d After 4 weeks, the flap is detached and the pedicle reimplanted.

e Result 2 years later.
   (The patient did not want any contouring of the flap.)

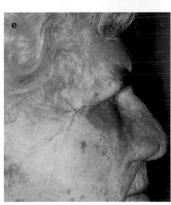

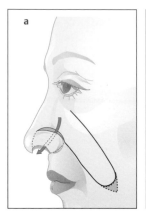
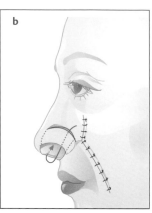
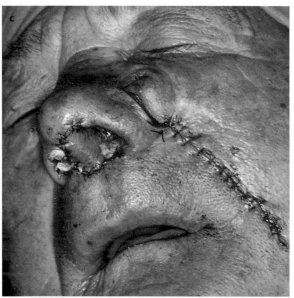
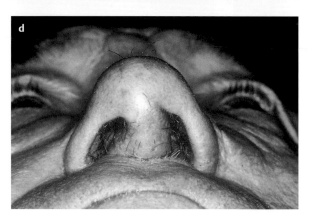

The Columella

Nelaton Flap
(Fig. 5.49)

Larger defects of the columella can be reconstructed with a Nelaton flap (nasolabial flap) in patients with scant facial hair (see p. 56). An incision is made through all three tissue layers in the alar groove, conforming to the width of the flap (**Fig. 5.49a**). The flap is then outlined to match the size of the defect, mobilized, and pulled into the nose through the incision in the alar groove. The necessary flap length should be measured with a paper or cloth strip, and an extra 1.5 to 2 cm of length added. The hair roots can be cut to a length of ~8 mm at the end of the flap. It may be necessary to reinforce the columella with auricular cartilage or with cartilage from the posterior nasal septum (**Fig. 5.49b, c**). In a second stage, ~16 to 20 days later, the flap is detached within the nose and pulled out of the incision, which is then closed. The end of the flap is inset into the alar groove at the incision site, and occasionally it must be completely detached (**Fig. 5.49d**). In some cases, the columellar area may require a later touch-up operation for thinning and scar revision. The nasolabial flap can also be swung around the ala for columellar reconstruction. In this case, a piece of silicone film is wrapped around the raw surface of the flap, to avoid maceration of the alar rim.

Frontotemporal Flap of Schmid and Meyer (1964)

This flap can occasionally be used for reconstructing the columella, especially when a concomitant nasal tip reconstruction is required (see **Fig. 5.18**).

Composite Graft
(Fig. 5.50)

Smaller defects of the columella can be reconstructed with a composite graft from the helix (see **Fig. 10.4**).

Fig. 5.49a–d Nelaton flap for two-stage reconstruction of the columella.
a Outline of the Nelaton nasolabial flap.
b, c The flap is pulled to the columella through an incision in the alar groove (arrow) and inset. In a second stage, the flap is detached and inset in the cheek area (see **Fig. 6.29c–f**).
d Result after 6 months.

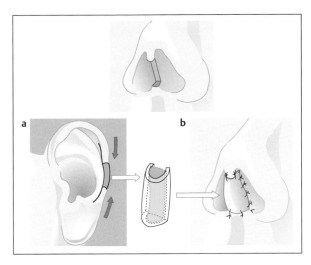

Fig. 5.50a, b **Columellar reconstruction** with a full-thickness composite graft from the helix.
a Donor site.
b Inset of the composite graft (see Gersuny's technique for resecting a helix tumor, **Fig. 10.24**).

Partial and Total Nasal Reconstruction

Median or paramedian forehead flaps (see **Figs. 5.15, 5.16, 5.51, 5.54**) can be effectively used for nasal reconstruction, depending on the size and location of the defect. In other cases, turnover flaps can be used in conjunction with nasolabial flaps (see **Figs. 5.12** and **5.40**) or bilobed flaps (see **Fig. 5.46**), or complex flaps may be required. Various flap combinations can be used in the reconstruction of large defects (see **Fig. 6.29**).

When a large forehead flap has been transferred (see **Figs. 5.16** and **5.51**), the upper two thirds of the donor defect can be closed by an H-advancement of the forehead skin (**Fig. 5.51e**), or with bilateral rotation flaps (**Fig. 5.51f**). If the scalp is hair covered, the superior flap incisions should be placed ~2 cm behind the hairline. The flaps should be securely coapted with absorbable subcutaneous sutures. Further details on these flaps are shown in **Fig. 5.15**. Oblique forehead flaps can also be used (see **Fig. 5.16**).

Converse Scalping Flap (Forehead-Scalp Flap)
(**Fig. 5.52**)

Use of the Converse scalping flap is illustrated for subtotal or total nasal reconstruction with partial reconstruction of the upper lip and cheek (**Fig. 5.52**). The neighboring esthetic units should be reconstructed prior to the nasal reconstruction (**Fig. 5.52a–e**). Soft-tissue expansion in the forehead (see **Fig. 5.16** and see also **Fig. 4.4**) may precede the reconstruction.

Stage I:
If necessary, a median forehead flap is used for nasal lining (**Fig. 5.52b–e**; see also **Fig. 5.15**). This flap is turned inferiorly (**Fig. 5.52**) and sutured to the residual nasal mucosa. Silicone stents or acrylate struts are inserted at this stage for structural support.

The incision for the forehead-scalp flap starts above the eyebrow, to the right or left of the median forehead flap, and is continued upward. For a total nasal reconstruction, this flap should be **at least 8 cm wide** and should span the full height of the forehead. Care is taken to preserve the frontal muscle as the flap is dissected upward (**Fig. 5.52d–f**). The scalping portion of the incision curves behind the hairline and ends behind the auricle on the opposite side. This large flap is supplied by numerous branches of the superficial temporal artery, along with the contralateral supraorbital vessels (**Fig. 5.53a, b**; see also **Fig. 2.8c**).

Following careful hemostasis, the entire scalp flap is brought downward with the well-perfused, relatively thin forehead flap. The forehead flap is folded to the desired shape and inset into the nasal defect (**Fig. 5.52f–i**). The galea and pericranium are preserved and are covered with impregnated gauze or film (**Fig. 5.52h**).

We allow the forehead defect to fill with granulation tissue. The soft granulations are repeatedly removed until a firm, stable granulating bed has reached the level of the surrounding forehead skin (**Fig. 5.52j**). Then the defect is grafted with full-thickness skin from the retroauricular and postauricular region on one or both sides, or with skin from the supraclavicular region (**Fig. 5.52i, k, l**). As a guide, we use a paper or foil pattern tailored to the size of the defect.

A full-thickness skin graft from the supraclavicular region can be used for nasal lining, as an alternative to the median forehead flap (this procedure can be done with the second stage). However, the somewhat thicker midline forehead flap provides a better framework for the cartilage strut that will be inserted later for structural support. We prefer to add supporting materials at a later time, rather than inserting cartilage grafts during the first operation (see pp. 71, 72, **Fig. 5.54**). If the forehead region has been expanded, large portions of the forehead defect can be closed in the initial sitting (see **Fig. 4.4**).

Stage II:
About 4 weeks later, the scalp flap can be incised and eventually detached from the reconstructed nose. The granulations on the scalp are removed, the edges of the flap freshened, and the unused portion of the flap is returned (**Fig. 5.52l**). At this time (no later!), the forehead defect is again freed of soft granulations

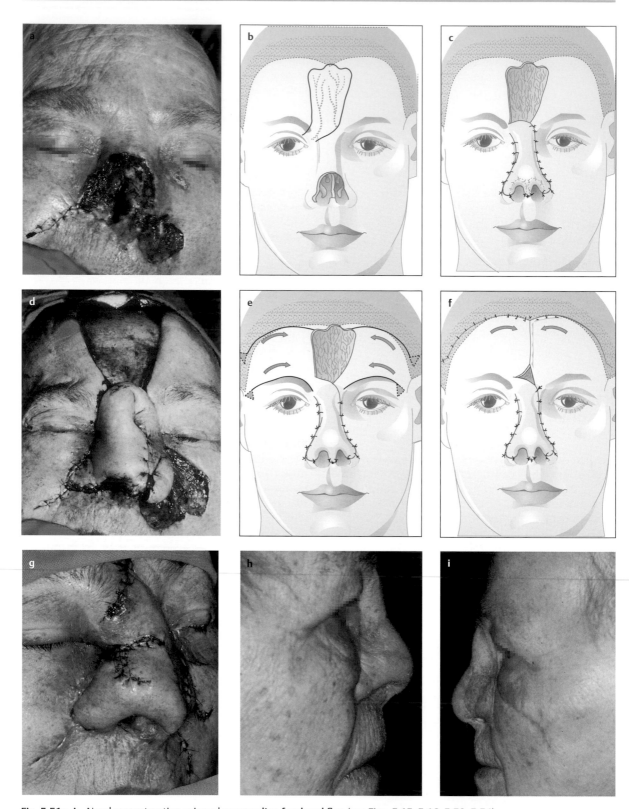

Fig. 5.51a–i Nasal reconstruction using a large **median forehead flap** (see **Figs. 5.15, 5.16, 5.50, 5.54**).

a Large subtotal defect of the nose and defects of the cheeks after tumor resection.

b The forehead flap is outlined. The nasal lining can be reconstructed with split-thickness skin, a nasolabial flap (see **Fig. 5.42**), or a sliding flap (see **Fig. 5.44**).

c, d Inset of the flap into the defects, the cheek defects are closed by mobilizing the surrounding skin and primary sutures (**a** right cheek, **d, i** left side).

e, f The donor defect can be closed with an H-flap (**e**) or bilateral rotation flaps (**f**) (see **Figs. 4.1–4.3**). A wedge-shaped defect is left between the eyebrows (**f**) (see **Fig. 5.47i**).

Second stage:

g After 4 weeks, the flap has been detached and its inset completed. The pedicle is reimplanted between the eyebrows (see **Fig. 5.15e**).

h, i Results 6 months later.

and grafted with full-thickness skin (**Fig. 5.52q–i**). Any necessary corrections such as defatting, scar revisions, or embedding cartilaginous supports (see **Fig. 5.54v–x**) are performed ~6 months later. Further

minor corrections can be added in later touch-up operations.

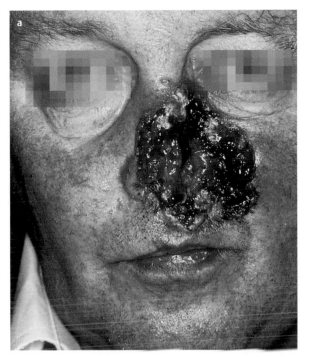

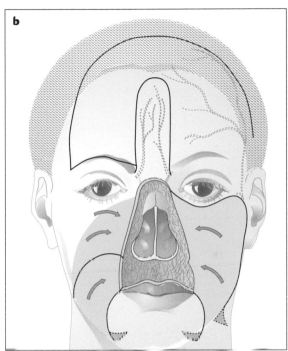

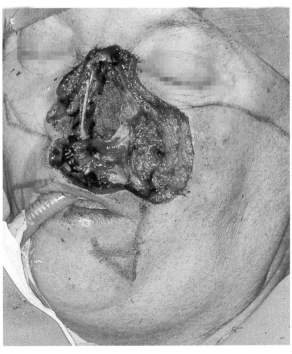

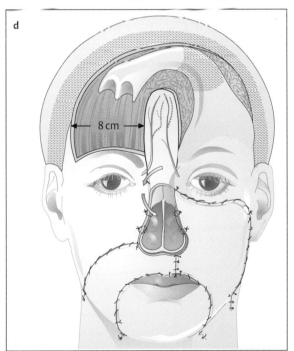

Fig. 5.52a–l   Converse scalping flap.
A patient with a large carcinoma of the nose, cheek and upper lip. The very fearful patient visited the doctor very late and did not want any refinement of the nose after tumor excision (**b**) and second stage of reconstruction (**l**).
Stage I:
a Patient with a tumor of the nose, cheek, and upper lip.
b, c Situation after tumor resection. The advancement flap (right) and cheek rotation flap are outlined to get an esthetic

unit. The lip is reconstructed with a modified Grimm flap (1966, see **Fig. 6.46**). The Converse scalping flap is outlined, laterally based, with a minimal width of 8 cm, and spans the full height of the forehead.
d, e The flap is incised to the galea and meticulous hemostasis is obtained. The median (paramedian) forehead flap is used for inner lining.

(Continued on next page) ▶

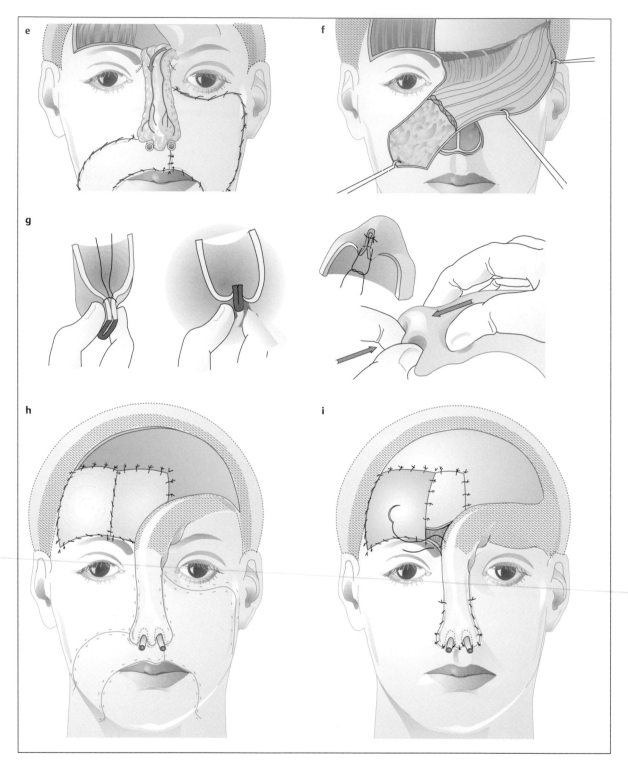

Fig. 5.52a–l   *(Continued)* **Converse scalping flap.**

f The scalping flap is elevated, the frontal muscle should be preserved in this technique (see Quetz p. 70, who elevates this flap with all layers).

g The distal portion of the flap is folded (see text).

h The new nose is inserted over silicone stents with an outer diameter of ~8 mm.

h, i The forehead, galea and epicranium defects are filled with granulation tissue, that should be conditioned (see text).

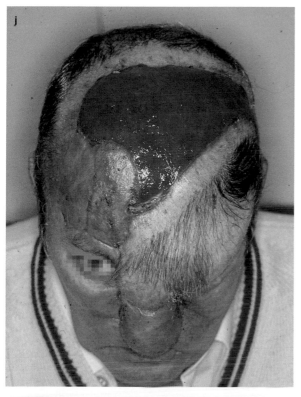

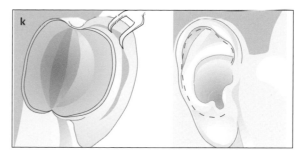

Fig. 5.52a–l   *(Continued)* **Converse scalping flap.**
Stage II:
j After ~4 weeks, the scalp flap can be incised, unfolded, and replanted. The forehead granulation tissue has been conditioned (see text) and grafted with full-thickness postauricular skin.
k Full-thickness postauricular skin of one or both sides (see text; see **Fig. 10.86**).
l The forehead reconstruction shows a good color match (and a good functional result because of preserving the forehead muscles). Further refinement of the nose was declined.

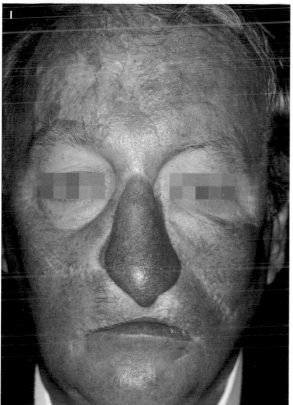

Total Nasal Reconstruction with the Sickle Flap (Farrior 1974)
(Fig. 5.53)

As in other reconstructions following total nasal loss, the forehead skin can be augmented by soft-tissue expansion for 6 to 8 weeks before the flap is incised (see **Fig. 4.4**).

Stage I:
The skin flap is taken from the median forehead, and its distal end is preshaped to form the ala and columella. As with the Converse scalping flap (see **Fig. 5.52**), the flap should not be made too narrow (**Fig. 5.53a**). It receives its blood supply from branches of the superficial temporal artery. The nasal lining is reconstructed with a thick split-thickness or full-thickness skin graft from the supraclavicular region. We stent the nostril openings with 8-mm silicone tubing (**Fig. 5.53b**). Incisions can be made over the eyebrow and in the scalp, in an attempt to reduce the size of the donor defect in the forehead or close it primarily (see **Fig. 5.51**; see also **Figs. 4.1** and **4.2**). As with the Converse flap, the pericranium is left intact and is covered with impregnated gauze or a similar dressing during healing of the reconstructed nose.

Stage II:
About 3 to 4 weeks after inset of the new nose, the pedicle is first partially incised on both sides and then divided, and the sickle flap is returned to the scalp.

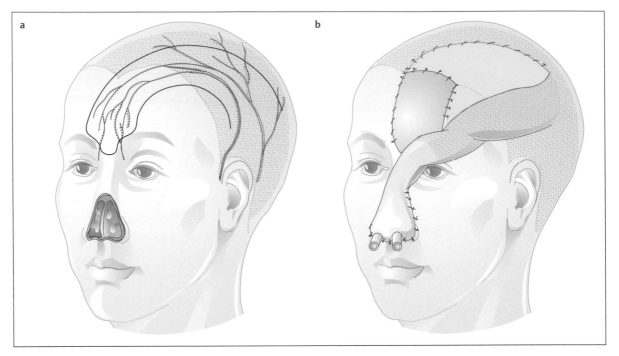

Fig. 5.53   Sickle flaps of Farrior (1974)

a The lower portion of the sickle flap is a median forehead flap at least 8 cm wide. It is supplied by a "transport flap" incised in the scalp and based on the superficial temporal artery (the galea remains intact).

b The forehead flap is inserted into the defect over silicone stents (reconstruction of the nasal lining; see text). Closure

of the donor defects is the same as with the Converse scalping flap (see **Fig. 5.52**).

The nasal lining is reconstructed with a thick split-thickness or full-thickness skin graft from the supraclavicular region. We stent the nostril openings with 8-mm silicone tubing (**Fig. 5.53b**).

- Residual defects in the forehead are grafted in the same sitting, with retroauricular or postauricular full-thickness skin (see **Fig. 5.51d, e**). Again, the granulation tissue should reach the level of the surrounding skin.
- If necessary, costal or auricular cartilage can be implanted at this stage, for intranasal support.

Stage III:

Approximately 6 months later, the flap is defatted and secondary scar revisions are performed.

Three-Stage Reconstruction of Total Nasal Defects (after Burget and Menick 1994, modified by Quetz 2011)

J. Quetz
(Fig. 5.54)

It is an ambitious surgical task to rebuild a nose so that it maintains good function and will not be recognized as a reconstruction. Even experienced surgeons are regularly confronted with complications and unfavorable results. A surgeon who is considering offering total nasal repair should critically review his own cases and demonstrate good results. Patients

should fully understand the extent of surgery involved, compared with procedures using modern implant-supported prostheses, which mostly ensure good camouflage, predictable results, fast rehabilitation, and an absence of donor-site morbidity (see **Fig. 2.20b, c**).

Some basic principles should be observed: the subunit principle (see **Fig. 2.20b, c**) has to be applied—in most cases defects within the nasal unit have to be enlarged (Burget and Menick 1985). The intranasal lining must be reconstructed without any gap, in order to be stable and provide the grafted cartilage with a good blood supply. Regional flaps beyond the nasal unit should not be used for regular repair of the intranasal lining, but should be preserved to manage any complications that arise. The nasal scaffold has to be strong enough to resist scar contraction, and the subsurface framework must be rebuilt by extensive non-anatomical cartilage grafting (Burget and Menick 1994) (**Fig. 5.54u–x**). The paramedian forehead flap (see **Figs. 5.16** and **5.49**) is by far the preferred choice for resurfacing the nose. It should be elevated as vertically as possible. The base of the pedicle should be unilateral and can be narrowed to less than 1.5 cm (**Fig. 5.54o–r**).

Our experiences in the past two decades have led to the following procedure, which has remained unchanged since 2005. We combine the bipedicle composite septal pivot flap (Burget and Menick 1994) with a full-thickness forehead flap, using, e.g., skin grafts for the inner lining (Quetz 2009). This forms a standard first step. For optimal safety and better control, we use free cartilagenous grafts in the second stage, thus dividing the whole reconstruction procedure into three regular stages (Quetz and Ambrosch 2011; see **Fig. 5.54s–x**).

Stage I:

This stage involves formation of a septal pivot flap, intranasal lining, and full-thickness paramedian forehead flap (**Fig. 5.54a–r**).

Septal pivot or rotation flap: at the first stage, we rotate the remaining nasal septum forward, if it is available. This was described by Burget and Menick 1989, as a bipedicle composite septal pivot flap (**Fig. 5.54a–h**). The upper edge of the flap is cut from the anterior skull base with straight scissors; the dorsal edge is then perforated with a 60°-angle blade and a curved chisel, and then the septal pivot flap is freed completely. Finally, the lower edge is ventrally severed, using a scalpel and chisel, by maintaining a 10- to 15 mm-wide mucosal bridge (**Fig. 5.54a, b**). The septal branches of the superior labial artery allow almost the entire septum to be elevated. After harvesting bony cartilagenous wedges of different sizes from between the mucosal bridges (**Fig. 5.54a, h**), the whole septal composite flap can be rotated anteriorly out of the pyriform aperture (**Fig. 5.54b–f**). The base of the flap is usually fixed sufficiently by the twisted pedicles in the spine area. In most cases, there is now enough protection supporting the lining and the paramedian forehead flap, while at the same time guaranteeing sufficient projection of the nasal tip. Excess bone and cartilage are removed from between the bilateral mucosal flaps, to achieve the desired nasal profile (**Fig. 5.54e, h**). When turned laterally, the mucosal flaps can contribute more or less lining to the nasal domes and vestibules (**Fig. 5.54e–h**). When a septal pivot flap is not available, minor changes are made to the standard procedure: most of the intranasal lining will be repaired by skin grafts. The design of the columella segment of the paramedian forehead flap is changed in such a way that it can wrap the columella strut completely. The missing support of the septal pivot flap is compensated, e.g., by modified silicone tubes and gauze swabs, until the second stage. In the second stage, we reinforce the dorsal strut in the shape of a T-beam, by wiring an additional segment to the underside.

The **intranasal lining** (**Fig. 5.54j–n**) is built according to the individual conditions. In most cases, it can be partly restored by excess mucosa of the septal pivot flap (**Fig. 5.54j–l**). Remnants of the former nose can often be used as turnover flaps and add some

vital skin to the intranasal lining. In subtotal defects, there may be enough residual skin to restore essential parts of the intranasal lining by turning the cover inside. In total or supratotal nasal defects, the intranasal lining is built almost completely with full-thickness skin grafts (**Fig. 5.54m**). In some cases, the excess mucosa of a large septal pivot flap is sufficient to repair almost the whole intranasal lining (**Fig. 5.54n**). However, in most cases, restoration of the intranasal lining results in a patchwork of excess mucosa of the septal pivot flap, turnover flaps from the remains of the former nose, and full-thickness skin grafts. During reconstruction, the intranasal lining is supported by bent aluminum foils or gauze swabs.

The **paramedian forehead flap** (see **Figs. 5.16** and **5.54**): a three-dimensional model of the new nose is prepared, according to the defect, dimension of the reconstructed intranasal lining, and desired shape of the new nose; this is mostly done by cutting and bending an aluminum foil (**Fig. 5.54o, p**). We use an ideal pattern as illustrated by Burget and Menick (1994), which is modified, slightly oversized, and then reduced according to the defect. When flattened into two dimensions, it serves as a template on the forehead. Its position is chosen as vertically as possible, reaching into the hair-bearing scalp in most cases. The base of the pedicle is narrowed to less than 1.5 cm. A full-thickness paramedian forehead flap is elevated with all the layers above the periosteum. Subcutaneous fat and frontal muscle are only removed along their distal edges, in order to form a columella and the nostril rims. After undermining the forehead, the donor site is minimized by using strong resorbable sutures to carefully approximate the wound edges. The intranasal lining is fixed to the forehead flap by quilting sutures: skin grafts are fixed tightly and vascularized flaps loosely. We prefer to use dry cotton wool for a tight tamponade, to exert gentle pressure on the tissue. It stays in place and absorbs secretions (**Fig. 5.54q**). The surface area on the forehead that remains open is allowed to heal gradually, under permanent semi-occlusive dressing. Over the course of a few weeks, the sutures are overgrown and resorbed, and the granulation tissue eventually reaches the level of the surrounding skin (**Fig. 5.54r**).

When all layers of the nose have healed properly, the second stage can be performed. If healing does not proceed as expected, an intermediate operation may be necessary, i.e., regrafting full-thickness skin to a necrotic area of the intranasal lining, or repairing a larger defect with a local or regional flap. If the septum and lining are not in perfect condition, the standard second step is postponed.

Stage II:

This stage involves re-elevation of the paramedian forehead flap, thinning of its layers, and reconstruc-

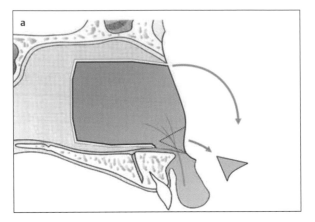

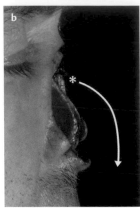

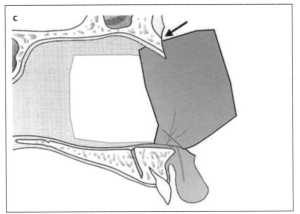

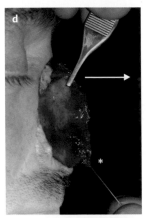

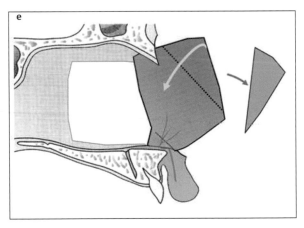

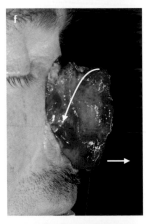

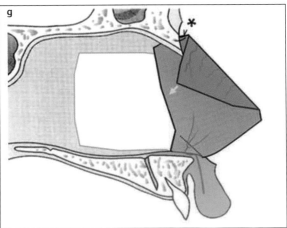

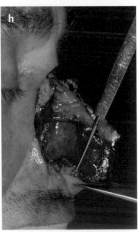

Fig. 5.54a–h   Three-stage-reconstruction of total nasal defects.

a–r   First stage of total nasal reconstruction with a septal pivot flap, and repair of the intranasal lining by mucosa from the SPF (= Septal Pivot Flaps) and skin grafts. The outside surface of the new nose will be reconstructed by a full-thickness paramedian forehead flap.

a–h Preparation and mobilization of the septal pivot flap for repair of septum and part of the inner lining.

a, b The flap is supplied by branches of the superior labial artery within a mucosal bridge that is less than 15 mm wide. The other edges are severed totally. A bony cartilagenous wedge is removed from between the mucosal bridges to allow rotation of the flap. The ventrocranial end of the septum (white asterisk) is transfixed by a suture (see d, f).

c, d Rotation is done by bending the flap, chiseling a groove into the nasal bone if necessary (black arrow), and pulling it out of the nasal cavity and downwards, with additional help of forceps. The former ventrocranial end of the septum is thus shifted to the spine area (white asterisk) and the portion from the skull base now forms the new ventral edge. The former dorsal edge of the flap is pulled out of the nasal cavity (long white arrow).

e, f The lower part of the neoseptum is gently pulled out, avoiding tension on the mucosal bridges (short white arrow). After the mucosa is separated on both sides of the upper septum as far as necessary for the trimming (curved white arrows), the profile is created by removing a bony cartilaginous segment.

g, h The neoseptum is normally blocked by itself. A suture (black asterisk) through the nasal bone may secure the position of the rotation flap. Further trimming of the bony cartilagenous neoseptum, e.g., in the spine area, is usually required.

Fig. 5.54i–n   ▶

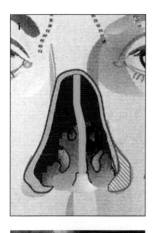

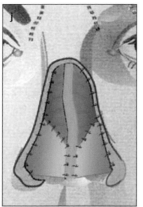

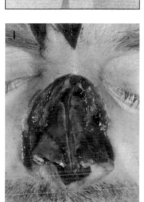

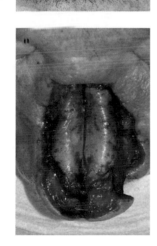

Fig. 5.54i–n Repair of the **inner nasal lining** following trimming of the neoseptum.

i The shape of the defect has to be modified according to the esthetic unit and subunits of the nose (see **Fig. 2.20**), in this case by removing a remnant of the left ala. The septal pivot flap is then rotated.

j The inner nasal lining is partly restored by excess mucosa of the septal pivot flap (red; see **n**), partly with full-thickness skin grafts (gray). If available, turnover flaps built from remnants of the old nose can be integrated into the patchwork. During reconstruction, the inner nasal lining is supported by bent aluminum foils or gauze swabs.

k The excess mucosa of the septal pivot flap serves as partial repair of the inner nasal lining. It has been separated from the upper neoseptum as far as necessary for trimming to the desired profile. Missing segments of the inner nasal septum are amended by skin grafts. The final shape of the inner surface is formed and supported by aluminum templates made, e.g., from suture packages.

l Front view of **k**: a deviation of the septum is negligible because the nasal dorsum will later be leveled by the fatty tissue from the paramedian forehead flap and defined by a dorsal strut from rib cartilage (**k**, **l**; see also **h**). (Balanced cartilage graft see p. 208)

m, n Two further examples for repair of the inner nasal lining.

m Supratotal defect: small wings of excess mucosa from the septal pivot flap have contributed to the new inner nasal lining. They are hidden under the reconstructed nasal bone built from calvarial bone grafts. Most parts of the inner nasal lining are restored by skin grafts (same patient as **r**, **t**, **v**, **y3–y5**).

n Subtotal defect: excess mucosa of the huge septal pivot flap is sufficient for repair of almost the whole inner nasal lining, completed by small turnover flaps from the tip area (same patient as **y1**, **y2**).

Fig. 5.54o–r ▶

tion of the nasal framework using autogenous rib cartilage (**Figs. 5.54s–x**; see also **Fig. 11.2**) and is performed after an interval of ~4 weeks.

Rib cartilage is harvested (see p. 207 and 208ff.) at the start of the operation, to allow the necessary time for further processing, shaping, and observation of this material. We take fascia from the adjacent muscles and perichondrium at the same time. Immediately after being harvested, two 5-cm-long pieces of rib cartilage are split into curved chips and straight struts of various dimensions. These are stored in saline solution and observed, carved, and observed again until they are used, in order to minimize the risk of warping and becoming deformed (see **Fig. 11.2**).

At the same time, the entire delayed paramedian forehead flap is easily and safely **re-elevated** in an unscarred subcutaneous plane, and **soundly thinned**. The area near the pedicle, the distal wings of the flap, and the redissected columella are thinned conservatively. The patchwork of skin grafts, mucosal flaps, and turnover flaps is thus completely separated from the overlying skin cover, forming a soft and homogeneous surface, coated by the fat of the forehead flap (**Fig. 5.54s**, **t**). This surface is also carefully thinned and trimmed to form a symmetric, well-proportioned and reliably vascularized recipient site for the cartilage grafts.

The **subsurface framework** is built by extensive and non-anatomically correct cartilage grafting. The

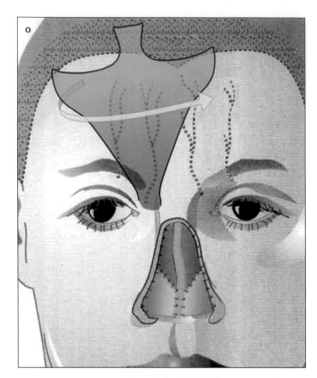

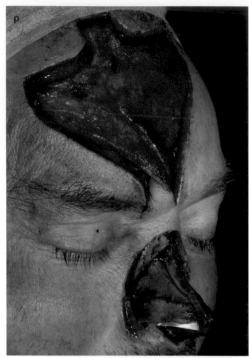

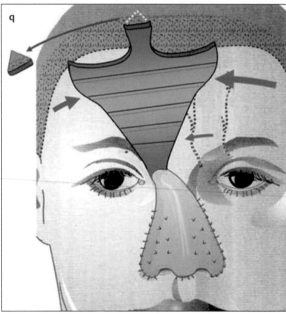

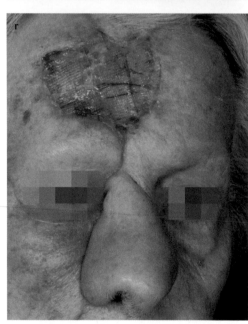

Fig. 5.54o–r   Reconstruction of the outside surface by a full-thickness paramedian forehead flap.

o A three-dimensional model of the new nose is prepared by an aluminum foil. Flattened out on the forehead, it serves as a template, with the position as vertical as possible, and base of the pedicle narrowed to less than 1.5 cm. A full-thickness paramedian forehead flap is elevated with all layers above the periosteum and will be twisted.

p The distal edges of the paramedian forehead flap are thinned to be able to form a columella and nostril rims (note the burns after thinning and cauterization). The flap is twisted 180° and will be turned down to cover the prepared inner lining .The thick subcutaneous layer, later firmly attached to the new inner nasal lining, will nourish the free skin grafts and fill up and smoothen the uneven surface of the inner nasal lining (same patient as **a–h, l, m**).

q The paramedian forehead flap has been turned down 180° and is sutured to its final position. The inner nasal lining is fixed to the paramedian forehead flap by quilting sutures to obliterate the dead space: skin grafts are fixed rather tightly and vascularized flaps loosely, supported by dry cotton wool tamponade. The mobilized wound edges of the donor site are approximated by strong resorbable sutures. The remaining defect will heal secondarily under permanent semi-occlusive dressing.

r Three weeks after the operation: granulation tissue has almost completely filled up the defect and overgrown the sutures. The aim of the first stage—basic stability and supply of soft tissue and surfaces—has been achieved. Projection, profile, and shape still have to be refined. The paramedian forehead flap will soon be re-elevated, thinned, and shaped by cartilage grafts in the second step (same patient as **k, l, t, v, y3–y5**).

Fig. 5.54s–x   ▶

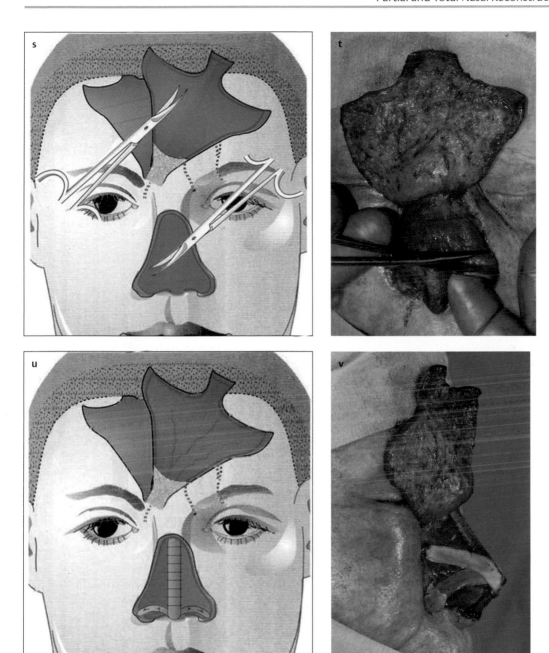

Fig. 5.54s–x　Second stage after ~4 weeks: **re-elevation** of the paramedian forehead flap, **thinning** and **shaping** of the intranasal lining, and **reconstruction of the nasal framework** using autogenous rib cartilage (same patient as **m, r, y3–y5**).

s, t　The entire delayed paramedian forehead flap is re-elevated in the unscarred subcutaneous plane as a thin layer. The inner nasal lining, a patchwork of skin grafts, mucosal flaps, and turnover flaps, is thus completely separated from the overlying skin, coated by the fat of the paramedian forehead flap. The inner nasal lining is also carefully thinned and trimmed to a symmetric, well-proportioned and reliably vascularized recipient site for the cartilage grafts.

u, v　The subsurface framework is built by extensive cartilage grafting: a dorsal strut is the most dominant element, tied down to the septal pivot flap by multiple thin sutures (7-0). A separate strut defines the exposition of the columella (not visible in the frontal view), and alar battens shape and stabilize the nostrils. Elements replacing the lateral portions of the alar cartilages define and reinforce the nasal tip and the supratip area.

Fig. 5.54w–x　　▶

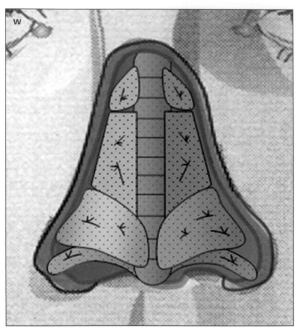

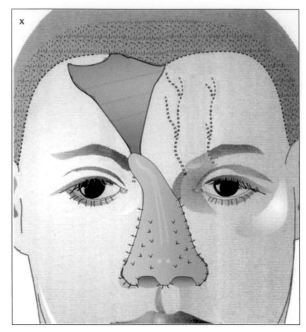

Fig. 5.54w–x

w The remaining unprotected surfaces of the sidewalls also have to be splinted **with thinly sliced pieces of cartilage**. The nasal tip mostly needs an extra cover of fascia or perichondrium.

x The paramedian forehead flap is resutured to its final position, and excess skin regularly trimmed. The inner nasal lining is carefully fixed to the paramedian forehead flap, with thin quilting sutures running in between and through the grafts. A tight dry cotton wool tamponade helps obliterate the dead spaces. The remaining defect of the forehead is kept under permanent semi-occlusive dressing.

Fig. 5.54y ▶

straight and curved cartilaginous pieces are carved in multiple steps until the desired shapes are achieved (**Fig. 5.54u–w**). The dorsal strut will be fixed to the dorsal edge of the septal pivot flap. In most cases, the strut has to have a concave underside that precisely matches the convex roof of the septal pivot flap. A columella strut defines the columella show. Alar battens are made, e.g., from elastic strips of rib cartilage bearing perichondrium on one side. They should extend into the soft triangle region, to give support to the nostril margins and are sutured to the caudal end of the intranasal lining (**Fig. 5.54u, v**). Replacement of lower lateral cartilages reinforces the cover and shape of the nasal tip and the supratip area. Conchal cartilage is best suited to this end; alternatively, thin elements of rib cartilage can be carved and assembled but they should be covered by a perichondrial layer at the end. The remaining unprotected surfaces of the sidewalls must be splinted with thinly sliced pieces of rib cartilage. All the small gaps and cavities must be filled with adequate pieces of cartilage and perichondrium. In particular, the nasal tip sometimes needs an extra cover of fascia or perichondrium (**Fig. 5.54w**).

The paramedian forehead flap is now repositioned and fixed onto the recipient bed, using lightly tied mattress quilting sutures to close the dead spaces. These sutures must be removed a few days later, to avoid marks in the skin (**Fig. 5.54x**). If the transplants and cover have healed and the symmetry and shape meet expectations, the third stage can be performed. Otherwise, an intermediate operation is necessary, e.g., for modifying and repositioning the grafts or for repair. Division of the pedicle is postponed until there is no further possibility of major revision (cartilage should be preserved in the thoracic wound, see **Fig. 10.53**).

Stage III:

After a minimum of 6 weeks, the following steps are taken: division of the pedicle, incorporation of its proximal and distal ends (**Figs. 5.15e** and **5.16c**), minor corrections where necessary, and, sometimes, closure of the residual skin defect in the forehead with a skin graft (**Fig. 5.54y5**; see also **Fig. 5.50**).

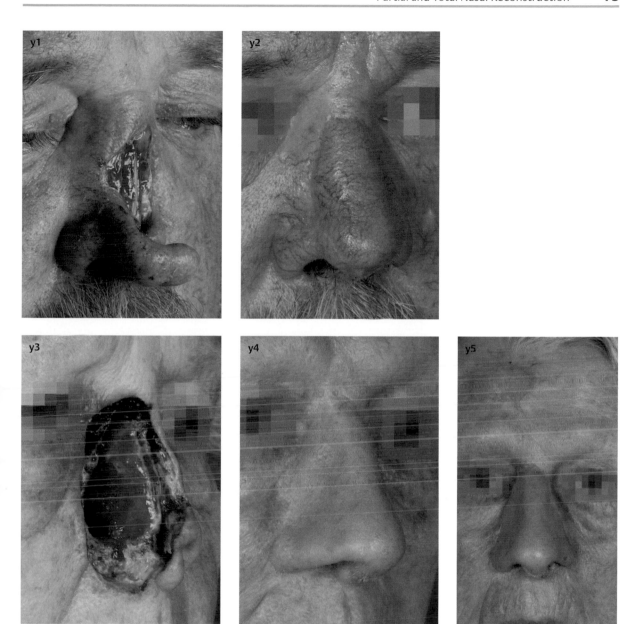

Fig. 5.54y   Primary defects and late follow-up after **three-stage-reconstruction of** large nasal defects.

y1   Subtotal defect (Same patient as n): Some soft tissue and skin on the right side has been preserved.

y2   Two years after the third stage: inconspicuous nose with fairly good scar formation and stable form and profile. The skin of the paramedian forehead flap blends in well. Nasal breathing and olfaction are normal.

y3   Supratotal defect (same patient as **m, r, t, v**): left nostril intact; part of the left cheek, the upper lip on the right side, and most of the nasal bone is destroyed.

y4   Three years after the third stage: good form and scar formation. The skin blends in well—it looks a bit "younger" than the rest of the face. Nasal breathing and olfaction are normal.

y5   Frontal view. Note the important symmetric position of the nostrils. The remaining harvesting defect on the forehead was, in this case, partly covered with a thinned full-thickness skin graft from the postauricular region (see **Figs. 5.52k; 10.86**).

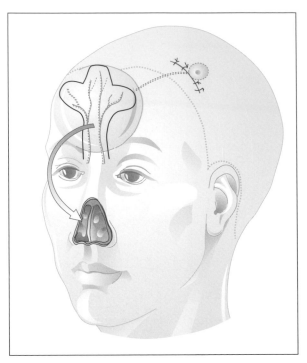

Fig. 5.55 Broad median forehead flap following preliminary soft-tissue expansion with a 200-mL expander. A small incision in the scalp gives access for inflating the envelope. The flap is dissected from the galea and periosteum in a subcutaneous plane, preserving the frontal muscle (oblique forehead flap, see **Fig 5.16**). We can get better results, without a rigid scar, with lateral expansion (see **Fig. 4.4**).

Median Forehead Flap with Soft-Tissue Expansion
(**Fig. 5.55**)

In this technique, the median forehead skin is expanded with a 200-mL envelope for 6 to 8 weeks, and then a forehead flap is incised to match the nasal defect (**Fig. 5.55**; Siegert et al. 1992; Siegert and Weerda 1994; see also **Fig. 5.51** and **Fig. 5.16**, oblique forehead flap).

Nasal Reconstruction with Distant Flaps

It is unusual today for surgeons to use distant flap techniques such as the upper arm flap (Tagliacozzi) or "jumping" a flap to the face via the wrist or upper arm. Free flaps such as the radial forearm flap (see **Fig. 14.1**) may give a poor color and texture match for nasal reconstructions, and are used only in exceptional cases where donor sites close to the defect are unavailable.

Defect-prostheses are an acceptable alternative specially for aged patients (see **Fig. 6.19h**).

Perforations of the Septum

Small Perforations

Small septal perforations can be managed with small unilateral or bilateral U-advancement flaps, which can be elevated in one or two layers (**Fig. 5.56**). Small

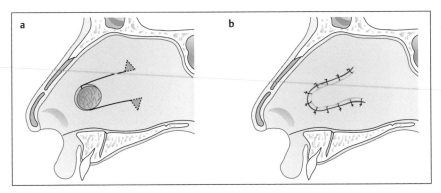

Fig. 5.56a, b   U-advancement flap.

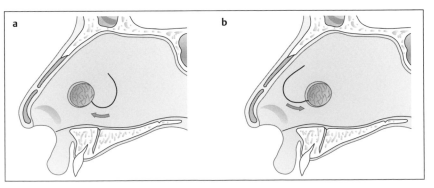

Fig. 5.57a, b   A rotation flap may be incised anterior or posterior to the defect.

Fig. 5.58a, b Bipedicle flap.

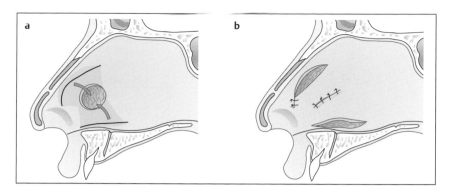

Fig. 5.59a, b
a Posteriorly (or anteriorly) based flap from the inferior turbinate (may include a piece of bone).
b Meyer's (1988) intraoral mucosal flap. The flap is precut and pre-lined with a cartilage graft. Two weeks later, it is delivered through a tunnel to the nasal septum. The wound is closed in two layers, and the flap is detached at 3 weeks.

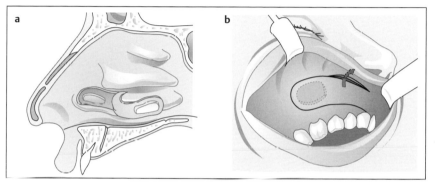

unilateral or bilateral rotation flaps (**Fig. 5.57**) and bipedicle flaps (**Fig. 5.58**) may also be considered. We have also used anteriorly or posteriorly based mucosal flaps from the inferior nasal turbinate, in which case a small piece of turbinate bone may be transferred with the flap (**Fig. 5.59a**). A second operation is needed for dividing the flap and insetting it into the anterior or posterior wound margin in the septum.

Large Defects

Oral Mucosal Flap of Meyer (1988)
(**Fig. 5.59b**)

Meyer described a technique in which a medially or laterally based mucosal flap is first dissected from the oral vestibule and lined with mucosa or a composite graft matching the size of the defect. In a second stage, the flap is brought upward to the defect, through a tunnel in the vestibule and septal mucosa, where it is sutured into place. If necessary, the entire anterior nose can be opened up for this operation. The pedicle is later divided.

Nasolabial Flap of Tipton (1975)
(**Fig. 5.60**)

In 1975, Tipton suggested using the Nelaton flap for larger defects. The ala is detached for its full thickness, and the Nelaton flap is sutured into the defect (**Fig. 5.60a**). The upper edge of the flap can be de-epithelialized prior to inset. The second side can be left

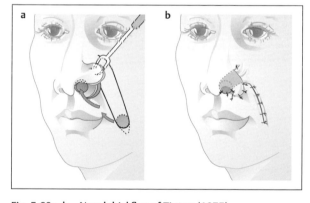

Fig. 5.60a, b Nasolabial flap of Tipton (1975).
a The ala is detached, and the Nelaton flap is raised.
b The Nelaton flap is swung into the septal defect and inset, and the ala is returned to its original position and sutured into place. (In a second stage, the flap is detached and the alar groove is closed.)

to granulate. Three weeks later, the flap is detached and the ala returned to its original position (see **Fig. 5.49**).

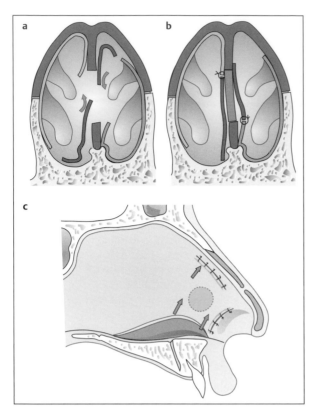

Fig. 5.61a–c   Bilateral bipedicle flap technique of Schultz-Coulon (1989).

a The septal mucosa around the defect is mobilized through a hemitransfixion incision, and the entire mucosa is mobilized past the nasal floor to the inferior turbinate (here, on the right side). The mucosa on the left side is separated past the nasal dorsum. The mucosa on the right side is incised below the turbinate and mobilized, and the mucosa on the left side is incised dorsally and mobilized. (These flaps can also be incised superiorly or inferiorly on both sides.)

b Bilateral coverage of the septal defect.

c Closure viewed from the right side.

Bipedicle Flap of Schultz-Coulon (1989) (**Fig. 5.61**)

First the mucosa on both sides of the septal defect is undermined from the front through a transfixion incision, and the defect is freshened. The entire mucosa on one side is then mobilized down to the nasal floor and inferior turbinate, divided (**Fig. 5.61a**, right), and advanced toward the defect (**Fig. 5.61b**, right). On the opposite side, the mucosa above the defect is mobilized past the sidewall and dorsum, and divided (**Fig. 5.61a**, left). The mucosal flap is then pulled down over the defect like a roller shade, and the defects are closed (**Fig. 5.61c**). This can also be done with mucosa that is mobilized only superiorly or only inferiorly.

6 The Lips

All operations on the lips should restore both the esthetic appearance of the lips and their function, i.e., their ability to maintain oral continence during eating and drinking. Our suture material of choice for approximating muscle stumps about the lips is 4-0 or 5-0 absorbable, and we prefer 6-0 or 7-0 monofilament for the mucosa.

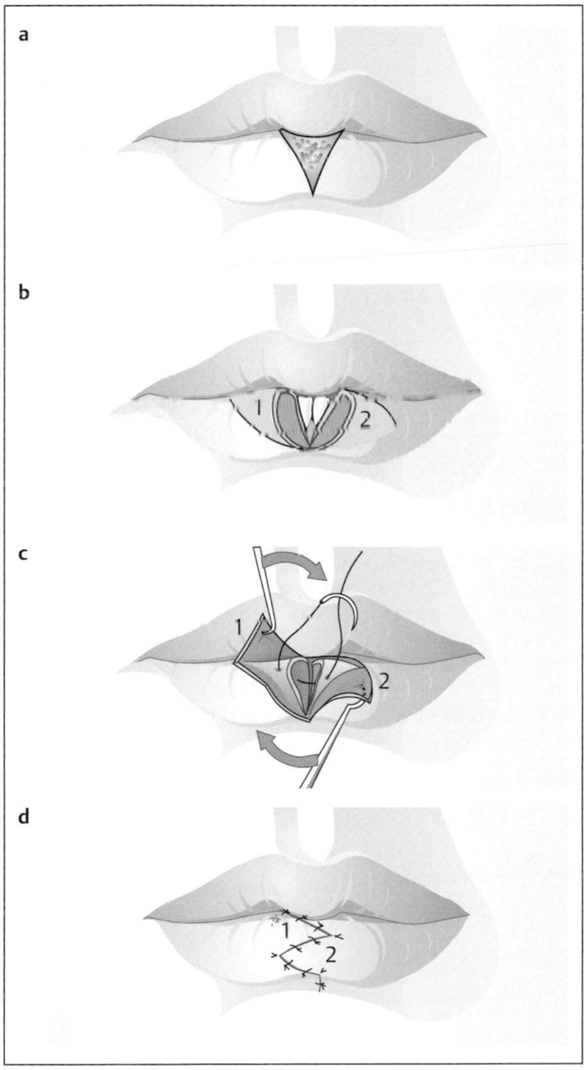

Mucosal Defects

Wedge-Shaped Defects
(Fig. 6.1)

Small scars or defects can be excised (**Fig. 6.1a**) and closed using a Z-plasty technique (**Fig. 6.1b–d**; Dufourmentel et al., after Converse 1977).

Large Superficial Defects
(Fig. 6.2)

Vermilion defects involving up to one third of the length of the lip can be repaired with a sliding flap (**Fig. 6.2a**), or the entire myomucosal stump can be mobilized as an advancement flap, as described by Goldstein (1990). The natural elasticity of the lip mucosa permits good coverage of the defect (**Fig. 6.2b**; see also **Fig. 6.52**). These techniques can also be combined with the methods described by Blasius (1840)(see **Figs. 6.25** and **6.26**).

Fig. 6.1a–d **Wedge-shaped defect** in the vermilion of the lower lip.
a The defect is excised.
b Inferiorly and superiorly based mucosal triangles are cut in preparation for a Z-plasty.
c The triangles are transposed, and the muscular wound is closed.
d The small skin defects are closed.

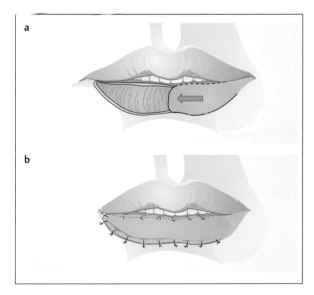

Fig. 6.2a, b **Large superficial mucosal defect in the right lower lip** (involving less than one third of the lip).
a The intact lip mucosa is mobilized and advanced to cover the defect.
b The flap is sutured in place (see **Fig. 6.54**).

Upper Lip

Median Deficiency
(**Fig. 6.3**)

A small median notch or deficiency in the Cupid's bow of the upper lip can be corrected by advancing the adjacent vermilion toward the midline, using the V-Y method (**Fig. 6.3a, b**).

Thin Upper Lip
(**Figs. 6.4–6.6**)

Unilateral thinness of the upper lip (or lower lip) can be corrected by measuring the deficit (**Fig. 6.4a**), excising a strip of skin, and advancing the mobilized vermilion (**Fig. 6.4b**). If median deficiency is present, a V-Y advancement from the lateral vestibule (**Fig. 6.5a, b**) can add fullness to the lip. This incision is

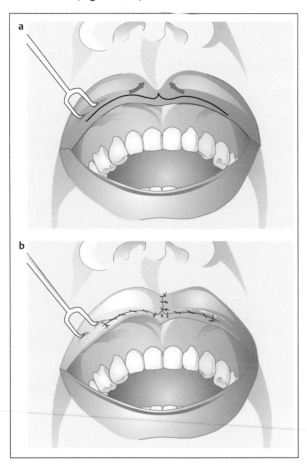

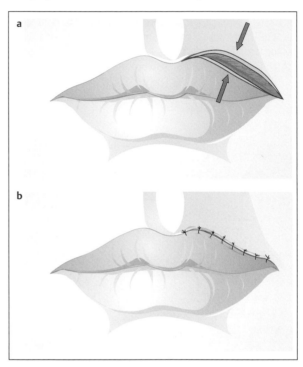

Fig. 6.4a, b   Widening the upper lip on one side.
a The lip height is measured on the opposite side and drawn on the affected side. A strip of skin is excised, and the vermilion is slightly mobilized.
b The incision is closed (with 6-0 or 7-0 monofilament) to create a new vermilion border. This type of operation can be used for total advancement of the upper lip area.

Fig. 6.3   V-Y advancement for adding median fullness to a thin upper lip.

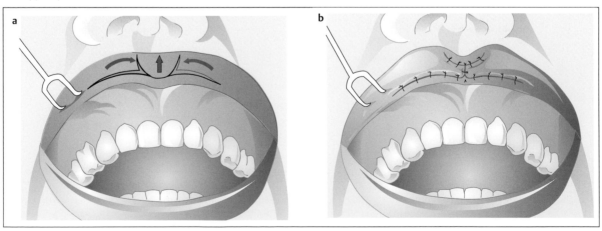

Fig. 6.5a, b   V-Y advancement for adding upper lip fullness and improving the shape of the Cupid's bow.
a The flap incisions are made, skirting the Cupid's bow.   **b** The V-Y advancement is completed.

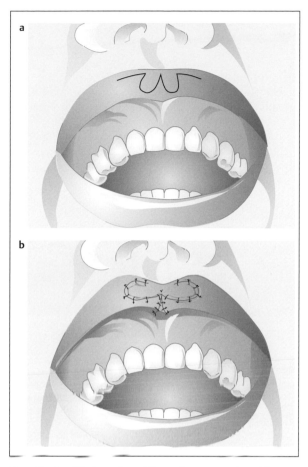

carried farther laterally than in **Fig. 6.3**. We can also use a W-plasty (**Fig. 6.6**).

Thin Upper Lip and Full Lower Lip
(**Fig. 6.7**)

A bipedicle flap can be used to add substance to the upper lip in a patient with a full lower lip, and vice-versa (**Fig. 6.7a, b**). The pedicle is divided ~3 weeks after the initial transfer.

Fig. 6.6a, b   W-plasty for adding substance to the mid-upper lip.
a The W-shaped incision is made around the vestibular mucosa and is carried laterally into the upper lip.
b The small flaps are transposed to close the defects.

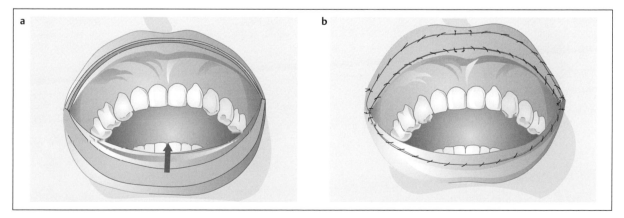

Fig. 6.7a, b   Augmenting the upper lip from a full lower lip.
a A bipedicle flap is cut from the lower lip, and the upper lip is incised.

b The bipedicle flap (mucosa or myomucosa) is transferred to the upper lip. The donor defect is closed (the flap base is divided and inset 3 weeks later).

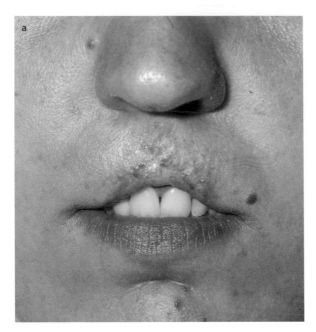

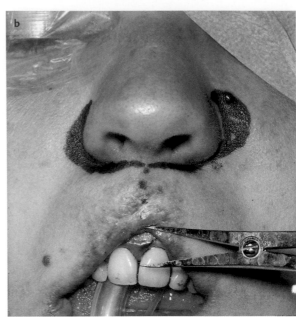

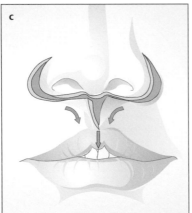

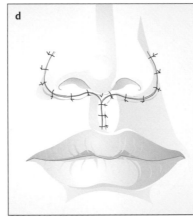

Fig. 6.8a–f   Correction of upper lip contracture following a cleft repair.
a Upper lip contracture.
b The incision and excisions are outlined, the shortening of the lip is measured.
c Crescent-shaped excisions are made lateral to the alar groove, and the scar is excised. The lip is mobilized and brought down to a normal position.
d, e All defects are closed.
f Result.

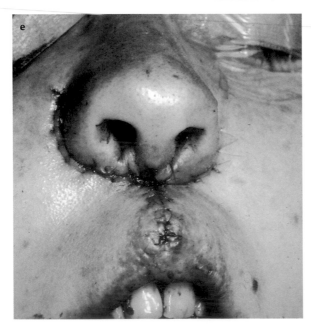

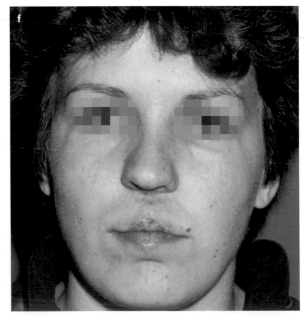

Fig. 6.9a, b   A Z-plasty can be added to **adjust the position of the vermilion** (see **Fig. 6.8**).

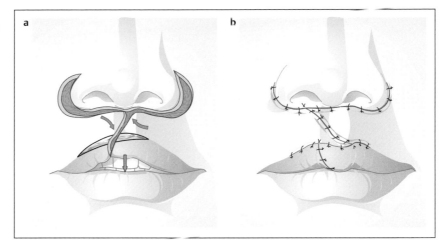

Fig. 6.10a, b   **Distortion of the vermilion** owing to scar contracture.
a The scar is excised, and releasing incisions are made in the nasolabial folds.
b The vermilion is brought downward, and the defects are closed (see also **Fig. 6.28**).

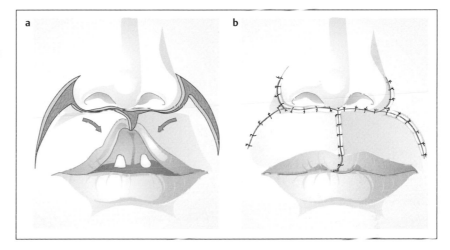

Median Scars and Upper Lip Defects

In cases where the central portion of the upper lip is retracted upward due to scarring after a cleft repair, burn, or irradiation of a hemangioma (**Fig. 6.8a, b**), the lip can be reconstructed using a method first described by Celsus in about 25 AD (Weerda 1994). A two-layer, crescent-shaped excision is made lateral to the alar groove on each side, and extended along the nasal base. A portion of the scar can be excised (**Fig. 6.8b, c**). Both upper lip stumps are then rotated and carefully sutured together to bring down the retracted vermilion (**Fig. 6.8d–f**). The muscle stumps

are carefully approximated with 4-0 or 5-0 absorbable suture material.

After the vermilion scar has been divided and excised, a Z-plasty can be incorporated to add fullness to the upper lip and lower the vermilion (**Fig. 6.9**). With greater upward retraction of the upper lip, the incision along the nasal base and alar groove can be extended at an approximate right angle along the nasolabial fold. The flaps are then rotated toward the midline to restore a natural-appearing upper lip (**Fig. 6.10**). The lip muscles are reapproximated separately in this type of operation.

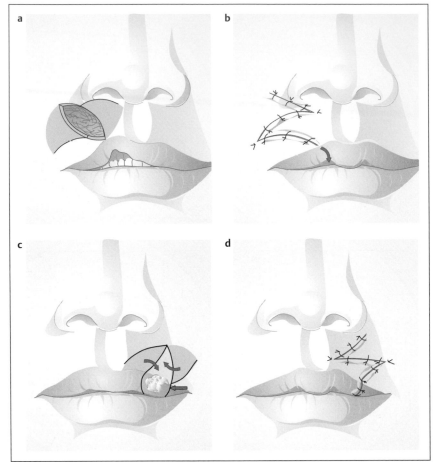

Fig. 6.11a–d **Tumor or scar** in the upper lip.
a, c The tumor is excised, and the Z-plasty incision is made.
b, d The scar is dispersed. The lip defect is closed.

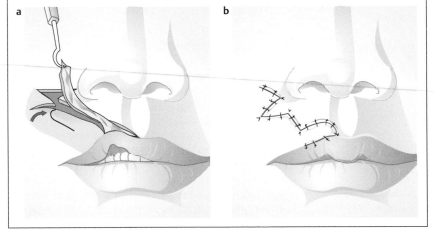

Fig. 6.12a, b **Scar contracture causing lateral distortion of the upper lip.**
a The scar is excised. A small flap is mobilized, and a Z-plasty is performed (see **Fig. 6.11**; see also **Fig. 2.16**).
b The completed repair.

Scar Revisions

Small Contractures
(**Fig. 6.11**)

In cases where the upper lip has been retracted upward on one side by a small scar, the scar is excised and then dispersed with a Z-plasty. This adds length in the direction of the scar and restores a normal shape to the upper lip. A similar technique is used after excision of small tumors (**Fig. 6.11c, d**; Härle 1993).

Larger Contractures
Burns, caustic injuries, and scar contractures can cause severe distortion of the upper lip. The revision technique is as follows:

1. The scar is excised down to muscle, and the vermilion is mobilized.
2. A pattern is made out of paper, cloth, or aluminum foil.
3. The pattern is used to harvest a full-thickness retroauricular skin graft.

Fig. 6.13a, b Scar contracture with distortion of the commissure.
a The scar is excised, and a triangular-shaped flap with a lateral base is outlined in the upper lip.
b The flap is transposed and inset, raising the commissure to a normal level.

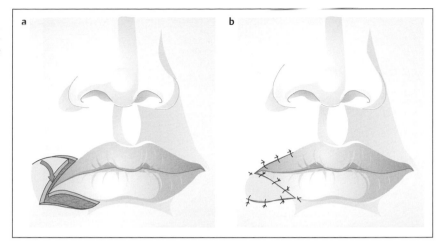

Fig. 6.14a–f
a, b Inferiorly based transposition flap.
c The defect is closed.
d Result after 4 weeks.
e Advancement flap (see **Fig. 3.2**).
f A large, inferiorly based nasolabial flap can be used to repair a defect in the nasal vestibule. A small flap covers the defect in the columella.

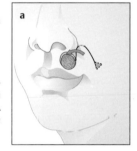
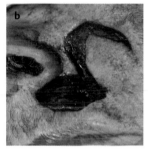
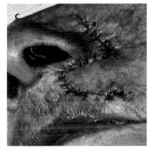
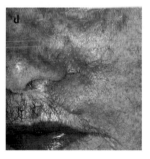
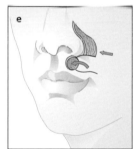
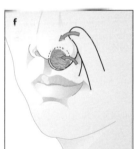

4. The full-thickness skin graft is inset using fibrin glue and 6-0 or 7-0 sutures. Alternating sutures are left long.
5. The long sutures are tied over a foam bolster or Vaseline gauze dressing for 6 to 7 days.

Larger Scar Contractures Causing Lip Retraction
(**Figs. 6.12** and **6.13**)

The scar is excised, and the defect adjacent to the vermilion is repaired with a small transposition flap (**Fig. 6.12a, b**).

With contracture and distortion of the oral commissure, the scar is excised (**Fig. 6.13a**) and the angle of the mouth is raised with a Z-plasty (**Fig. 6.13b**).

Defects in the Nasal Floor and Upper Lip

Transposition Flap from the Nasolabial Fold
(**Fig. 6.14**)

Smaller defects in the nasal floor and upper lip can be covered with a small superiorly based or inferiorly based (**Fig. 6.14a, b**) flap. Large, inferiorly based transposition flaps provide better reach for reconstructing the nasal vestibule and portions of the columella (**Fig. 6.14f**).

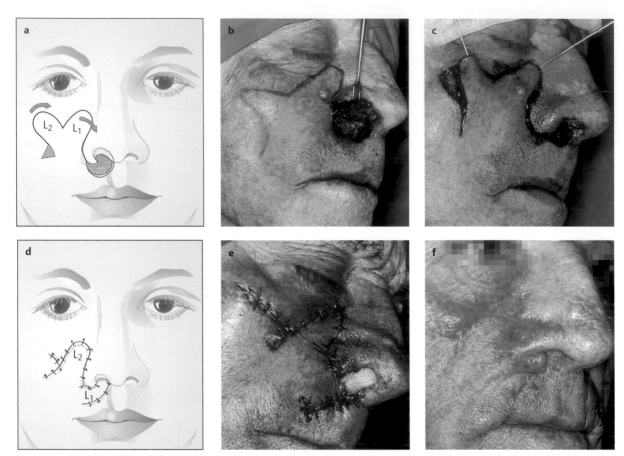

Fig. 6.15a–f   Inferiorly based bilobed flap for repairing a defect in the **upper lip and nasal vestibule** (after Weerda and Härle 1981).
a, b Outline of the flap.
c The flap is incised.

d, e The flap is rotated into place, and all defects are closed. The ala is located between lobes L1 and L2.
f Result.

Bilobed Flap
(Fig. 6.15)

Larger defects in this area are repaired with an inferiorly based bilobed flap from the cheek. The first lobe of the flap should cover the nasal floor and upper lip, and the ala should be correctly positioned without tension in the angle between the first and second lobes (**Fig. 6.15a**). A larger defect in the upper lip can be repaired with a full-thickness sliding flap (**Fig. 6.16**) or advancement flap (**Fig. 6.17e**). In the latter case, a crescent-shaped skin excision is made in the alar groove above the upper lip defect, the cheek skin is mobilized, and the flap is advanced into the defect (**Fig. 6.17a, b**).

For larger defects in the upper lip area, the incision can be extended along the orbital margin and down past the angle of the mouth to create a kind of U-flap (**Fig. 6.18a**) for covering the defect (Weerda and Härle 1981; Weerda and Siegert 1990; **Fig. 6.18b**; see also Imre cheek rotation in **Fig. 5.25** and Imre–Esser cheek advancement in **Figs. 8.2** and **8.4**).

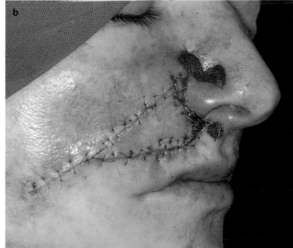

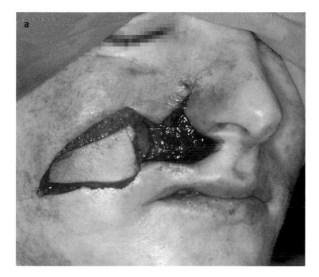

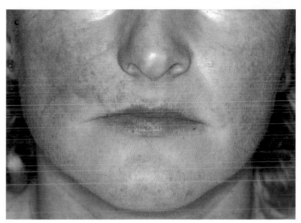

Fig. 6.16a–c   Nasolabial sliding flap of Barron and Emmett (1965) (see **Figs. 3.11, 5.7, 5.44**).
a Defect of the upper lip after tumor excision. The sliding flap is incised.
b The defects are closed.
c Result 2 years later.

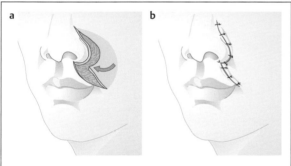

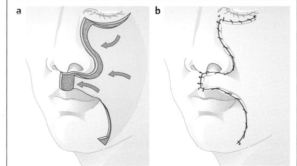

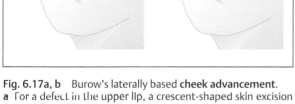

Fig. 6.17a, b   Burow's laterally based **cheek advancement**.
a For a defect in the upper lip, a crescent-shaped skin excision is made in the alar groove.
b The cheek flap is advanced and all defects are closed.

Fig. 6.18a, b   Modified **cheek advancement** of Weerda and Härle (1981) and Weerda and Siegert (1990).
a The flap is cut and the cheek is mobilized, aided by a crescent-shaped excision in the area of the alar groove and lateral nose.
b The completed repair (see **Figs. 6.29a, b**).

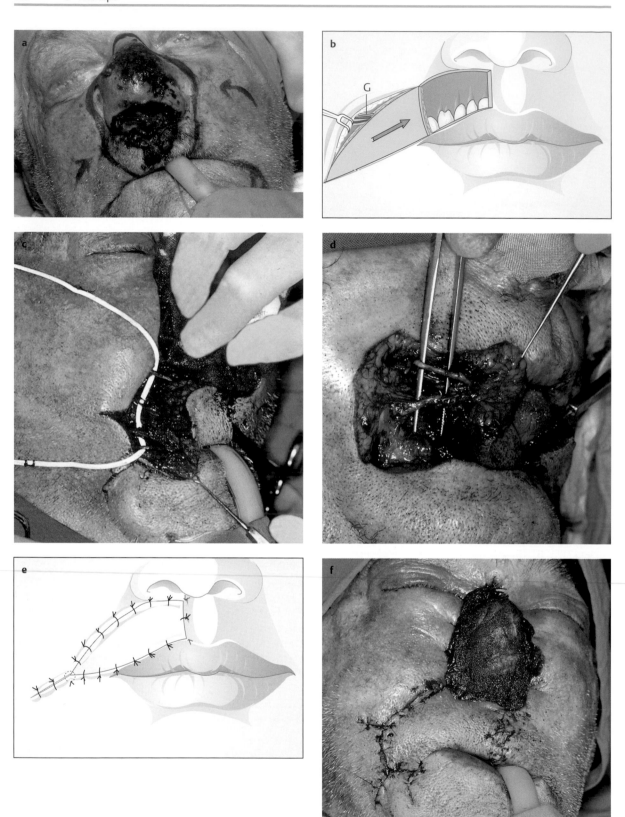

Fig. 6.19a–h   Neurovascular island flap from the lower cheek (after Weerda 1980d) in an 81-year-old patient.
a Tumors of the nose and upper lip, the flaps are outlined.

b–d The two-layered flap is advanced on a neurovascular pedicle (G = blood vessels plus a branch of the facial nerve).
e, f The completed repair of the lip (see **Fig. 6.28**).

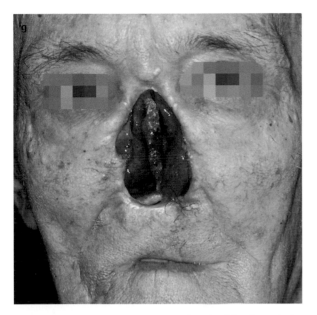 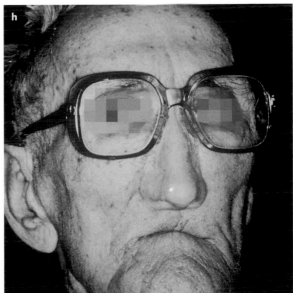

Fig. 6.19a–h   *(Continued)* Neurovasular island flap from the lower cheek in an 81-year-old patient.
g Situation 1 year after tumor excision and reconstruction.   **h** the nasal defect was covered with a defect prosthesis.

Neurovascular Island Flap from the Lower Cheek (after Weerda 1980d Figs. 6.19 and 6.28)

In this 81-year-old patient, we found a carcinoma of the nose and upper lip (**Fig. 6.19a**). The resulting cheek defects were closed by cheek advancement (see **Fig. 5.52a, b**). To close the large defect of the upper lip, a two- or three-layered neurovascular island flap of the cheek is incised (**Fig. 6.19b–d**). The vessels and the branch of the facial nerve were preserved (**Fig. 6.19b d**). The lip defect could be closed (**Fig. 6.19e, f**). The remaining defect of the nose (**Fig. 6.19g**) was covered with a defect prosthesis (**Figs. 6.19h** and **6.28**).

Central Defects of the Upper Lip
(Fig. 6.20; see Fig. 6.8)

As noted earlier (see **Figs. 6.18** and **6.19**), the classic reconstruction described by Celsus (ca. 25 AD) and Bruns (1859) (**Fig. 6.20**) can also be used to repair full-thickness defects of the upper lip. A perialar skin crescent is excised (**Fig. 6.20a, b**), and the mobilized cheek flap is shifted medially into the defect (**Fig. 6.20c–e**).

Celsus Method Combined with an Abbé Flap
(Fig. 6.21; see also Figs. 6.20 and 6.22)

Large defects of the upper lip can be repaired by closing or reducing the central defect by the Celsus method (**Figs. 6.20** and **6.21a**) and then using a three-layered Abbé flap from the lower lip (**Figs. 6.21b, c** and **6.22**) to replace the central part of the upper lip (**Fig. 6.22a, b**). In a second stage ~3 to 4 weeks later, the turnover flap is detached from the lower lip and the wounds in the upper and lower vermilion are closed (**Fig. 6.21c**).

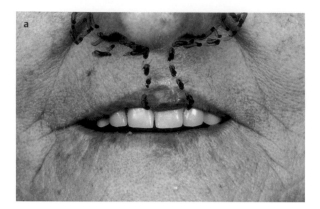

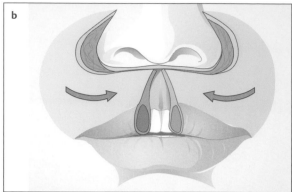

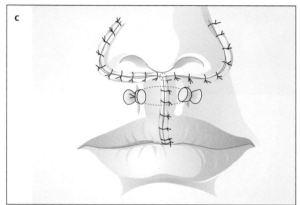

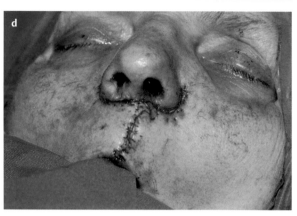

Fig. 6.20a–e   **Upper lip reconstruction** by the method of Celsus (ca. 25 AD) and Bruns (1859).
a Tumor of the middle part of the lip.
b A two-layer, crescent-shaped excision is made lateral to the alar groove, and the incision is extended along the nasal base (for larger defects, the mucosa is mobilized) (see **Fig. 6.8**).
c, d The completed repair.
e Result 3 years later.

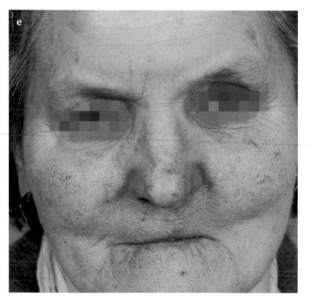

Classic Reconstructive Techniques in the Upper Lip

Abbé Flap (1898, reprinted 1968)
(**Fig. 6.22**)

Moderate-sized defects of the upper lip can be repaired by transposing a wedge-shaped flap from the lower lip, based on the inferior labial artery. The Abbé "lip switch" is particularly useful for reconstructing defects associated with a cleft lip, or excision of a medially located tumor (**Fig. 6.22a, b**). About 16 to 20 days after the flap has been inset, its vascular pedicle is divided (see **Fig. 6.21b, c**). A prong-shaped flap can also be designed (**Fig. 6.23**; Converse 1977). A Z-plasty can be added to disperse the scar in the lower lip area (see **Fig. 6.24d, e**).

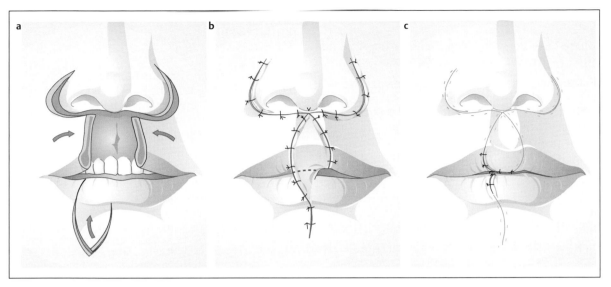

Fig. 6.21a–c **Upper lip reconstruction** by the method of Celsus (ca. 25 AD) and Abbé flap (1898, reprinted 1968).
a Mobilization of the upper lip (see **Fig. 6.20**) and three-layered incision of the Abbé flap (see **Fig. 6.22**).
b The Abbé flap is rotated into the upper lip defect.
c About 20 days later, the pedicle is divided and the small lip defects are closed.

Fig. 6.22a, b Three-layered Abbé flap (1898, reprinted 1968) from the lower lip (see also **Figs. 6.23** and **6.24**).
a Incision of the three-layered Abbé flap in the lower lip.
b Rotation of the Abbé flap into the upper lip defect. The flap is divided ~20 days later.

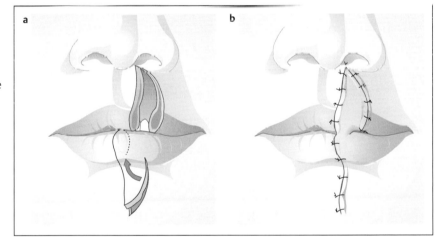

Fig. 6.23a, b **Modification of the Abbé flap** (Converse 1977; see **Figs. 6.22** and **6.24**).

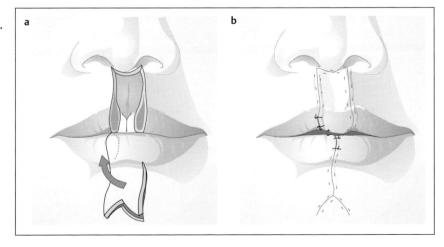

Estlander Flap (1872) (Figs. 6.24; 6.40)

A three-layer lip-switch flap similar to the Abbé flap can be used in the area of the oral commissure.

1. The flap is based on the commissure and is outlined in the lower lip area (**Fig. 6.24a**). It is rotated 180° and sutured into the wedge-shaped defect in the upper lip (**Fig. 6.24b, c**).
2. The pedicle is divided ~16 to 20 days later. If desired, revision of the rounded commissure can be done as a secondary procedure (**Fig. 6.24d**). Bilateral Estlander flaps can also be used.

Upper Lip Reconstruction with a Rotation Flap (Blasius 1840)
(**Fig. 6.25**)

A two-layer rotation flap can be cut from the cheek to reconstruct portions of the upper lip (**Fig. 6.25a**). The vermilion in that area can also be restored by presewing the slightly mobilized mucosa of the upper oral vestibule to the flap (Weerda and Härle 1981; see **Fig. 6.25b**). A modification of this method is shown in **Figs. 6.26** and **6.27**.

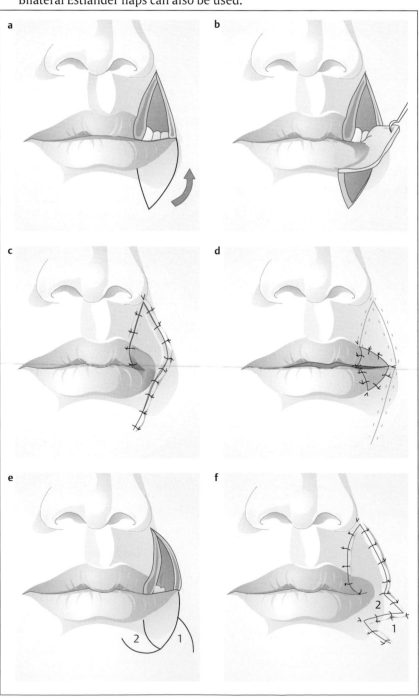

Fig. 6.24a–f The Estlander flap (1872) is similar to the Abbé flap, used at the angle of the mouth. The wedge-shaped flap, based on the inferior labial artery, is rotated around the angle of the mouth into the defect.

a The Estlander flap is cut through all layers of the lower lip.
b The flap is rotated into the upper lip defect.
c All defects are closed.
d About 16 to 20 days later, the pedicle is divided, the triangular mucosal flaps are mobilized, and the lip is closed (see **Fig. 6.56**).
e, f A Z-plasty can be added for closure of the donor site. The Estlander flap can also be used for lower lip reconstruction (see **Figs. 6.40, 6.41**).

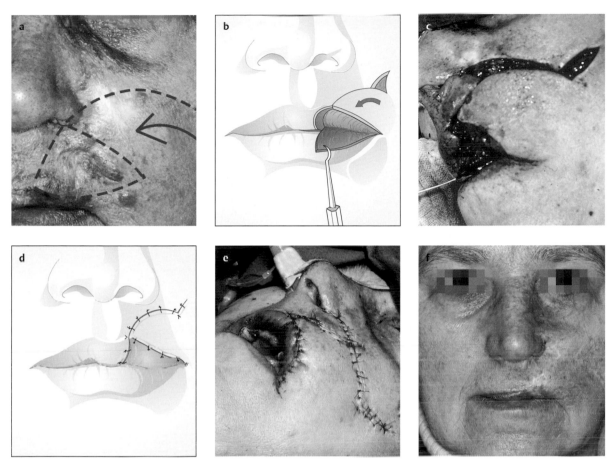

Fig. 6.25a–f   Cheek rotation of Blasius (1840).
a   Tumors after hemangioma radiation years ago in childhood.
b, c   A two-layer rotation flap is cut from the cheek. The flap is slightly de-epithelialized in the area of the upper lip.

d, e   The flap is rotated into the defect, the vestibular mucosa is mobilized and sutured to the new upper lip (see **Figs. 6.26** and **6.29**).
f   Results 3 years later.

Fig. 6.26a, b   Rotation flap of Blasius (1840). The vermilion is reconstructed by advancing the upper lip vermilion of the intact side.
a   Cutting the rotation flap and the mucosa of the lip stump.
b   The completed repair. The rotation flap is epithelialized by advancing the upper lip vermilion (see **Figs. 6.2, 6.25, 6.29, 6.54**).

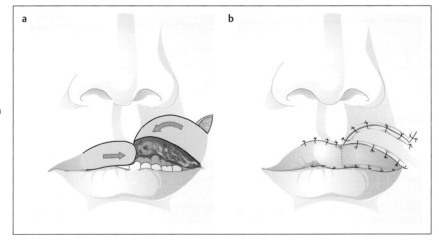

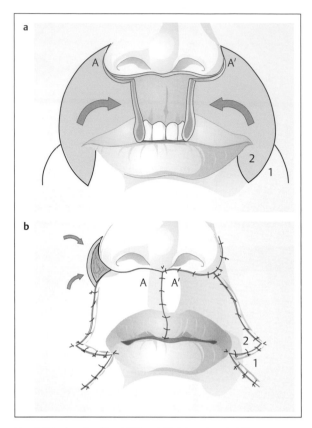

Fig. 6.27a, b   Fan flap (Gillies 1976) (see **Fig. 6.45**).
a The flap contains the orbicularis oris muscle. It is dissected
  bluntly to preserve the superior and inferior labial vessels (see
  Fig. 6.29).
b The completed repair (see text).

Gillies Fan Flap (1976)
(**Fig. 6.27**)

This is a three-layer nasolabial flap cut around the ala
(**Fig. 6.27a**). It provides enough tissue to fully reconstruct the lip. The flap is nourished by the labial vessels. The Gillies flap is usually cut in two layers, and
the mucosa is mobilized toward the midline. The
muscular ring around one or both commissures is
rotated medially and closed (**Fig. 6.27b**, see also **Fig.
6.45**). A lateral Z-plasty gives the Gillies flap sufficient
mobility (**Fig. 6.27b**). With a large defect, elongation of
the oral fissure (see pp. 102–104) may be done 3 to
4 weeks later as a secondary procedure (see **Fig. 6.54**).

Neurovascular Skin–Muscle–Mucosal Flap of Weerda
(1980d, 1990)
(**Figs. 6.19** and **6.28**)

This flap is incised in two or three layers (**Fig. 6.28a**).
The inferior labial artery and vein are dissected laterally in the cheek, then, if necessary, the mucosa is
divided. The facial nerve branches are dissected and
preserved. The three-layer skin–muscle–mucosal
flap is then slid into the upper lip defect on its vasc-

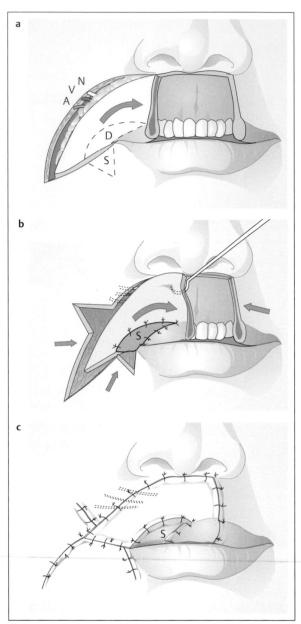

Fig. 6.28a–c   Neurovascular myocutaneous island flap of
Weerda (1980d) and Weerda and Siegert (1990) (see **Fig. 6.19**).
a The flap can be cut in two layers (with mobilization of the
  cheek mucosa) or three layers, preserving its neurovascular
  pedicle (see **Fig. 6.45a**). A = superior labial artery; D = de-
  epithelialized area; N = facial nerve; S = mucosal flap from the
  oral vestibule; V = vein.
b The flap is advanced into the upper lip defect, and Burow's
  triangles are excised.
c The completed repair.

uar pedicle, and the secondary wound is closed by
mobilizing the surrounding skin (**Fig. 6.28b, c**). If part
of the upper lip remains, the flap is incised downward at the commissure, portions of the upper lip
mucosa are advanced medially, and the flap mucosa
is flattened out to form the lateral mucosa of the

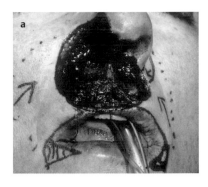
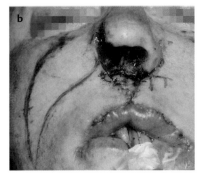
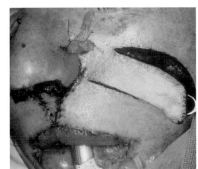

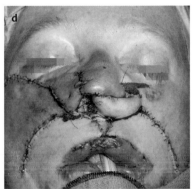
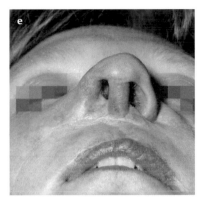
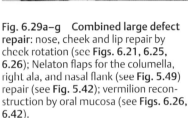

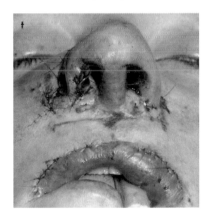
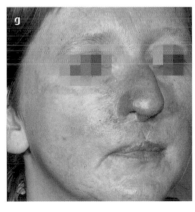

Fig. 6.29a–g **Combined large defect repair:** nose, cheek and lip repair by cheek rotation (see **Figs. 6.21, 6.25, 6.26**); Nelaton flaps for the columella, right ala, and nasal flank (see **Fig. 5.49**) repair (see **Fig. 5.42**); vermilion reconstruction by oral mucosa (see **Figs. 6.26, 6.42**).

a Defect of the upper lip, cheek, nasal ala, and columella following a tumor resection. The cheek rotation is outlined.

b, c **Stage 2:** appearance after reconstruction of the upper lip with two cheek rotation flaps. The outline for the Nelaton flap is drawn on the right side (**b**) and incised (**c**) on the left side. The vestibular mucosa was mobilized to reconstruct the lip (see **Figs. 6.25b, e**).

d The Nelaton flaps are inset into the nasal ala and columnella, and the secondary defects are closed after mobilizing the surrounding skin (using a cheek advancement flap on the right side) (see **Fig. 8.4**).
Stage 3: the flaps are deseted, thinned, and sutured into place. Situation 4 weeks after the operation.

e, f Before and after correction and refinement.

g Result 4 years after tumor resection.

upper lip(s). If cheek mobilization is not sufficient to close the secondary defect, Burow's triangles are excised to facilitate the closure (**Figs. 6.19** and **6.28b**).

Combined Defect Repair of the Ala, Columella, Cheek, and Upper Lip
(Fig. 6.29)

Multiple carcinomas occurred after hemangioma radiation treatment in childhood. In this specific care, excision resulted in a large defect (**Fig. 6.29a**). The cheek rotation is outlined (see **Fig. 6.19**; see also **Fig. 5.52**) to close the defect of the cheek and the upper lip (**Fig. 6.29a**). The vestibular mucosa is mobilized (**Fig. 6.25b**) to reconstruct the vermilion border (**Fig. 6.29b, c**). The right ala and nasal flank are restored by a cheek transposition flap (**Fig. 6.29b–d**). The resulting defect is closed with a modified Imre cheek advancement (**Fig. 6.29d**; see also **Fig. 8.4**). The columella is reconstructed with a nasolabial (Nelaton) flap (**Fig. 6.29c–e**) in a second stage. In a further third step, the nose is modeled, the nasal groove is refined, and the vermilion border is corrected (**Fig. 6.29e, f**). The result after 4 years is shown in **Fig. 6.29g**.

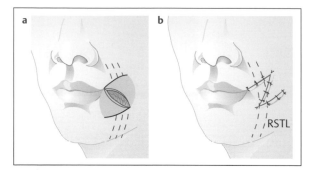

Fig. 6.30a, b   Excision of a **scar at the commissure**. A Z-plasty is used to disperse the scars and place them in the RSTLs.

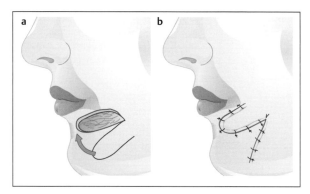

Fig. 6.31a, b   **Defect closure** with a transposition flap.

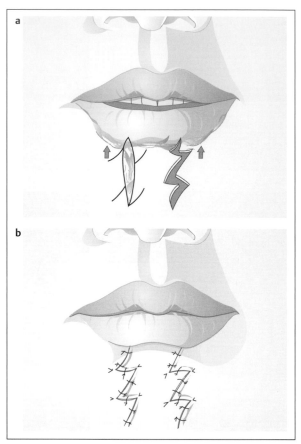

Fig. 6.32a, b   The vermilion is stretched out to its normal length by excising the scars and performing multiple Z-plasties.

Lower Lip

Scar Contractures and Small Defects

Small Contractures
(**Figs. 6.30** and **6.31**)

A small scar contracture can be managed by excising the scar and using a Z-plasty to disperse the new scars and orient them along RSTLs (**Fig. 6.30**). If contracture is not present, the defect can be repaired with a small transposition flap (**Fig. 6.31**).

Larger Contractures
*Burn with ectropion of the lower lip (***Fig. 6.32***):*
A small contracture causing ectropion of the lower lip can be dispersed with one, two, or more Z-plasties, to lengthen the lower lip and restore the everted vermilion to a normal position (**Fig. 6.32b**).

Severe burns:
A more severe contracture with fixation of the lower lip and destruction of the underlying skin can be managed much as in the upper lip, by excising the scar and then mobilizing the vermilion and shifting it upward. After making a pattern, we cover the defect with a full-thickness retroauricular skin graft.

The repair should be immobilized with a tie-over dressing for ~1 week.

Small Defects
In small defects with scar contracture (**Fig. 6.33a**), the scar is excised and the defect closed by the V-Y method. The first suture (**Fig. 6.33a**) is used to obtain precise coaptation of the skin–vermilion border. The result is shown in **Fig. 6.33c**.

Lip Reduction
Protuberant lips can be reduced by an intraoral mucosal resection (**Fig. 6.34a, b**) to decrease the size of the visible vermilion and thus narrow the lips. Since the scars are intraoral, they cannot be seen (**Fig. 6.34c**).

Sliding Flaps in the Vermilion
A kind of V-Y advancement can be used within the vermilion to repair defects of varying shapes (**Fig. 6.35**). Bilateral advancements can also be used (**Fig. 6.36**). The angle of the mouth can be moved upward by transposing a Z-flap (**Fig. 6.37**).

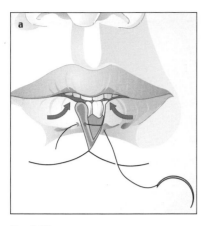
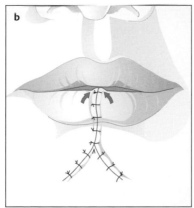
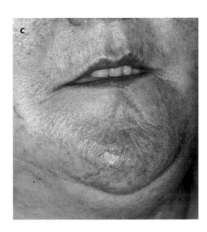

Fig. 6.33a–c
a, b Small defect of the lower lip with scar contractures repaired by a V-Y closure. Excess tissue should be provided in the vermilion area to prevent formation of a new defect after the scars have contracted.
c Result.

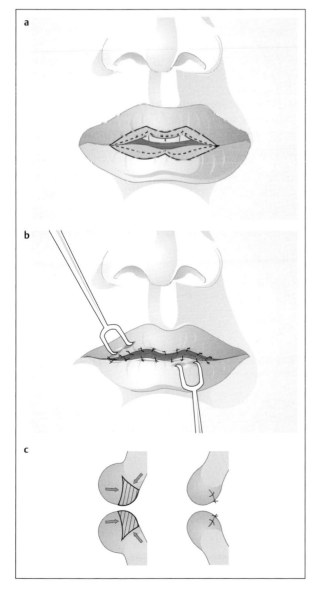

Fig. 6.34a–c Lip reduction.
a Mucosa and some muscle tissue are excised intraorally from the protuberant lips.
b All defects are closed, thinning the lips.
c Cross-sectional view.

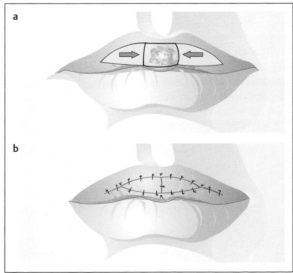

Fig. 6.35a, b V-Y closure of a small lip defect using sliding flaps.

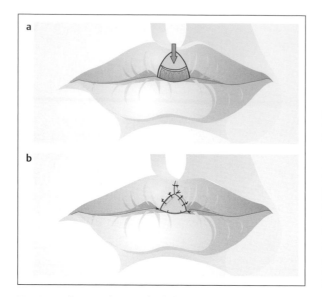

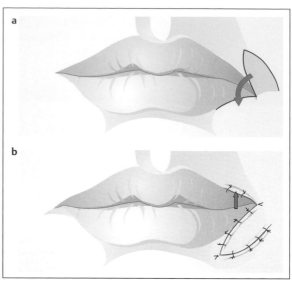

Fig. 6.36a, b   **V-Y closure** of a defect using a sliding flap.

Fig. 6.37a, b   **Z-plasty** used to raise the angle of the mouth.

Classic Lower Lip Reconstructions

Approximately 90% of all lip tumors occur in the lower lip. It is important, therefore, to obtain a good esthetic and functional result when repairing small and large defects of the lower lip.

Wedge Excision
(**Fig. 6.38**)
Tumors (**Fig. 6.38a**) that require excision of up to one third of the lower lip can be removed by a wedge excision. The sides of the excision should curve outward (**heart-shaped excision**, Fig. 6.38b, c); this creates a slight tissue excess along the suture line that will prevent notching after the scar has matured. The wound is closed from inside to outside (**Fig. 6.38d**),

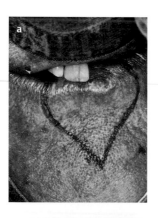

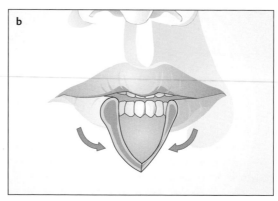

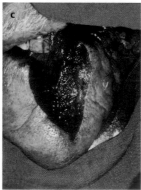

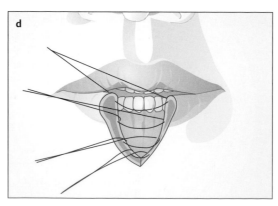

Fig. 6.38a–g   **Heart-shaped wedge excision** from the lower lip (up to one third).
a Tumor of the middle part of the lower lip.
b, c Excision of the tumor.
d The mucosa is closed first.

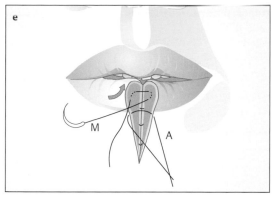

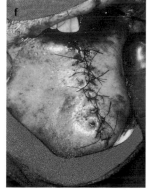

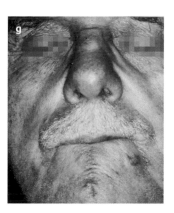

Fig. 6.38a–g (Continued) **Heart-shaped wedge excision** from the lower lip (up to one third).
e Then the muscle edges are approximated with absorbable sutures (M). A coapting suture is placed at the skin–vermilion border (A).

f The defect is closed.
g Situation 1 year after tumor resection.

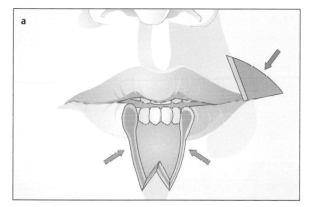

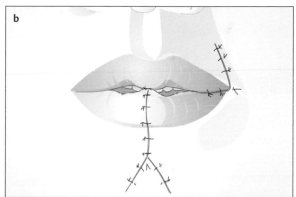

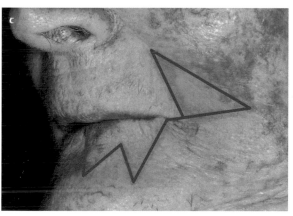

Fig. 6.39a-d Modifications of the wedge excision.
a, b Outline of the W-shaped excision and closure of the defect. A Burow's triangle is excised in the nasolabial fold.

c, d Additional advancement of the lateral lip to close the defect. (**c**) Excision of a large Burow's triangle in the nasolabial fold. (**d**) Closure of all defects.

using a special stay suture (**Fig. 6.38e**, A) to coapt and align the vermilion. The muscle stumps are approximated separately with absorbable sutures (**Fig. 6.38e**, M). The skin is closed with monofilament suture 5-0 or 6-0 **Fig. 6.38f**). The result is shown in **Fig. 6.38g**. Various types of incision can be used to close these defects (**Fig. 6.39**).

Estlander Flap (1872)
(Fig. 6.40)

Lateral defects can be covered with a three-layer Estlander flap based on the superior labial artery. The flap is raised from the upper lip and rotated around the angle of the mouth. This transfer shortens the oral fissure, especially when bilateral flaps are used, making it necessary to elongate the oral fissure as a secondary procedure (see **Fig. 6.24**; see also **Figs. 6.54** and **6.57**). The Estlander technique can be used in a variety of modifications and combinations (see **Fig. 6.44, 6.45**).

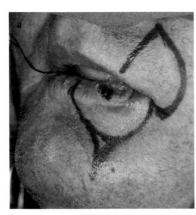
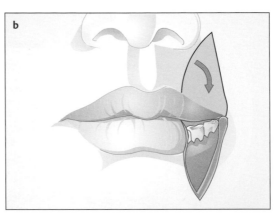
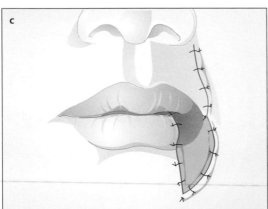
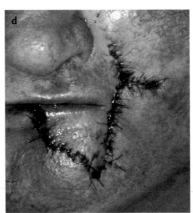
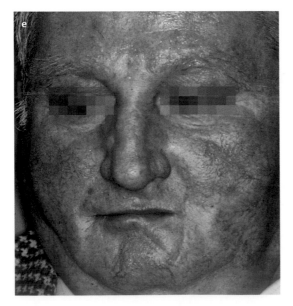

Fig. 6.40a–e   Lateral lower lip reconstruction of Estlander (1872).
a Tumor of the lateral lower lip, the Estlander flap is outlined.
b A three-layer triangular flap is outlined in the upper lip down to the vermilion border, preserving the superior labial artery of the other side. The medial limb of the flap is convexly curved. The lateral limb extends to the commissure roughly along the nasolabial fold.
c, d The Estlander flap is rotated into the defect, bringing the lateral vermilion downward, and sutured in three layers (see **Fig. 6.38**). Revision of the rounded commissure may be necessary as a secondary procedure (see **Figs. 6.24** and **6.54–6.57**).
e Result after 4 months (Weerda and Härle 1981).

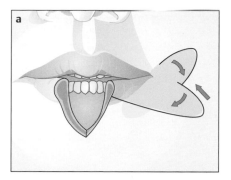

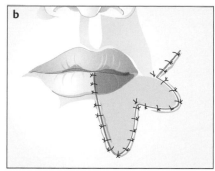

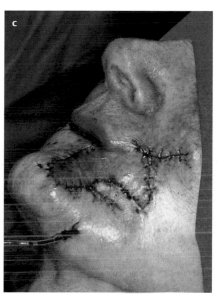

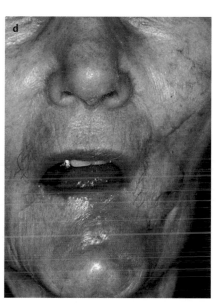

Fig. 6.41a–d Modification with a bilobed Estlander flap (Weerda 1980); tumor of the lateral lower lip (see **Fig. 6.40**).
a The bilobed flap is outlined, the tumor is excised and the flaps are incised.
b, c The wounds are closed (see **Fig. 6.40c, d**).
d Result (an elongation of the oral fissure should follow (see **Figs. 6.54–6.57**).

Bilobed Estlander Flap
(**Fig. 6.41**)

After tumor resection of the lower lateral lip (**Fig. 6.41a**) we incised a bilobed Estlander flap **Fig. 6.41b, c**).

Vermilion Reconstruction by the Method of von Langenbeck (1855)
(**Fig. 6.42**)

The usual treatment for actinic damage of the lower lip with premalignant changes is to remove the entire vermilion of the lower lip. The mucosa lining the oral vestibule is then mobilized and advanced to resurface the lip, with an excellent cosmetic result. The skin–vermilion border is carefully restored using 6-0 or 7-0 monofilament, which is removed on the fifth or sixth day (**Fig. 6.42b**). In all lip reconstructions, the mucosal surface of the lip should be coated with petroleum jelly to keep it from drying out. The resurfaced lip shows an initial livid discoloration that looks dangerous but is usually harmless and should clear within a few days.

Tongue Flap
(**Fig. 6.43**)

The resected vermilion can also be replaced with a tongue flap. This flap may be raised from the tip of the tongue (**Fig. 6.43a, b**) or tongue margin and is sutured to the skin resection margin of the lip. Its pedicle is divided 17 to 20 days after the initial transfer.

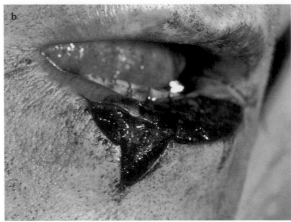

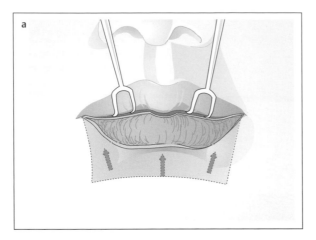

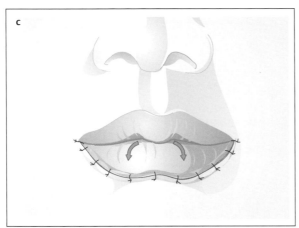

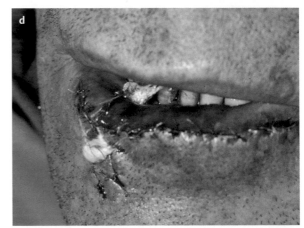

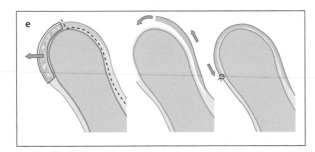

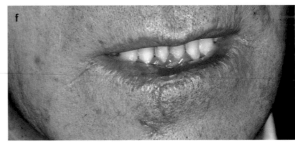

Fig. 6.42a–f   Vermilion reconstruction by the method of von Langenbeck (1855).

a, b, The premalignant vermilion has been completely resected. The mucosa of the oral vestibule is mobilized, advanced over the raw surface, and sutured into place.

c, d Closure of the defect.

e Cross-sectional view of the operation (see **Figs. 6.25** and **6.29**).

f Result (the scar was refined by a z-plasty; see **d** and **f**).

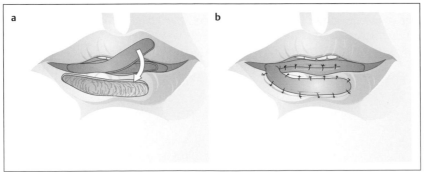

Fig. 6.43a–f

a, b The tongue flap.

a A mucosal flap from the anterior margin of the tongue, based on the right or left side, is swung into the defect.

b The lip and tongue defects are closed. The pedicle is divided ~3 weeks later, and the residual defects in the lip and tongue are closed.

Fig. 6.43a–f *(Continued)*
c, d Other potential donor sites for tongue flaps.

Fig. 6.44a–f   Modified Estlander flap (Brown 1928; Kazanjian and Converse 1974).

a Large median defect of the lower lip. The lateral lower lip is incised through all three layers. Note the outline of the Estlander flap, which is incised just to the mucosa inferiorly, where a small mucosal flap (S) is raised.

b The lateral lip segment is slid medially into the primary defect and sutured in three layers (see **Fig. 6.38**). D = defect (new vermillion).

c The lateral lip defect is closed with the Estlander flap (see **Fig. 6.40**), which is rotated into place. The small vermilion defect is covered with the mucosal flap (S).

d All defects are closed.

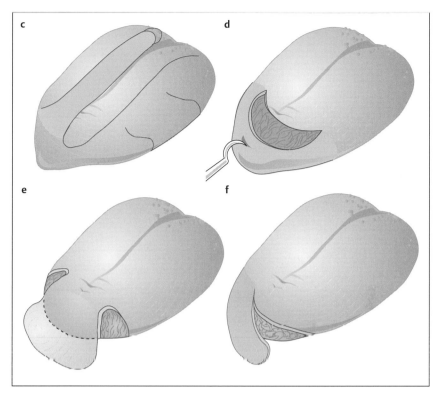

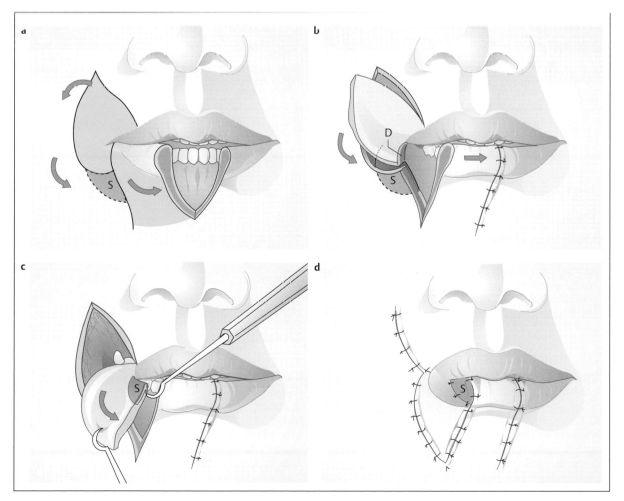

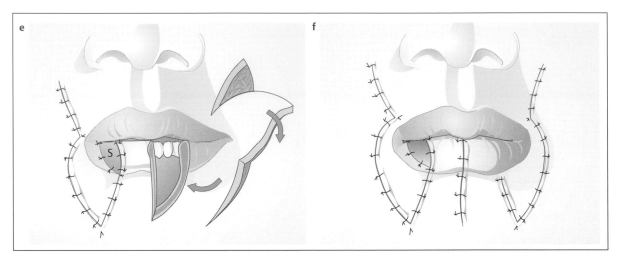

Fig. 6.44a–f   *(Continued)* e, f Modification preserving the angle of the mouth (left side; Weerda and Härle 1981).

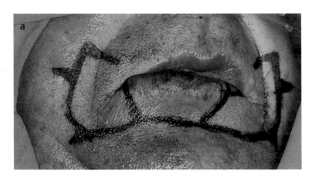

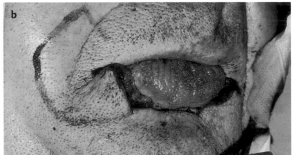

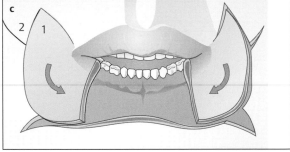

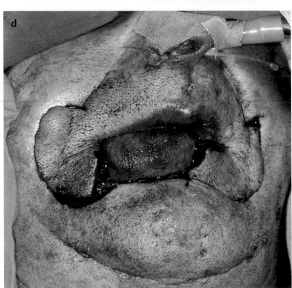

Fig. 6.45a–j   **Unilateral and bilateral** Gillies fan flap (1957) (modified) in subtotal or total tumor resection.

a, b Tumor and outline after tumor excision. The fan flap is basically a large two-layered Estlander flap that is rotated around the orbicularis muscle, if possible maintaining its neurovascular supply (see **Figs. 6.17** and **6.28**).

a The flaps are outlined.

b Subtotal resection of the lower lip, the fan flap is outlined.

c, d The flaps are incised (see **Fig. 6.53f, g**).

Brown Modification of the Estlander Flap (1928)
(**Fig. 6.44**)

An Estlander flap can also be used for larger medial defects involving more than one third of the lower lip. The defect created by the wedge excision (**Fig. 6.44a**) is covered by making a three-layer incision through the lower lip at the commissure, and advancing the lip into the defect (**Fig. 6.44a, b**). A superior Estlander flap is then used to close the remaining lateral defect (**Fig. 6.44c, d**).

Unilateral or Bilateral Gillies Fan Flap (1957)
(**Fig. 6.45e–j**)

As in the upper lip (see **Fig. 6.28**), a large defect of the lower lip can be reconstructed by rotation of the orbicularis oris muscle as originally suggested by Bruns (1859) and Ganzer (1917) (**Fig. 6.45a**). This flap, called the **Gillies fan flap**, is raised by incising through the full thickness of the oral vestibule, then upward into the cheek, and back toward the commis-

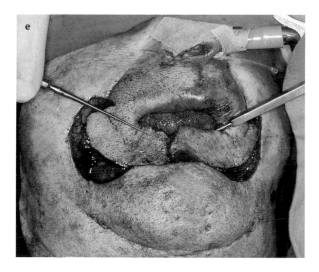

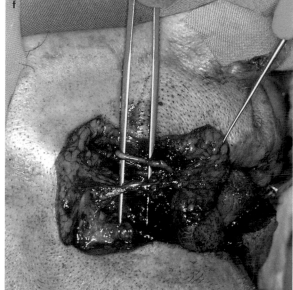

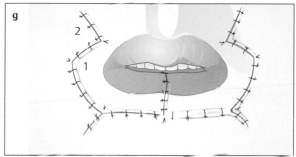

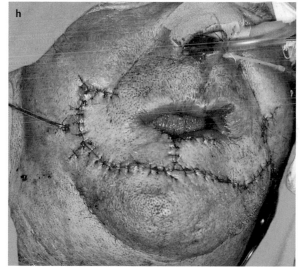

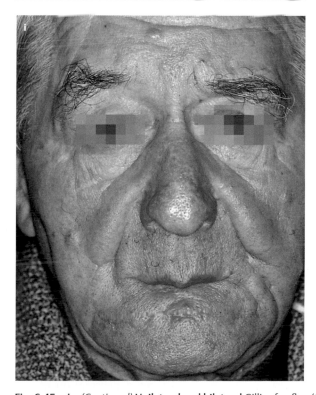

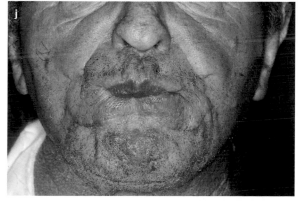

Fig. 6.45a–j   *(Continued)* **Unilateral and bilateral** Gillies fan flap (1957)

e The flaps are rotated into the defect.

f The vessels and the branch of the facial nerve are preserved.

g, h Appearance after flap rotation and closure of the defects (Z-plasty at the end of the flaps; **c, g:** 1, 2). The mucosa is

closed first (see **Fig. 6.38**). The mucosa of the oral vestibule was mobilized to close the raw surface of the lip.

i Esthetic result.

j Functional result after 8 months.

sure, so that the upper portion resembles a short Estlander flap (**Fig. 6.45a**, 1). Z-flaps at the top of the flap are transposed, and the whole flap is rotated into the defect (**Fig. 6.45b–h**).

The wound is then closed in layers from inside to outside, using separate sutures to approximate the orbicularis oris muscle (see **Figs. 6.28** and **6.38**). As in other procedures, care is taken to avoid a stepoff at the skin–vermilion border of the lower lip. When bilateral flaps are used, the angles of the mouth will have to be revised in a later sitting (see **Figs. 6.55** and **6.57**). We like to use a binocular loupe for prepara-

tion. We see a good esthetic (**Fig. 6.45i**) and functional result (**Fig. 6.45j**).

Universal Method of Bernard (1852), Grimm (1966), and Fries (1971)
(**Fig. 6.46**; unilateral or bilateral)

Bernard (1852) described an operation, which has been repeatedly modified during the past century, for unilateral or bilateral reconstruction of the lower lip. Placing the incisions and Burow's triangles in the lines of the esthetic units yields a very good cosmetic result,

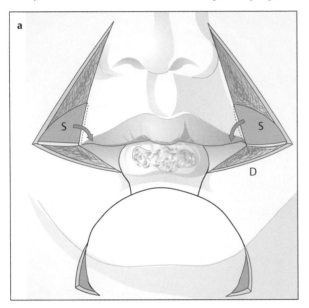
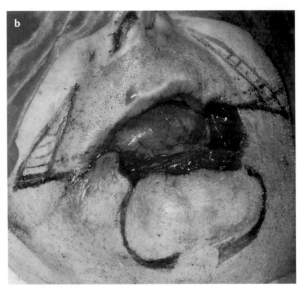
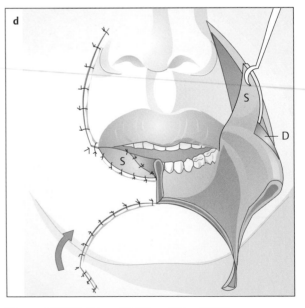

Fig. 6.46a–g   Lower lip reconstruction by the **universal method** of Bernard (1852), Grimm (1963), and Fries (1971).

a, b For a subtotal defect of the lower lip, the lateral cheek is mobilized by incising the commissure and excising two-layer Burow's triangles lateral to the commissures. A portion of the cheek U-flap is de-epithelialized (D) and resurfaced with a mucosal flap (S) from the cheek. Using a more medially cut Burow's triangle, we can achieve a slightly better cosmetic result.

c The tumor has been resected. The cheek U-advancement flap has been raised, on the left side the mucosal flap (S) is raised, and on the right side it has been sutured into place.

d The right side has been closed and the left side mobilized.

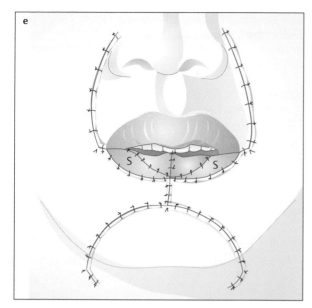

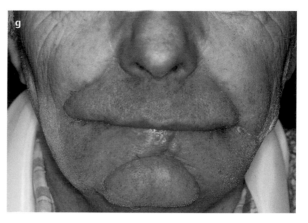

Fig. 6.46a–g   *(Continued)* Lower lip reconstruction by the **universal method** of Bernard (1852), Grimm (1963), and Fries (1971).
e, f The completed repair.
g Result (slightly better cosmetic results can be gained if the inercious are carried out near the angles as can be seen in the drawings).

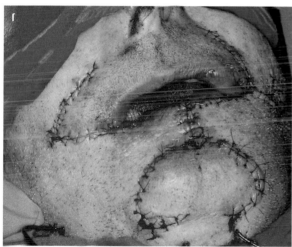

with acceptable mobility and width of the reconstructed lip. A turnover flap of cheek mucosa (**Fig. 6.46a–c**, S) is raised to restore the vermilion on the opposing de-epithelialized portion of the reconstruction flap (**Fig. 6.46a–c**, D). Cutting along the nasolabial folds can give the mouth a froglike appearance, however, and so we prefer to cut from the angle of the mouth to the alar groove (**Fig. 6.46c, d**; see also **Fig. 6.40**). Meyer (1962) described a modification of the technique (**Fig. 6.47a, b**). The defect can be closed in a one-stage procedure with good esthetic and functional results (**Fig. 6.46g**; see also **Fig. 6.47**).

Fig. 6.47a, b   **Meyer's modification.**
a The triangles are cut lateral to the upper lip, and the cheek mucosa is incised and mobilized to cover the upper lip defects. Burow's triangles are excised in the cheek skin, and turnover flaps of the cheek mucosa (S) are incised to restore the lateral vermilion defects.
b The completed repair.

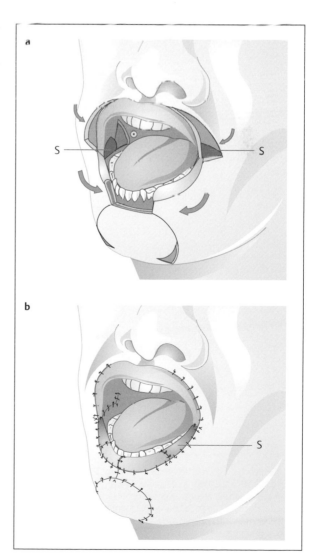

Reconstruction of the Lateral Lip and Commissure

Burow's Method of Reconstructing the Lateral Upper Lip (1855)
(Fig. 6.48)

Following the wedge excision of a tumor of the lateral upper lip (**Fig. 6.48a**), that part of the lip and the commissure can be reconstructed by a simple advancement technique following excision of a Burow's triangle next to the lower lip. A mucosal flap raised adjacent to the lower lip (**Fig. 6.48a**, S) is used to resurface the de-epithelialized area (**Fig. 6.48a**, D) on the reconstruction flap. This restores an accept-able length to the oral fissure and yields a good cos-metic result (**Fig. 6.48b**; Zisser 1970). Brusati (1979) proposed a similar reconstruction for both commissures (**Fig. 6.49**).

Reconstruction of the Commissure by the Method of Rehn (1933), as Modified by Fries (1971) and Brusati (1979)
(Fig. 6.50)

When the commissure must be resected along with portions of the lateral upper and lower lip (**Fig. 6.50a**), the incisions are placed on a roughly semicircular segment in the cheek above and below the lips. The secondary defects can be closed by excision of Burow's triangles. The commissure is restored by

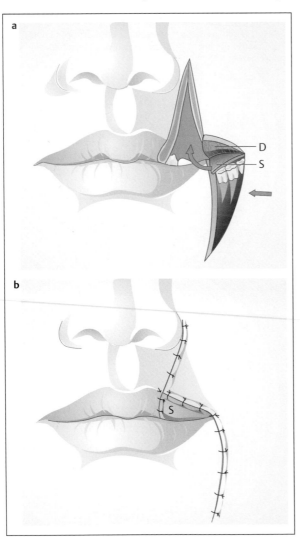

Fig. 6.48a, b   Lateral lip reconstruction by the method of Burow (1855) and Zisser (1970) (see **Fig. 6.39**).
a Burow's triangle after tumor excision. The flap is transposed by cutting a three-layer Burow's triangle lateral to the lower lip. D = de-epithelialized area.
b As in previous reconstructions, a flap of cheek mucosa (S) is used to resurface the de-epithelialized area.

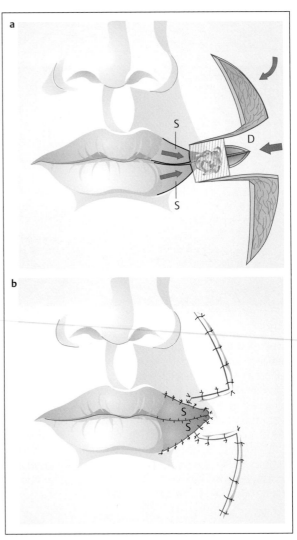

Fig. 6.49a, b   Reconstruction of the commissure by the method of Brusati (1979).
a The commissure is resected. Two Burow's triangles are excised from the cheek, and the cheek U-flap is advanced medially. A small area of the flap at the commissure is de-epithelialized (D).
b The lip mucosa is mobilized and advanced (S) into the de-epithelialized area (D).

suturing small triangular mucosal flaps (**Fig. 6.50**, S) to corresponding de-epithelialized sites on the flap (**Fig. 6.50**, D). (Vermilion advancement can also be used; see **Fig. 6.55**.)

Reconstruction of Large Commissural Defects
(**Fig. 6.51**)

As in the previous reconstruction, a two-layer trapezoidal flap is cut above and below the defect, and the vermilion is restored by turning a mucosal flap (**Fig.**

6.51a, b, S) over a corresponding de-epithelialized area (**Fig. 6.51a**, D). If mucosa is not available on the cheek flap, a mucosal flap can be taken from the side of the tongue, or the remaining vermilion can be advanced to cover the defect (see **Fig. 6.55**).

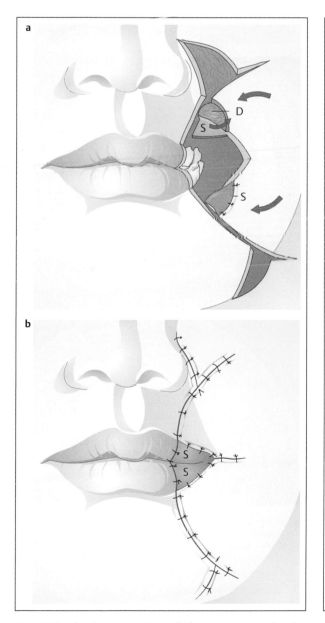

Fig. 6.50a, b **Reconstruction of the commissure** by the method of Fries (1973) and Brusati (1979). If intraoral mucosa is not available, the vermilion can be mobilized and advanced (see **Fig. 6.55**).

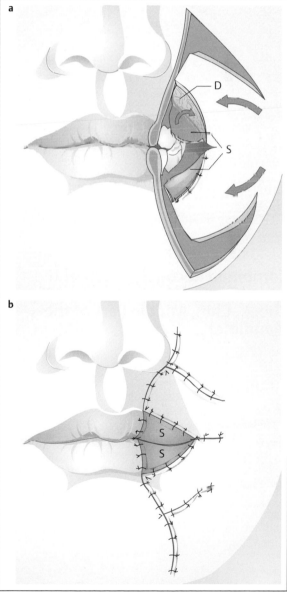

Fig. 6.51a, b **Reconstruction of the commissure** by dual V-Y advancement. Vermilion reconstruction (see **Figs. 6.48–6.50**). D = de-epithelialized area; S = cheek mucosa.

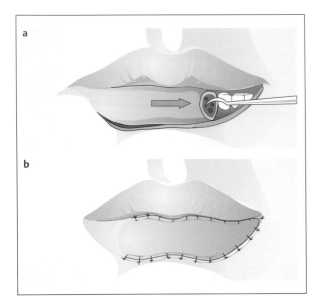

Fig. 6.52 **Vermilion advancement** of Goldstein (1984).
a The vermilion is incised through all three layers along the skin–vermilion border, preserving its attachment to the labial artery.
b The flap is advanced over the defect and sutured into place.

Vermilion Defects

Vermilion Advancement of Goldstein (1990)
(**Fig. 6.52**)
The defect is closed by mobilizing the lip at the vermilion border (**Fig. 6.52a, b**).

Combined Reconstruction of the Lower Part of the Face (Lower Lip, Cheek, Chin, Middle Part of the Mandible)

(**Fig. 6.53**)

Stage I:
In a 74-year-old patient, the lower part of the face had to be resected (**Fig. 6.53a, b**).

The mandible was reconstructed by a graft of the iliac crest (see **Fig. 15.4**, p. 235) and a plate (**Fig. 6.53c, d**). The cheek, the chin, and parts of the neck were reconstructed with a free pectoralis major island flap (see Chapters 12 and 14, **Fig. 6.53e**).

Stage II:
Four weeks later, the lower lip was reconstructed with a Gillies fan flap on both sides (**Fig. 6.53f**).

Stage III:
After elongation of the oral fissure (**Figs. 6.53g** and 6.54), we see the result 4 years later (**Fig. 6.53h**).

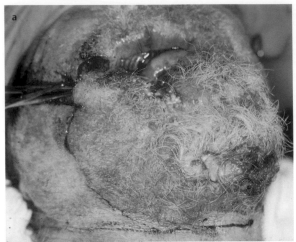

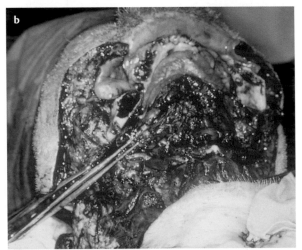

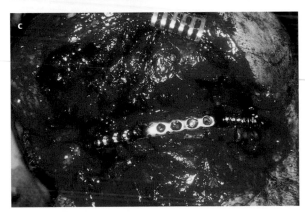

Fig. 6.53a–h Resection of the lower lip, chin and parts of the cheeks with partial resection of the mandibula.
a **Stage I: tumor** of the lip, chin, and parts of the cheeks.
b Resection of the tumor and parts of the mandible.
c, d Reconstruction of the mandible.

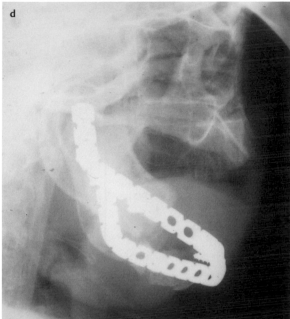

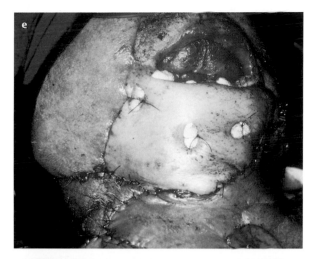

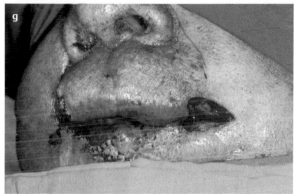

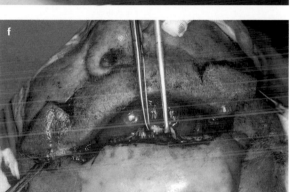

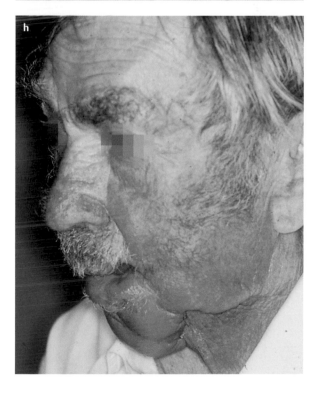

Fig. 6.53a–h   *(Continued)* **Resection of the lower lip, chin and parts of the cheeks with partial resection of the mandibula.**
e   Reconstruction of the cheeks and chin with a free pectoralis flap.
f   **Stage II:** Gillies fan flap (see **Fig. 6.45**) for reconstruction of the lower lip.
g   **Stage III:** elongation of the oral fissure (see **Fig. 6.54**).
h   1 year after tumor resection with a good functional result.

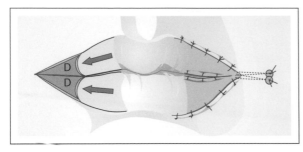

Fig. 6.54   Elongation of the oral fissure by the method of Converse (1959). Right side: the epithelium is excised following measurement of lip length. The vermilion is incised and mobilized. Left side: closure of the defects (D).

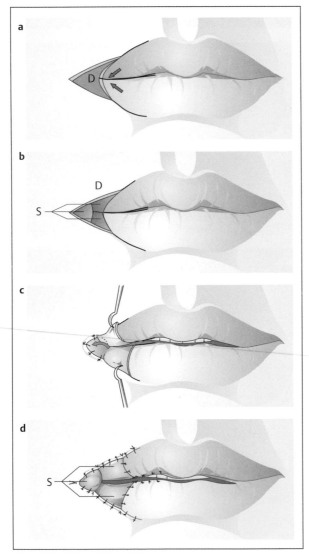

Fig. 6.55a–d   Elongation of the oral fissure (Converse 1977).
a The lip length is measured. A triangle of epithelium (D) is excised down to the mucosa, which is left intact. The existing commissure is incised (arrows).
b T-shaped incisions are made in the exposed mucosa, to create three mucosal flaps (S).
c The three mucosal flaps are turned.
d The completed repair.

Elongation of the Oral Fissure

The various Estlander lip reconstructions (see **Figs. 6.24, 6.41, 6.44**) and other methods (see **Fig. 6.45**) cause a shortening of the oral fissure that requires secondary correction.

Method of Converse (1959) (Weerda 1983)
(**Fig. 6.54**)

The center of the lip is determined, and the length of vermilion is measured on the healthy side. For a bilateral elongation of the oral fissure, an average is taken. A horizontal incision is made laterally in the direction of the oral fissure, and the epithelium above and below the incision is removed (**Fig. 6.54**, D, right). The mucosa of the lip stump is mobilized, pulled laterally into the angle of the mouth, and secured with tie-over bolster sutures (**Fig. 6.54**, left).

Method of Converse (1977)
(**Fig. 6.55**)

After the lip length is measured, an ipsilateral triangle of skin and subcutaneous tissue is excised, exposing the oral mucosa (**Fig. 6.55a**, D). The medial portion of the mucosa is incised, and a smaller vertical incision is made in the commissure itself (**Fig. 6.55b**). The three resulting mucosal flaps (S) are turned upward, down-

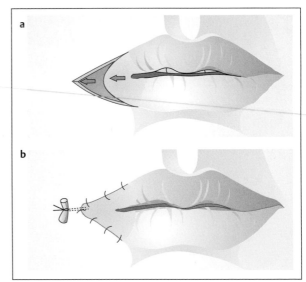

Fig. 6.56a, b   Elongation of the oral fissure by the Ganzer (1921) method.
a An epithelial triangle is excised following measurement of lip length. An incision is made around the vermilion without dividing it.
b The entire vermilion is advanced laterally and sutured into the defect.

ward, and laterally, and are sutured to the skin edges with 7-0 monofilament material (**Fig. 6.55c, d**).

Method of Ganzer (1921)
(**Fig. 6.56**)

If the mucosa in the angle of the mouth is sufficiently mobile, it may be possible to remove an epithelial triangle at the appropriate site and advance the entire commissure laterally (**Fig. 6.56a, b**).

Method of Gillies and Millard (1957)
(**Fig. 6.57**)

A vermilion flap is outlined on the upper or lower lip (**Fig. 6.57a**), according to the degree of elongation required. A two-layer excision is made at the commissure, sparing the mucosa on the inner aspect of the lower lip, which is raised as a flap (**Fig. 6.57b, c**). That flap is sutured to a de-epithelialized area, to reconstruct the vermilion of the lower lip (**Fig. 6.57d**). The vermilion flap is rotated laterally to restore the upper vermilion at the commissure. The mucosal flap may have to be mobilized slightly toward the oral vestibule.

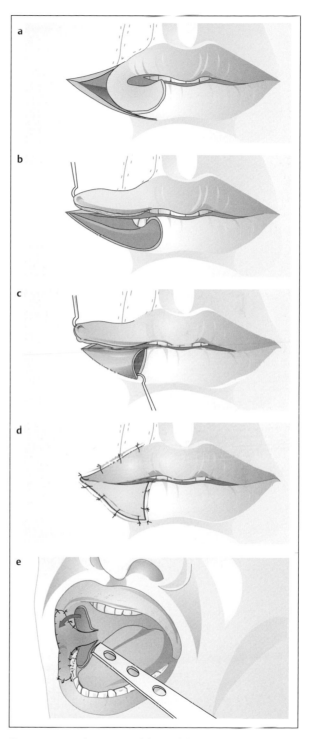

Fig. 6.57a–e Elongation of the oral fissure by the method of Gillies and Millard (1957).
a After the necessary elongation is determined, a triangular segment of skin is excised lateral to the rounded commissure, and a vermilion flap is raised from the lower (or upper) lip.
b The vermilion flap is rotated laterally, and the remaining tissue is excised down to the oral mucosa.
c The mucosal flap is mobilized to form the vermilion of the lower lip.
d Both flaps are sutured into the upper and lower lip defects (using 6-0 or 7-0 monofilament).
e Two-part mucosal flap from the cheek.

7 The Chin

Coverage of Small Defects in the Chin Area

(See also Scar Revision pp. 10–15; 21, 22)

Advancement Flap
(**Fig. 7.1**)

Small defects in the chin area can be covered by advancement of the lateral inferior cheek (**Fig. 7.1**). The incision is placed below the mandibular border, and a Burow's triangle is excised at the mandibular angle for closure of the secondary defect.

Bilobed Flap
(**Fig. 7.2a, b**)

A submental bilobed flap provides a very simple method for repairing this kind of defect.

Fig. 7.1a, b Burow's hook-shaped cheek advancement flap, used here to resurface a defect on the chin.

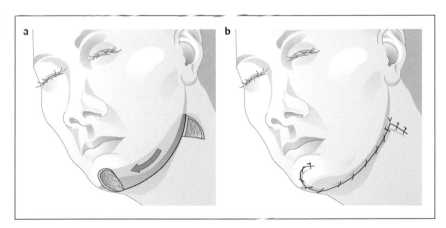

Fig. 7.2a, b Defect repaired with a bilobed flap.

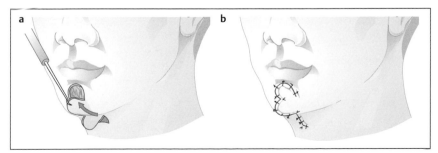

8 The Cheek

Medial Cheek Defects
Upper Medial Cheek

Esser Cheek Rotation (1918)
(**Fig. 8.1**)

The Esser cheek rotation can be used to reconstruct portions of the nose, as well as the medial cheek (see also **Fig. 5.52a**). From the defect, the incision extends along the lower eyelid and up into the temporal area, then curves down in front of the ear, where it may run a short distance back below the earlobe if necessary. It then proceeds downward and forward behind the mandibular angle (**Fig. 8.1**). The circumscribed flap is mobilized in the fat plane and rotated forward. Ectropion is prevented by fixing the flap to the periosteum of the infraorbital region. Burow's triangles

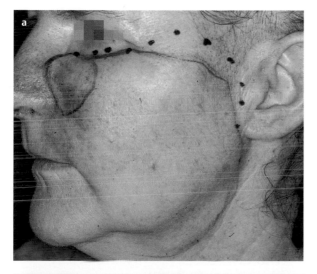
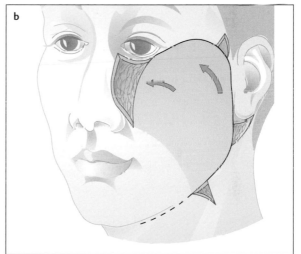
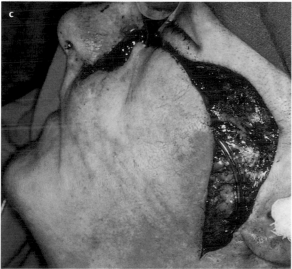
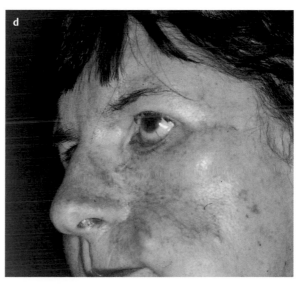

Fig. 8.1a–f Esser cheek rotation (1918).
a Tumor of the sinus and medial cheek, the cheek rotation is outlined.
b The flap is cut somewhat higher in the temporal area to provide excess tissue at the lower lid (to prevent ectropion). It is fixed to the periosteum of the orbital rim, and the cheek skin is mobilized (sparing the branches of the facial nerve).
c The flap is rotated, Burow's triangles are necessary to close the defect (see b).
d Result with ectropion after 1 year.

(Continued on next page) ▶

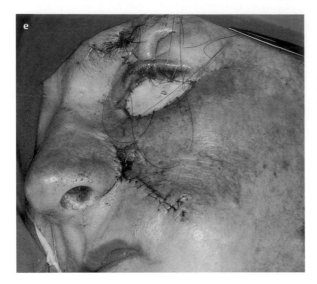

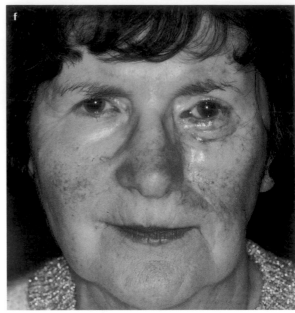

Fig. 8.1a–f *(Continued)* **Esser cheek rotation** (1918).
e Full-thickness skin graft from the retroauricular region for correction of the ectropion.
f Result 3 years after reconstruction.

are excised to close the secondary defect. If greater rotation is needed, the submandibular limb of the incision can be extended. The surgeon should not dissect too deeply in the fat, especially in the temporal area, as this could damage intact facial nerve branches.

Cheek Reconstruction Combining the Methods of Esser (1918) and Imre (1928) (Weerda 1980)

(Fig. 8.2)

For defects of the medial cheek and lower eyelid area, it may be necessary to combine the Esser flap with a nasolabial advancement. We have obtained good overall cheek mobility by combining the Esser rota-

Fig. 8.2 Cheek reconstruction combining the Esser and Imre techniques (Weerda 1980; see **Fig. 8.4**). A crescent-shaped excision in the nasolabial fold is added to the Esser rotation (see **Fig. 8.1**). The flap is mobilized in the fat plane to avoid facial nerve injury (see **Fig. 9.10**).

Fig. 8.3a, b
a Burow's cheek advancement.
b The scars are located in the nasal flank and nasolabial fold (see **Fig. 5.22**).

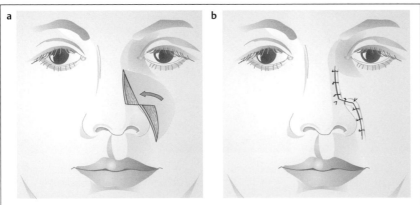

Fig. 8.4a, b
a Modified **Imre** cheek advancement.
b The scars are located at the boundaries of the esthetic units and in the RSTLs (nasolabial fold) (see **Figs. 5.48a, b** and **9.10**).

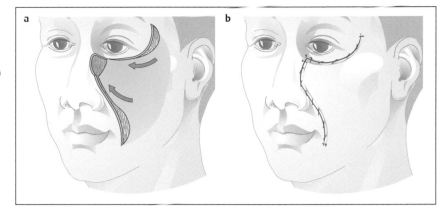

tion with a two-layer crescent-shaped excision in the nasolabial fold.

Small Cheek Defects

Small defects are repaired with transposition or rotation flaps, and small bilobed flaps can also be used (see pp. 21, 25, 46–48; **Figs. 3.1b** and **3.22**). Defects in the nasal flank area can be closed by a Burow-type cheek advancement with a Burow's triangle (**Fig. 8.3**) or by excising a skin crescent in the nasolabial angle (see Fig. **8.4**).

Imre Cheek Advancement Flap (After Haas and Meyer 1973, modified)
(**Figs. 8.4** and **8.5**)

Defect in the Medial Canthus
(**Fig. 8.6**)

A medial defect can be repaired with an Imre cheek rotation flap combined with a rotation flap from the forehead (see **Figs. 5.2–5.8**).

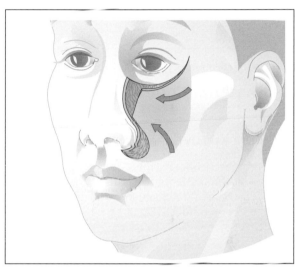

Fig. 8.5   Modified Imre flap. The scar is located in the alar groove. (see **Fig. 5.51**).

Fig. 8.6a, b   Imre cheek rotation combined with a small forehead flap to repair a defect involving the cheek and medial canthal area (see **Figs. 5.2–5.8**; see also **Fig. 8.2**).

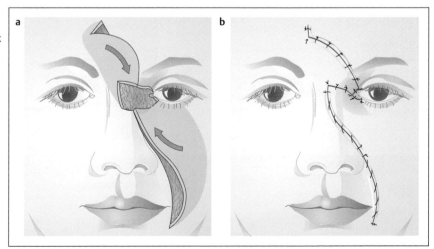

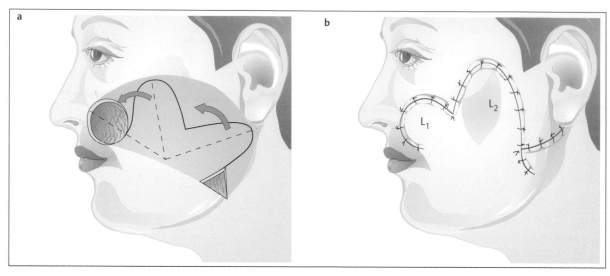

Fig. 8.7a, b   Inferiorly based bilobed flap.

Mid-Anterior Cheek
(Fig. 8.7)

Pedicled Bilobed Flaps

Inferiorly based bilobed flaps are particularly suitable for elderly patients (Dean et al. 1975; Weerda 1983). The secondary lobe may be placed behind the ear or in the upper neck (**Fig. 8.7a, b**).

Large Inferiorly/Anteriorly Based Bilobed Flap
(Fig. 8.8)

In modern oncosurgery, we normally reconstruct this defect with a free forearm flap (see **Fig. 14.1**). Sometimes, this bilobed flap can be used in older patients (**Fig. 8.8a**). The anterior sinus wall and orbital floor are reconstructed with temporal muscle and fascia (**Fig. 8.8b–e**).

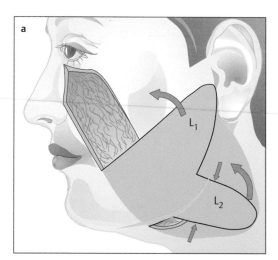

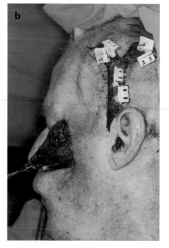

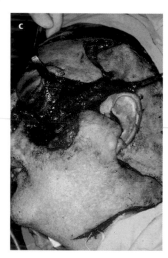

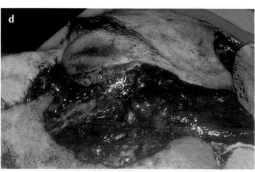

Fig. 8.8a–g   Large inferiorly based bilobed flap.
a Defect of the median cheek; the bilobed flap is outlined.
b To close the large defect of the anterior cheek, sinus wall, and orbital floor (see **c**), we harvest **temporalis muscle and fascia** (here another patient).
c The bilobed flap is incised anteriorly inferiorly, the orbital floor is reconstructed with rib and plates.
d The anterior wall and the orbital floor are covered with the temporal muscle, and the anterior wall of the sinus is reconstructed with bone.

Fig. 8.8e–g   ▶

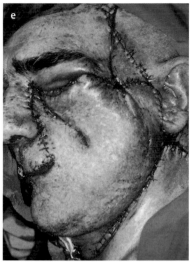

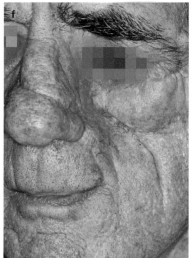

Fig. 8.8e–g
e The defects are closed and sutured.

f Result after 2 years.
g X-ray.

V-Y Advancement

(**Fig. 8.9**; see also **Fig. 3.9**)

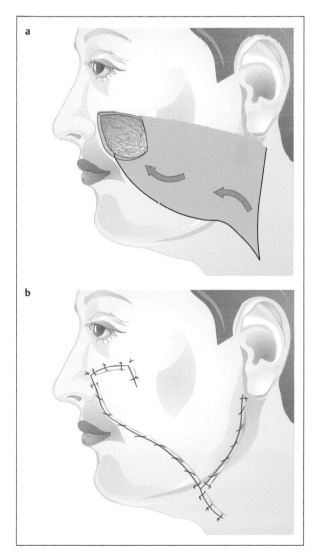

Fig. 8.9a, b V-Y advancement of the cheek.

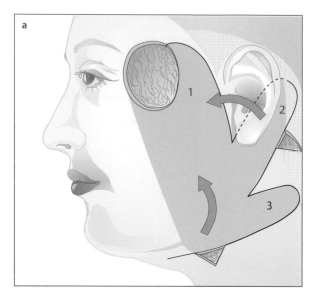

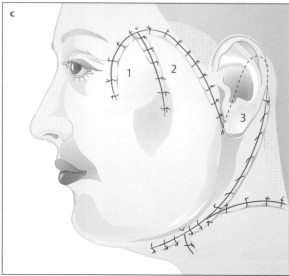

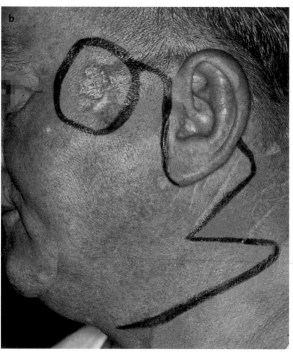

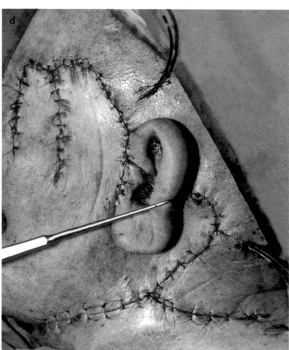

Fig. 8.10a–d   Trilobed flap of Weerda (1979).

a, b Trilobed flap for a defect in the temporal region consists of a preauricular lobe (1), a retroauricular lobe (2), and a neck lobe (3).

c, d The completed repair. All defects can be closed by excising Burow's triangles and mobilizing the surrounding skin.

Upper and Posterior Cheek

Trilobed Flap of Weerda (1979)
(**Fig. 8.10**)

Occasionally, a bilobed flap is insufficient for repairing a cheek defect, which requires one lobe between the ear and the defect (**Fig. 8.10a, b**), a second lobe behind the ear, and a third lobe in the lateral neck.

As in an Esser cheek rotation, the lower limb of the third lobe may be extended below the mandible. Clo-sure of the secondary defects may require excision of Burow's triangles (**Fig. 8.10c, d**).

Bilobed Flap
(**Fig. 8.11**)

A defect involving the lateral cheek or earlobe area can be repaired with a retroauricular bilobed flap (**Fig. 8.11a**). The somewhat smaller secondary lobe is raised from the side of the neck (**Fig. 8.11b**).

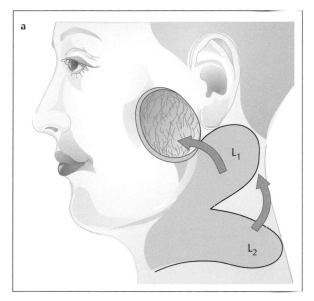

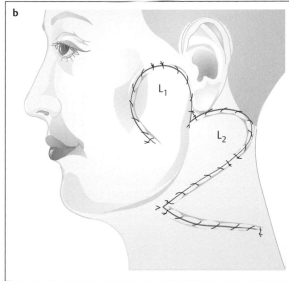

Fig. 8.11a, b   Bilobed flap from the side of the neck.

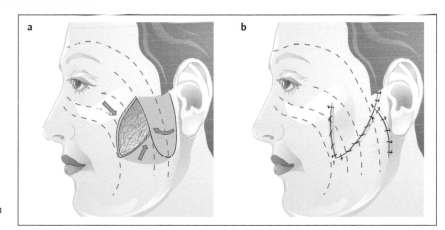

Fig. 8.12a, b   Small **preauricular transposition flap** (can be cut slightly smaller than the defect). Scar revision may be necessary as a secondary procedure.

Lateral Cheek Defects

Small Lateral Cheek Defects

These defects can be repaired with various flaps, such as transposition flaps (**Fig. 8.12**), the trapezoidal flaps described by Limberg (1967) or Dufourmentel (1962) (**Fig. 8.13**; see also **Figs. 3.24–3.27**), by flap advancement, or by Z-plasties (**Figs. 8.14** and **8.15**).

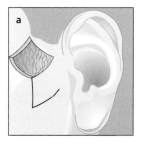

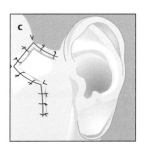

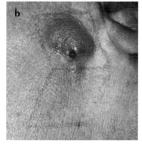

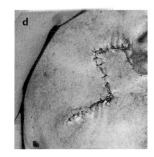

Fig. 8.13a–d
a, b Limberg flap (rhomboid flap; see **Figs. 3.24–3.27**) for the reconstruction of a preauricular cheek defect.
c, d The defects are covered.

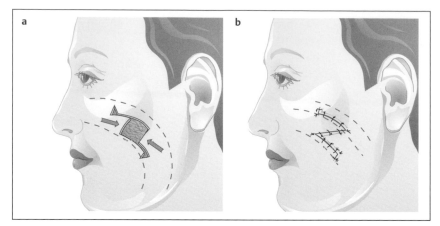

Fig. 8.14a, b   **Double advancement flap** (see **Fig. 3.1**).

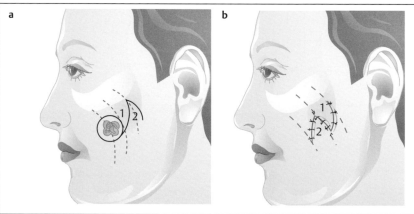

Fig. 8.15a, b   Small cheek defect repaired by a **Z-plasty** (see **Fig. 2.15** and **Plate 1** on page 31).

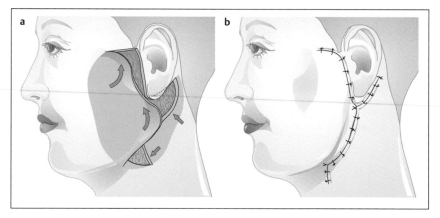

Fig. 8.16a, b   **Skin advancement** from the retroauricular area.

Small Preauricular Defects

Small preauricular defects can be covered by advancing tissue from the retroauricular neck area (**Fig. 8.16**).

Simple Skin Advancement and Rotation (Burow's Method)
(**Fig. 8.17a–d**)

Wedge-shaped defects of the lower lateral cheek can be repaired by a simple Burow skin advancement (**Fig. 8.17a, b**). For a round or oval defect, we use rotation flaps from the upper neck (**Fig. 8.17c, d**).

Opposing Transposition Flaps
(**Fig. 8.18**)

If the primary reconstruction flap can be raised in the preauricular area (**Fig. 8.18a**), the secondary defect can be closed with an inferiorly based retroauricular flap. The tertiary defect can then be covered by mobilization (**Fig. 8.18**), or with a thick split skin graft (e.g., from the buttock).

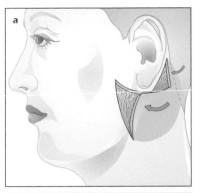

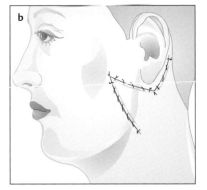

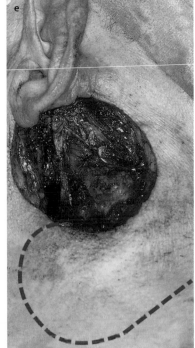

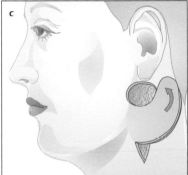

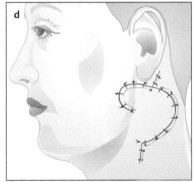

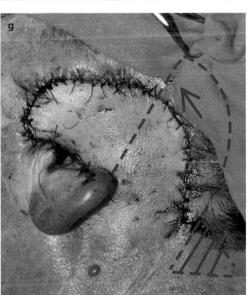

Fig. 8.17a–g   Burow's flap advancement and different rotation flaps.
a Wedge-shaped defect with a superior base. A retroauricular Burow's triangle is excised.
b The completed repair.
c A circular defect is covered with a rotation flap from the upper neck, anteriorly pedicled.
d The completed repair.
e, f Posteriorly pedicled rotation flap of the upper neck.
g Retroauricular, inferiorly pedicled transposition flap.

Fig. 8.18a, b
a **Cheek defect** is repaired with a preauricular transposition flap (1). A second, inferiorly based flap is also raised (2).
b The completed repair.

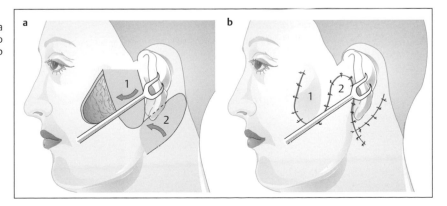

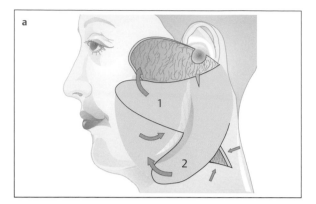

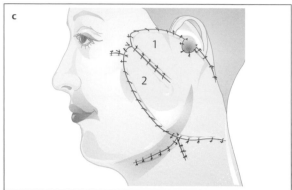

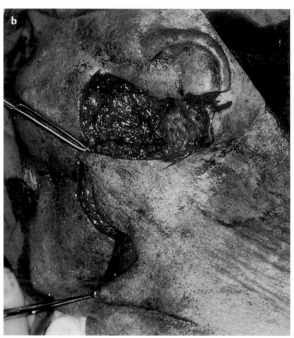

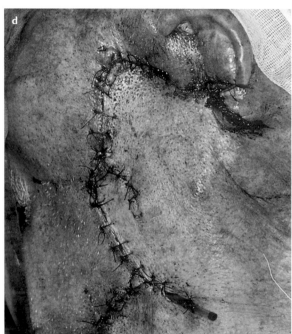

Fig. 8.19a–e Posteriorly based **bilobed flap from the cheek and submandibular region** (Weerda 1978c, 1980c).

a, b Large defect involving the posterior upper cheek and the auricle. One lobe of the flap (1) is outlined below the defect. A second lobe (2) is outlined in the submandibular area. Burow's triangles are excised to close the secondary defects.

c, d The completed repair.

e Result 6 months later.

Large Defects Involving the Auricle

A large defect involving the auricle can be repaired by transposing a posteriorly based bilobed flap with a submandibular secondary lobe (**Fig. 8.19**).

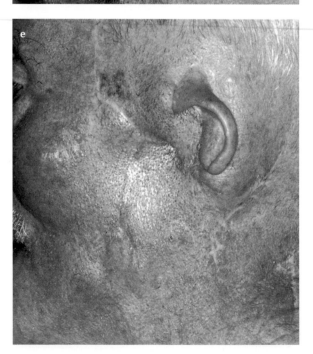

Fig. 8.20a, b Lateral cheek rotation of Weerda (1980c).

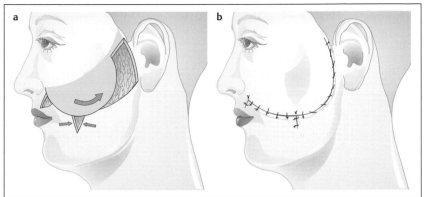

Fig. 8.21a–d High or low lateral cheek defect repaired with a transposition flap from the neck.
a The superiorly based transposition flap is outlined in a rhomboid-like design.
b, c All defects are closed by V-Y advancement (with neck dissection).
d Result after 3 weeks.

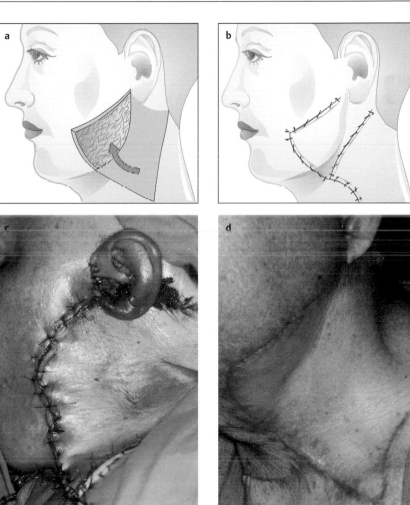

Lateral Cheek Rotation of Weerda (1980c)

(Figs. 8.20 and 8.21)

Moderate-sized preauricular cheek defects can be repaired with a superiorly based cheek rotation flap (Fig. 8.20). A transposition flap with V-Y advancement can be used in the inferolateral cheek area (Fig. 8.21). Large defects can alternatively be covered with

island flaps (see Chapters 12, 13) or with free flaps (see Chapter 14).

Pedicled Transposition Flaps

(Figs. 8.22 and 8.23)

Defects of the concha and preauricular region may sometimes require a flap that does not follow the RSTLs, especially in the case of elderly patients, where

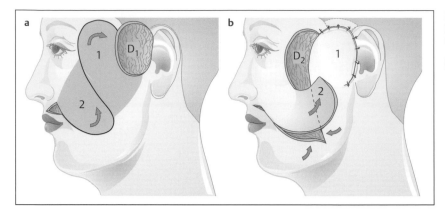

Fig. 8.22a, b   Defect in the upper preauricular region (D₁).
a Inferiorly based transposition flap (1).
b The secondary defect (D₂) is closed by lateral cheek rotation (2).

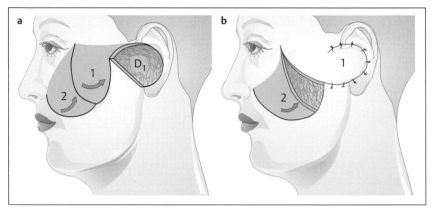

Fig. 8.23a, b   Defect involving the ear (D₁).
a Superiorly based preauricular flap (1).
b The secondary defect is closed by lateral cheek rotation (2).

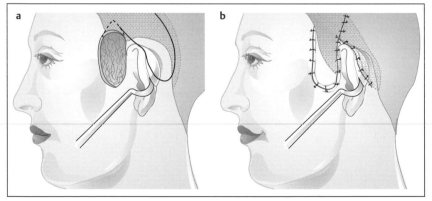

Fig. 8.24a, b   Preauricular hair loss corrected with a superiorly based **retroauricular transposition flap**.
a Outline of the transposition flap, which is hair bearing in its lateral portion.
b The completed repair.

swift treatment and rehabilitation are a priority. We have repaired these cases with an inferiorly based (**Fig. 8.22**) or temporally based transposition flap (**Fig. 8.23**, 1), using an anteriorly based cheek rotation to close the secondary defect (**Figs. 8.22** and **8.23**, 2).

Preauricular Hair Loss
(**Fig. 8.24**)

Preauricular defects can be covered with restoration of hair, by transposing a superiorly based retroauricular flap whose upper portion is hair bearing. The lower portion of the flap is designed to transfer hairless skin to the cheek. The specific flap design will depend on whether the patient is male or female (see **Fig. 8.18**).

Inferiorly Based Retroauricular Transposition flap (Weerda 1978b)
(**Fig. 8.25**)

A large defect involving the auricle and preauricular region can be covered with a large inferiorly based retroauricular flap. The secondary defect is closed by rotating the surrounding skin. Hair can be transferred with the flap if desired.

Fig. 8.25a, b Use of multiple flaps to close a large defect of the lateral cheek (D$_1$). An inferiorly based transposition flap (1) from the side of the neck is combined with rotation flaps (2, 3) to close the defects.

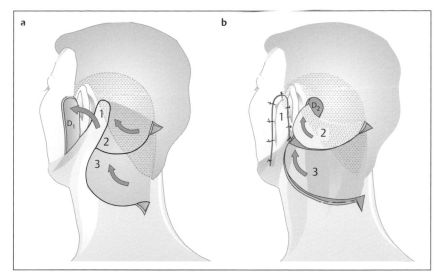

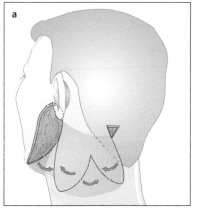

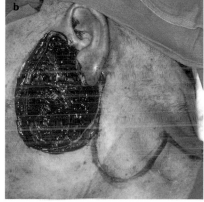

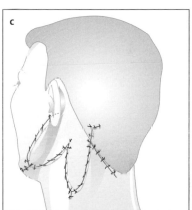

Fig. 8.26a–e Use of a posterosuperiorly based **bilobed flap** to close a defect in the lower cheek (see **Fig. 8.19**).
a, b Outline of the superiorly based bilobed flap.
c, d The completed repair.
e Result 8 weeks later.

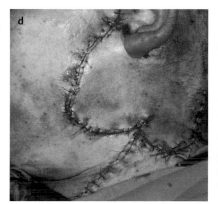

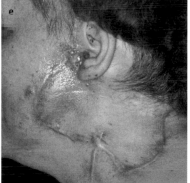

Large Bilobed Flap from the Neck (Weerda 1980b)
(**Fig. 8.26**)

We cover large defects of the lower lateral cheek and neck with a posteriorly based bilobed flap from the submandibular or neck–shoulder region. With extensive defects, the flap should be delayed. We prefer a myocutaneous flap in older patients, i.e., a mucocutaneous pectoralis major island flap or latissimus dorsi flap. If a skilled team is available, a radial forearm flap can be transferred to the recipient site by microvascular anastomosis (see **Fig. 14.1**).

9 The Eyelids

Upper Eyelid
Direct Closure
(Fig. 9.1)

Direct closure is suitable for defects that involve up to one quarter (~8 mm) of the eyelid margin (semicircular flap closure, **Fig. 9.1**).

Semicircular Flap Closure of Beyer-Machule and Riedel (1993)
(Fig. 9.2)

Larger defects involving up to one half of the lid margin can be closed by advancing a semicircular skin flap medially (**Fig. 9.2a**). The lid margin is sutured first (**Fig. 9.1**). Next the tarsus and orbicularis muscle are approximated with 6-0 interrupted Vicryl sutures (Ethicon, Hamburg-Norderstedt, Germany), and the skin is closed with 7-0 interrupted monofila-

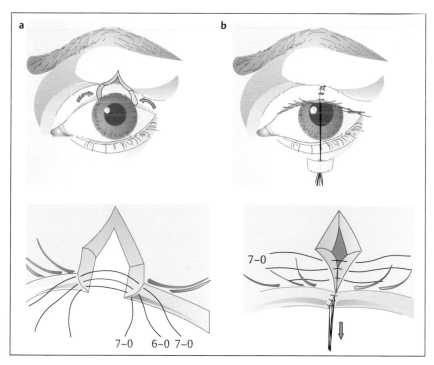

Fig. 9.1a, b Direct primary closure of an **upper eyelid defect** involving up to one quarter of the length of the lid margin (~8 mm).
- **a** The lid margin is closed with 6-0 or 7-0 PDS sutures. The tarsus and orbicularis muscle are then approximated with interrupted 6-0 absorbable sutures.
- **b** Continuous 7-0 monofilament suture. The ends of the adjacent deep intermarginal sutures are tied on the anterior lid margin to prevent them scratching the eye. Traction sutures are left long and taped to the cheek.

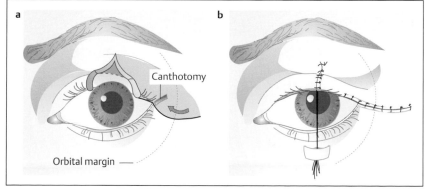

Fig. 9.2a, b Lateral semicircular flap closure of an upper eyelid defect involving one quarter to one half of the length of the lid.
- **a** A lateral canthotomy of the upper palpebral ligament is performed to facilitate advancement of the lateral skin.
- **b** All the wounds are closed (see **Fig. 9.1**). The same technique is used for the lower lid.

ment sutures (**Fig. 9.1a, b**). The lid margin is approximated with three stay sutures, two of which are placed deeply (close to the eyeball) and one more superficially (Beyer-Machule and Riedel 1993). Large upper lid defects are rare and should be repaired only by surgeons who are experienced in eyelid surgery.

Switch Flap
(**Fig. 9.3**)

Analogous to the Abbé lip switch, this flap can be rotated from the lower eyelid into a full-thickness upper eyelid defect involving up to one quarter of the length of the lid margin (**Fig. 9.3a, b**). The eye itself is covered with a special protector to prevent corneal

injury. The lower lid defect is closed directly with continuous 6-0 monofilament (**Fig. 9.3b**), followed by placement of both the upper lid sutures (**Fig. 9.3c**).

Upper Eyelid Reconstruction of Fricke and Kreibig
(**Fig. 9.4**)

Large portions of the upper (and lower) eyelid can be reconstructed with a narrow transposition flap that is raised above the eyebrow on a lateral pedicle. Thick split retroauricular skin grafts can also be used.

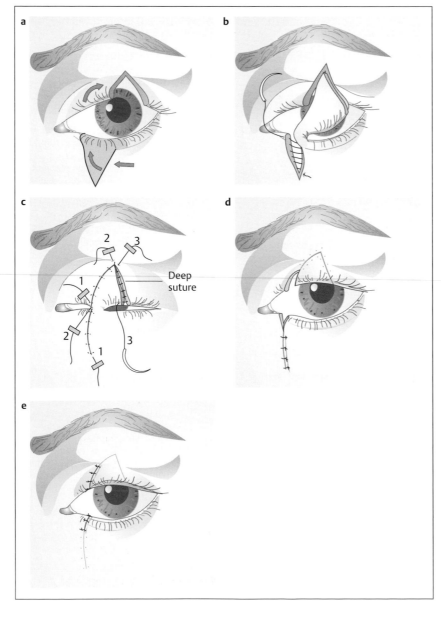

Fig. 9.3a–e Mustardé's technique of **upper eyelid reconstruction** using a laterally based full-thickness flap from the lower lid (after Beyer-Machule and Riedel 1993).
- **a** The full-thickness lower lid flap is outlined with a lateral pedicle.
- **b** The flap is swung into the upper lid defect, and the lower lid defect is closed.
- **c** A continuous suture line incorporates three interrupted sutures that close the defect and are taped to the skin.
- **d, e** About 3 weeks later, the pedicle is divided and the defects are closed.

Fig. 9.4a, b Transposition flap from the forehead described by Fricke and Kreibig for reconstruction of the upper eyelid (**a**) and lower eyelid (**b**).

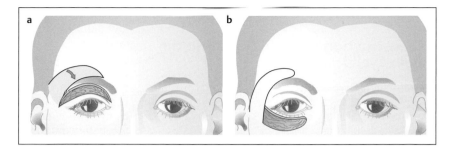

Fig. 9.5a, b Closure of **medial upper lid defects** with a bilobed flap (see **Figs. 5.3–5.7** and **5.24**).

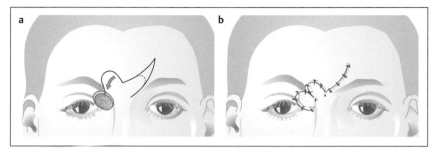

Fig. 9.6a–c Total upper lid reconstruction by Mustardé's two-step technique.

a A laterally based semicircular lower lid flap is used to reconstruct the upper lid (see **Fig. 9.2**). A chondromucosal composite graft is taken from the septum. The mucosal part of the graft is twice as large as the cartilaginous part.

b The composite graft is used to replace the lower lid.

c All defects are closed. Three weeks later the pedicle is divided and inset (see **Fig. 9.3d, e**) (after Beyer-Machule and Riedel 1993).

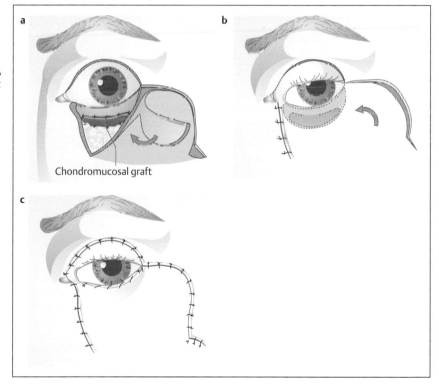

Chondromucosal graft

Bilobed Flap
(Fig. 9.5)

More medially situated defects of the upper eyelid can be repaired with a bilobed flap from the forehead. The secondary lobe should be slightly larger than the primary lobe. Rotation of the secondary lobe may cause skin bunching that requires correction in a second operation (**Fig. 9.5b**). A V-Y advancement can also be used (see **Figs. 5.2–5.7**).

Total Upper Lid Reconstruction by the Two-Stage Mustardé Technique (Beyer-Machule and Riedel 1993)
(Fig. 9.6)

Similar to the switch flap (**Fig. 9.3**), the entire lower lid is raised on a lateral pedicle (**Fig. 9.6a**). The semicircular flap is transposed medially and rotated upward into the upper lid (**Fig. 9.6b**). The lower lid is reconstructed with a composite graft from the septum (**Fig. 9.7**). The pedicle is divided ~3 weeks later (see **Fig. 9.3d, e**).

Reconstruction of the Lower Eyelid

Reconstruction of Small Defects in the Lower Eyelid

Small defects of the lower eyelid can sometimes be closed by direct suture (**Fig. 9.1b**) or, by transposing a flap from the upper lid (**Fig. 9.3**), analogous to the Abbé switch flap.

Large Defects
(**Figs. 9.6** and **9.7**)

As in the upper lid, the rotation-advancement technique of Mustardé (1980) can be used to close a large defect in the lower lid. The incision starts in the lateral canthus, curves upward, and ends in the preau-

ricular area. The skin is undermined in a fairly shallow plane, and the lid defect is incorporated into a wedge excision that points downward (**Fig. 9.7a**). A chondromucosal composite graft from the septum is used for inner lining. The cartilaginous part of the graft should be slightly smaller than the mucosal part. The septal cartilage is thinned to 1 to 1.5 mm, using a no. 11 scalpel blade or special cartilage knife. After the composite graft has been sewn into place (with the mucosa inward), the defect is closed by rotation-advancement of the lateral cheek skin (**Fig. 9.7b**). Special care is taken to reconstruct the lacrimal ducts (**Fig. 9.7c**).

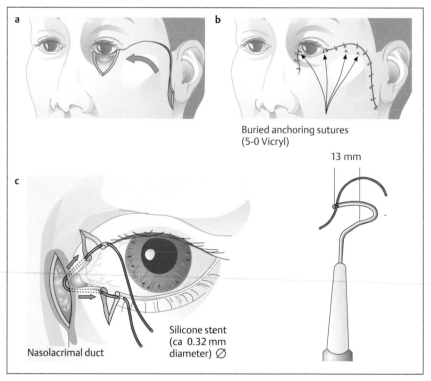

Buried anchoring sutures
(5-0 Vicryl)

13 mm

Silicone stent
(ca 0.32 mm
diameter) Ø

Nasolacrimal duct

Fig. 9.7a–c   Lower lid reconstruction using the rotation-advancement technique of Mustardé (1980).
a The mucosal defect is reconstructed with a composite graft from the septum. Note the curved flap incision in the temporal region (**Fig. 9.6**; see also **Figs. 8.1** and **8.6**).
b The reconstruction is completed.
c The lacrimal ducts are intubated with a pigtail catheter and splinted with a small silicone stent.

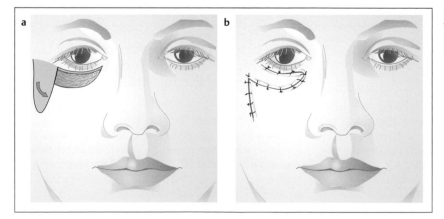

Fig. 9.8a, b   Transposition flap of von Langenbeck (1855) for repairing a lower lid defect and correcting ectropion.

Fig. 9.9a, b   Median nasolabial flap for repairing a lower lid defect or correcting ectropion.

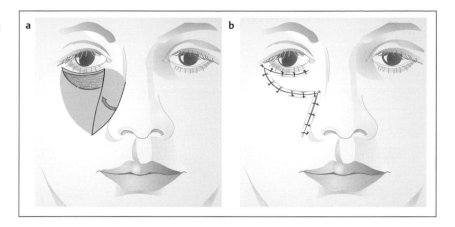

Fig. 9.10a,b   Imre cheek advancement for repairing a lower lid defect or correcting ectropion (see **Fig. 8.2**).

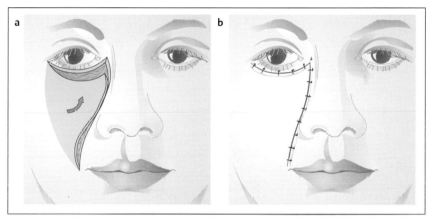

Fig. 9.11a, b   A simple mucocutaneous transposition flap (Tripier flap) from the upper lid is used to correct ectropion of the lower lid.

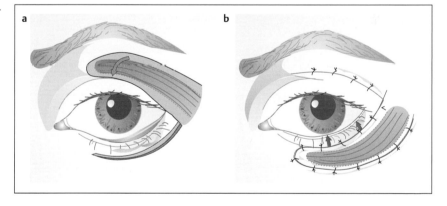

Reconstruction of the Lower Lid with Ectropion

Transposition Flap
(**Figs. 9.8 and 9.9**)

A superiorly based lateral transposition flap (as described by von Langenbeck 1855) is excellent for reconstructing a lower eyelid defect and also correcting ectropion due to scarring (**Fig. 9.8**). Larger flaps can be obtained medially (**Fig. 9.9**). A retroauricular full-thickness skin graft, or an Imre cheek rotation flap, are also good options for this type of reconstruction (**Fig. 9.10**; see also **Figs. 8.2** and **8.6**).

A few cases will also require use of a cartilage graft or chondromucosal composite graft from the nasal septum (see **Fig. 9.6**).

Total Lower Lid Reconstruction
(**Figs. 9.11 and 9.12**)

The entire lower lid can be reconstructed with a transposition flap (**Fig. 9.11a, b**) or a bipedicle flap (myocutaneous flap, **Fig. 9.12a, b**) from the upper eyelid (Tripier flap). As in other methods, a chondromucosal graft from the nasal septum can be used for lining (see **Figs. 9.6** and **9.7**). The lateral and medial pedicles are divided and inset in a later sitting.

Reconstruction of the Medial Canthus
(Figs. **9.13** and **9.14**; see also **Figs. 5.2–5.7**)

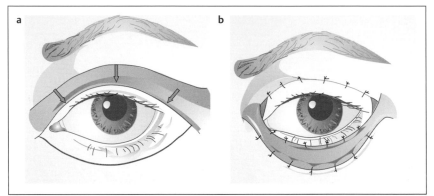

Fig. 9.12a, b   Double Tripier flap designed as a bipedicle flap.
a The flap is outlined in the upper eyelid as a myocutaneous flap.
b The flap is transposed, eliminating ectropion of the lower eyelid. About 3 weeks later, the lateral and medial pedicles are divided and inset (see **Fig. 9.3d, e**).

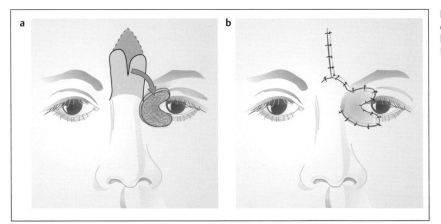

Fig. 9.13a, b   **Medial canthal defect** repaired with a **bilobed forehead flap** (see **Fig. 9.5**; see also **Figs. 5.3–5.7**).

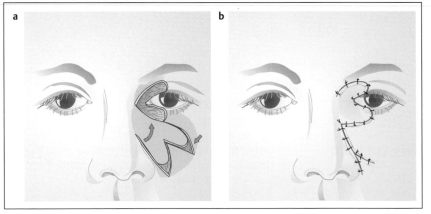

Fig. 9.14a, b   Use of a **bilobed cheek flap** with a superior and medial pedicle to repair a **medial canthal defect** (see **Figs. 9.5** and **9.13**; see also **Figs. 5.3–5.7**).

10 The Auricular Region

H. Weerda

Classification (Table 10.1) and Esthetic Units (Fig. 10.1)

Although there will inevitably be overlaps when attempting to classify auricular defects, we still regard it as worthwhile to classify the defects for didactic reasons, to offer a system of surgical reconstruction (Weerda 1980b, 1984, 1987, 1989c, 1994d, 2001; Weerda and Siegert 1999a; Mellette 1991) (**Table 10.1**). The esthetic units (**Fig. 10.1**) cannot always be taken into consideration, and reconstruction of the auricle is performed in accordance with surgical requirements (see Weerda 2004, pp. 1–3, 12).

Central Defects: Recommended Defect Coverage (Fig. 10.2)

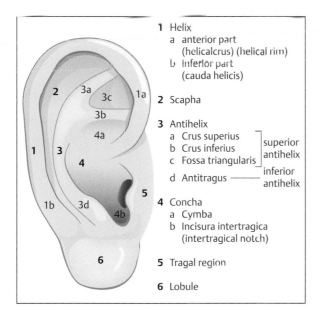

Fig. 10.1 Esthetic units and subunits of the auricle (Weerda 1980, 2001; Mellette 1991; see also Sherris and Larrabee 2009).
1   Helix (helical rim).
a   Anterior part (helical crus).
b   Inferior part (cauda helicis).
2   Scapha.
3   Antihelix.
a   Superior antihelix: crus superius.
b   Inferior antihelix: crus inferius.
c   Fossa triangularis.
d   Inferior antihelix: antitragus (see **Fig. 10.8**).
4   Concha.
a   Cymba.
b   Incisura intertragica (intertragical notch).
5   Tragal region.
6   Lobule.

Labels in Fig. 10.1:
1   Helix
  a   anterior part (helicalcrus) (helical rim)
  b   inferior part (cauda helicis)
2   Scapha
3   Antihelix
  a   Crus superius
  b   Crus inferius   } superior antihelix
  c   Fossa triangularis
  d   Antitragus   } inferior antihelix
4   Concha
  a   Cymba
  b   Incisura intertragica (intertragical notch)
5   Tragal region
6   Lobule

Table 10.1 Classification of auricular defects (Weerda 1980, 1987)

1.   Central defects
   • Conchal defects
   • Defects of the antihelix and combined central defects

2.   Peripheral defects
   • Helix reconstruction with auricular reduction
   • Helix reconstruction without auricular reduction

3.   Partial Reconstruction of the auricle
   • Upper-third auricular defects
     – Reconstruction with auricular reduction
     – Reconstruction without auricular reduction
   • Middle-third auricular defects
     – Reconstruction with auricular reduction
     – Reconstruction without auricular reduction
   • Lower-third auricular defects

4.   Reconstruction of the earlobe
   • Traumatic earlobe cleft
     – Reconstruction without preservation of the earring perforation
     – Reconstruction with preservation of the earring perforation
   • Defects of the earlobe
   • Loss of the earlobe

5.   Posterior defects
   • Postauricular defects
   • Retroauricular defects
   • Combined postauricular and retroauricular defects

6.   Subtotal defects

7.   Loss of the auricle
   • Fresh avulsion injuries
   • Auricular reconstruction following total amputation
   • Reconstruction of the ear or auricular region in patients with skin loss or burns
   • Reconstruction of defects of the auricular region after partial or total amputation

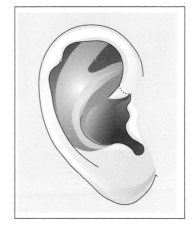

Fig. 10.2 Central defects: concha–antihelix–combined defects.

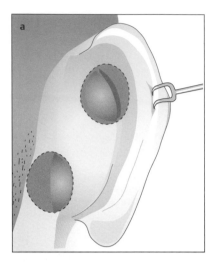

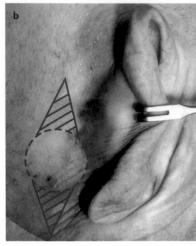

Fig. 10.3a–h Coverage of a central defect with full-thickness skin.

a–c Outline of a full-thickness skin graft harvested from the sulcus or mastoid region and fashioned by means of a template of aluminum foil (**c**) (suture wrapping material) or glove paper.

d Defect and full-thickness graft.

e, f Inset using a few approximation sutures (6-0 monofilament) and fibrin adhesive.

g Primary closure of the wounds.

h Result.

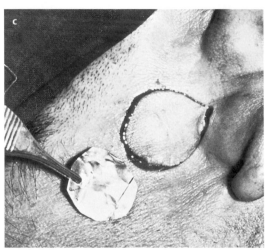

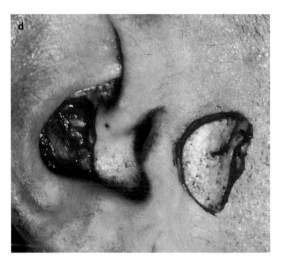

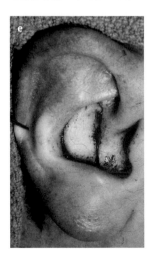

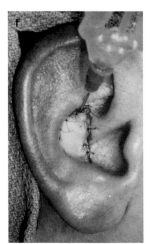

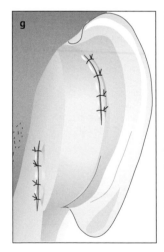

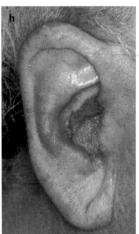

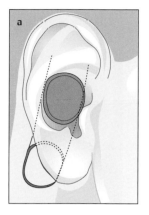
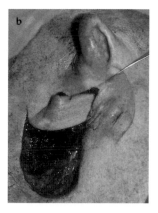
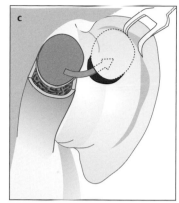
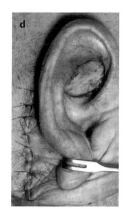

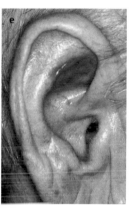
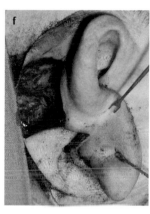
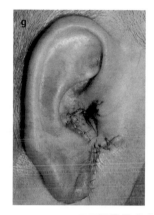
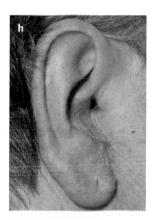

Fig. 10.4a–h Two-layer defect of the concha (a, b) or the triangular fossa: and cymba (c–e), coverage using a superiorly (a) or inferiorly (c) based transposition flap.

a, b Retroauricular, superiorly based transposition flap with de-epithelialized area located beneath the tunnel (**l in c**).

c Inferiorly based transposition flap (alternative technique to a).

d Inset into the defect, the retroauricular defect is closed.

e Result 6 weeks after excision of the pedicle.

f Inferiorly based transposition flap for reconstruction of the lower concha and the ear canal (see c).

g Inset of the flap.

h Result after 1 year.

Conchal Defects

Reconstruction with a Full-thickness Skin Graft
(**Fig. 10.3**)

Since large parts of the concha adjoin the mastoid region, full-thickness skin is an option for reconstructing the concha. Reconstruction with a full-thickness skin graft is shown in **Fig. 10.3a–h**.

Transposition Flap and U-shaped Advancement
(**Fig. 10.4**)

When the defects are situated somewhat higher, and extend into the antihelix, or into the auditory canal, it is possible to use superiorly or inferiorly based transposition flaps, de-epithelialized at the site that comes to lie beneath the tunnel when passed anteriorly (**pull-through technique; Fig. 10.4c**).

Reconstruction with Island Flaps
(**Figs. 10.5–10.7**)

"True" island flaps are flaps that are supplied by an artery but disconnected from the surrounding tissue (Kazanjian 1958; Weerda 1999b, 2004). The following techniques are used:

- Reconstruction of a two-layer defect using a **myocutaneous island flap** based posteriorly on the posterior auricular artery (Krespi et al. 1983; Weerda and Siegert 1999a; Weerda 2001; **Fig. 10.5a–f**).
- Zong-ji and Chao (1990) also use an island flap based posteriorly on the posterior auricular artery.
- Large **island flap based on a dermal pedicle** (as described by Masson 1972; Renard 1981; Koopmann and Coulthard 1982; Jackson 1985b; **Fig. 10.6a–g**)
- Island flap as described by Park et al. (1988; **Fig. 10.7a, b**).

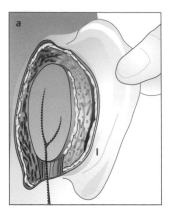
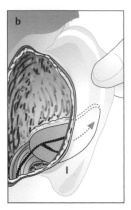
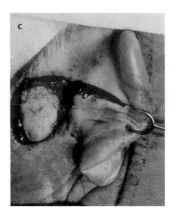
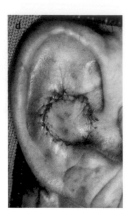

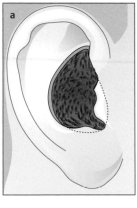
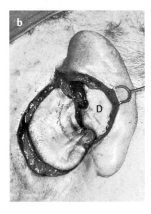

Fig. 10.5a–f   Two-layer central defect: coverage using a myocutaneous island flap based on the posterior auricular artery (Krespi et al. 1983).

a, b The flap is incised according to a template of the defect, while protecting the vessels arising from beneath, as well as the muscular pedicle.

c The postauricular skin is undermined as far as the anterior defect; I = tunnel.

d, e The flap is inset into the anterior defect and the posterior wound is closed.

f Result after healing onto the concha.

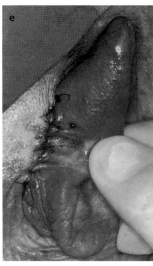
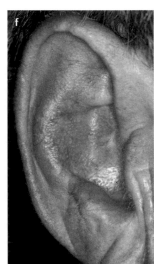
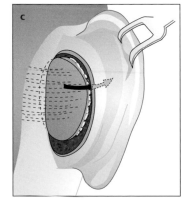

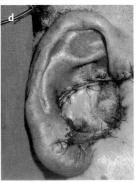
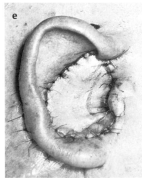
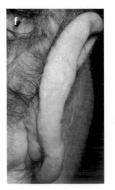
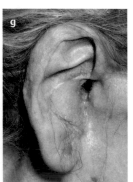

Fig. 10.7a–d

a, b Reconstruction of an anterior defect using a postauricular island flap as described by Park et al. (1988).

c, d The vessels are identified using Doppler ultrasound and the flap is elevated. The flap is brought out anteriorly and sutured onto the defect.

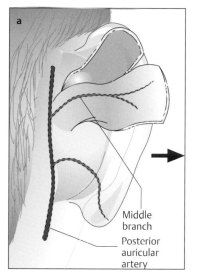

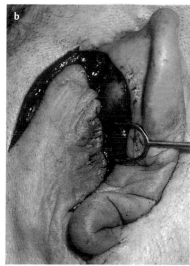

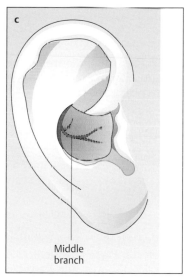

Middle
branch

Posterior
auricular
artery

Middle
branch

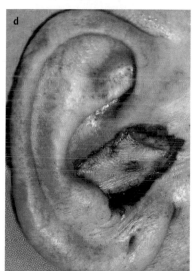

◄ **Fig. 10.6a–g   Coverage of a full-thickness conchal defect using a two-layer island flap based on a dermal pedicle.**

a Defect in the concha, antihelix. Advancement flap for tragal repair (d).

b Retro- and postauricular island flap, based on a dermal pedicle; D = defect in concha and antihelix.

c, d The island flap is brought out anteriorly onto the defect and sutured (anterior surface).

e, f Suture of the secondary defect (posterior surface); there is considerable reduction of the sulcus: the postauricular surface was sutured onto the defect on the mastoid surface (see **Fig. 10.80**, p. 184).

g Result after 2 years.

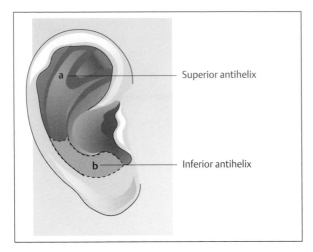
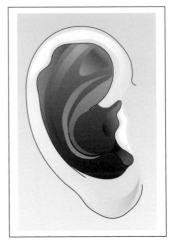

Fig. 10.8a, b   Antihelical defects (see Fig. 10.1).
(Transposition flap: see **Figs. 10.4** and **10.11**; island flap: see **Fig. 10.6**; U-shaped advancement flap: see **Fig. 10.12**).
a Superior antihelix.
b Inferior antihelix.

Fig. 10.9   Combined central defects.
Flaps as used for conchal and antihelical defects can be used (see **Figs. 10.1, 10.6, 10.14**).

Park and Chung (1989) have pointed out that the direction of blood flow is reversed after the flap is inset. The donor site is covered with a split-thickness or full-thickness skin graft.

Defects of the Antihelix and Combined Central Defects (Figs. 10.8 and 10.9)

In particular, posterior transposition flaps and island flaps based posteriorly on a dermal pedicle or on the posterior auricular artery can be used (see **Figs. 10.4–10.6**) for the reconstruction of defects in the antihelical region (**Fig. 10.8a, b**) or for more extensive central defects (combined central defects; **Fig. 10.9**), as previously described (see pp. 138, 139).

Converse and Brent's (1977) Three-stage Reconstruction of Full-Thickness Defects of the Antihelix (Fig. 10.10)
The flap can be extended onto the postauricular skin to cover large defects of the concha and antihelix (Jackson 1985b; see **Fig. 10.6**).

Superiorly or Inferiorly Based Transposition Flap (Fig. 10.11; see also Fig. 10.4)

Stage I:
A large, superiorly based, retroauricular transposition flap is raised, which, depending on the size of the defect, can be extended to the neck (**Fig. 10.11a**). The flap is de-epithelialized at the site where it is brought through, and then inset (**Fig. 10.11c**). Behind

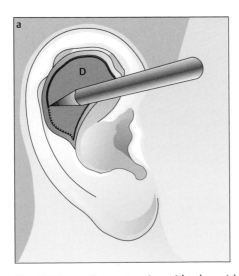

Fig. 10.10a–e   Reconstruction with a large island flap (Converse and Brent 1977).
Stage I:
a The defect (D) is outlined on the mastoid skin.

b Incision around the flap, with minimal mobilization of the margins of the flap and the mastoid skin (the flap remains pedicled to the mastoid). The mastoid skin is sutured to the skin of the posterior auricular defect.

Fig. 10.10c–g   ▶

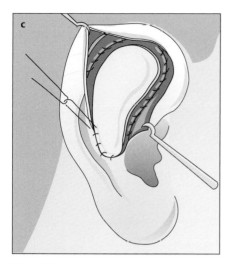
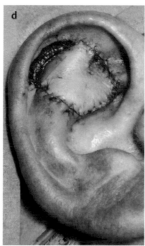
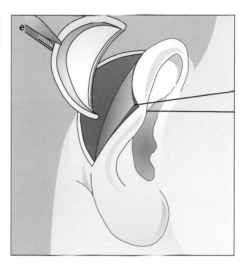

Fig. 10.10c–e
c, d The island flap is sutured to the margins of the anterior defect (see **Fig. 10.4e**).
Stage II:
Elevation after 3 weeks and insertion of a framework.
e Conchal cartilage from the ipsi- or contralateral side or from costal cartilage.

Stage III:
After a further 3–4 weeks, the framework, together with its fibrous coating, is elevated and the defect is covered with a split-thickness or full-thickness skin graft (see **Fig. 4.48d–f,** p. 164).

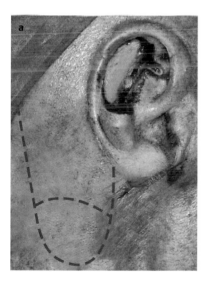
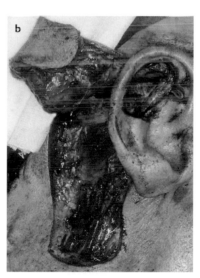
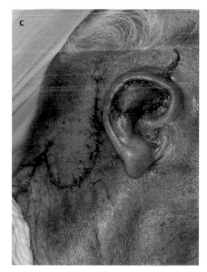
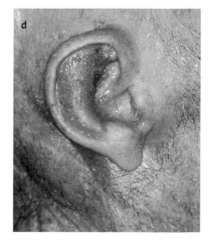

Fig. 10.11a–d   Single-stage coverage of a large central defect using a superiorly based transposition flap.
a, b The superiorly based transposition flap is outlined and de-epithelialized at the site that will come to lie beneath the tunnel when passed anteriorly.
c The flap has been set into the defect (see **Fig. 10.4**), the secondary defect is closed by a rotation flap).
d Result.

the ear, the flap may also be used to cover the postauricular defect (Weerda 1994b; see **Fig. 10.4**).

Stage II:

The flap pedicle can be divided after 3 weeks. The remnants of the pedicle are thinned out and incorporated into the mastoid surface, and the wound is closed in two layers. Full-thickness defects that are not too large can be covered on their postauricular

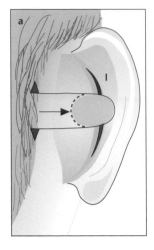

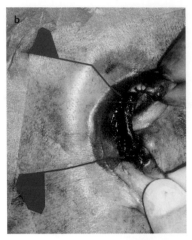

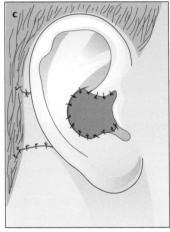

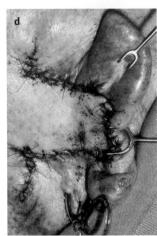

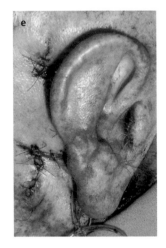

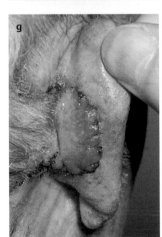

Fig. 10.12a–g U-shaped advancement flap as described by **Gingrass and Pickrell** (1968; see also **Figs. 10.57 and 10.59**).
a–c Defect in the concha, U-shaped advancement flap to be drawn anteriorly to close the defect and Burow's triangles; l = tunnel.
d, e Coverage of the conchal defect.
f Reconstruction of the fossa region and superior antihelical region.
g Postauricular region after reconstruction.

surface with a split-thickness or full-thickness skin graft. Double rotation (see also **Fig. 10.88** or transposition–rotation flaps (see also **Figs. 10.61, 10.86** and **10.87**) can be used for the single-stage resurfacing of particularly large central defects (see also pp. 137–141).

U-shaped Advancement Flap of Gingrass and Pickrell (1968) (Fig. 10.12)

After ~3 weeks, the pedicle is divided and the postauricular wound closed. This flap is also suitable for defects in the region of the posterior auditory canal and the antitragus.

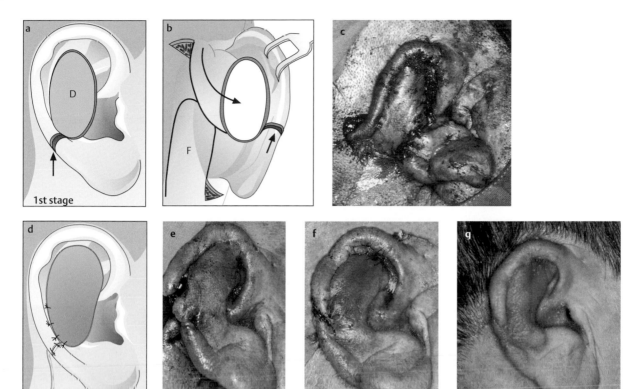

Fig 10.13a–g   Temporary repositioning of the helix for a large two-layer or full-thickness auricular defect (Weerda 1984; Weerda and Siegert 1999a).

Stage I:

a   Defect (D) and helix divided inferiorly above the earlobe (arrow).

b   Inferiorly based transposition flap (F) to cover the anterior surface, rotation flap to cover the posterior surface (a thick split-thickness skin graft may also be used here).

c   The flaps have been inset.

Stage II:

d–f   Separation of the transposition flap and replacement of the helix after ~3 weeks.

g   Appearance after healing.

Weerda's Reconstruction with a Transposition Flap and Temporary Repositioning of the Helix
(Fig. 10.13; Weerda 1984)

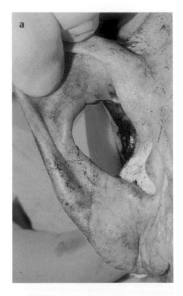
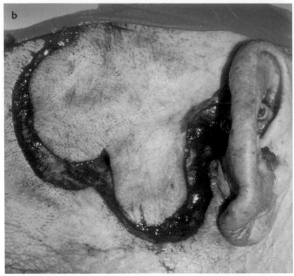
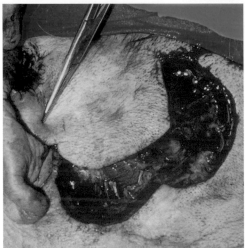
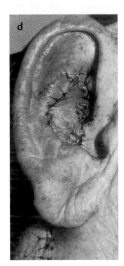
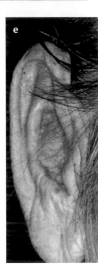
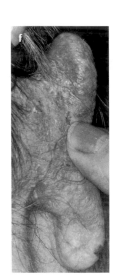

Fig. 10.14a–f   Reconstruction of large, full-thickness defects with a bilobed flap (transposition–rotation flap; Weerda and Münker 1981; Weerda 2001).

a Defect.

b Incision of the non-hair-bearing transposition flap (reconstruction flap 1) and hair-bearing rotation flap (transport flap 2).

c, d The flaps are inset after de-epithelialization beneath the helix, the cartilaginous strut is inserted, and the primary and secondary defects are closed.

e Result, anterior aspect; 1 = transposition (reconstruction) flap.

f Posterior aspect.

Weerda's Bilobed Flap as a Transposition–Rotation Flap

(**Fig. 10.14**; Weerda and Münker 1981)

As will later be described in detail, a bilobed flap (**Fig. 10.14b, c**) can also be used for larger, full-thickness antihelix–conchal defects (**Fig. 10.14a**). The flap is de-epithelialized below the helix and supported with cartilage (**Fig. 10.14d**).

Weerda's Scaphal Reconstruction with a U-shaped Advancement Flap

(**Fig. 10.15**)

Preauricular Flaps

Many authors use preauricular flaps for smaller central defects.

Tebbetts' (1982) Superiorly Based, Preauricular Flap for the Triangular Fossa

(**Fig. 10.16**)

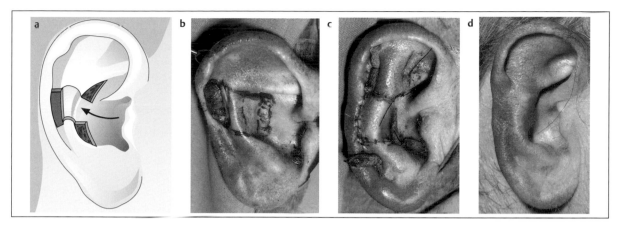

Fig. 10.15a–d   Weerda's technique of scaphal reconstruction using a U-shaped advancement flap from the concha.

a, b Defect in the scapha, skin incision over the antihelix, Burow's triangles in the concha, cartilage strut from the concha.

c The defect is closed by U-shaped advancement; the flap is adapted with mattress sutures (5-0 monofilament, P3 or PS 3 needle) tied over small cotton bolsters.

d Result.

Fig. 10.16a–c Technique by Tebbetts (1982) for coverage of the triangular fossa using a superiorly based preauricular flap.

a, b Elevation of the flap and deepithelialization at the site that will come to lie beneath the tunnel.

c The flap has been inset.

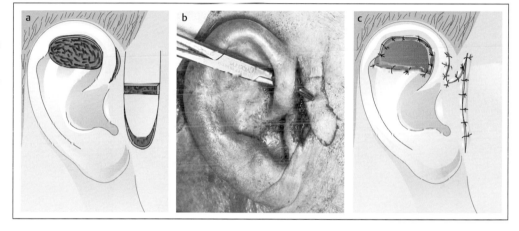

Fig. 10.17a–e Reconstruction of the helical crus (Weerda 1999a, 2004; 2007).

a, b Outline of the flap. Elevation of the flap adjacent to the helical stump.

c Transposition of the flap.

d, e Closure of the defects.

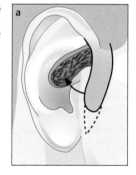
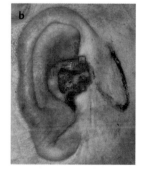
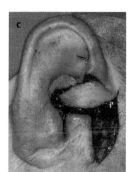

Mellette's (1991) Preauricular Flap Based Superiorly on the Helical Crus
(Fig. 10.17)

This technique is also suitable for reconstruction of the helical crus. The flap is pedicled on the ascending limb of the helical crus and can be used to cover defects in the region of the concha and the entrance to the auditory canal. Sometimes, improvements can be made to the helical crus in a second stage (Weerda and Siegert 1999a, 2001).

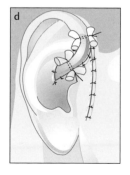
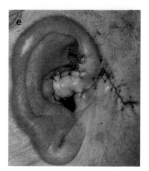

Subcutaneous Pedicle Flap of Barron and Emmett (1965) (Fig. 10.18)

Inferiorly Based Preauricular Flap
(Fig. 10.19)

An inferiorly based preauricular flap can be used for covering the intertragic notch and the inferior concha, for the posterior surface of the tragus and the lateral auditory canal.

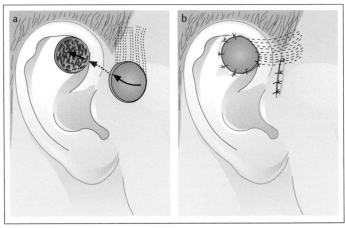

Fig. 10.18a, b   Subcutaneous island pedicle flap, as described by Barron and Emmett (1965).
a Elevation of the flap and development of a tunnel.
b Inset and closure of the secondary defect (Weerda).

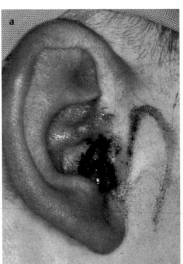
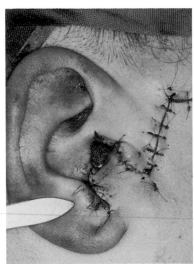
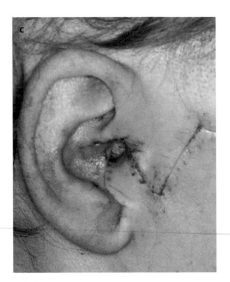
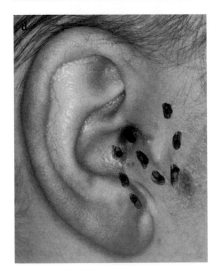
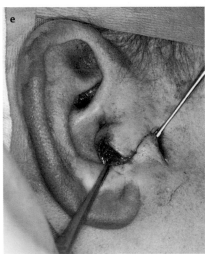

Fig. 10.19a–g   Reconstruction of the intertragic notch.
Stage I:
a–c Reconstruction of the intertragic notch, lower concha, and lateral auditory canal, using an inferiorly based transposition flap.
Stage II:
d, e After the notch has been widened in this way, it is subsequently reduced with the use of a Z-plasty.

Fig. 10.19f–g   ▶

Fig. 10.19f–g
f Result.
g Tragus reconstruction with a superiorly
  based pretragal flap.

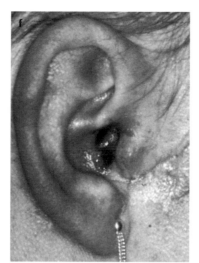
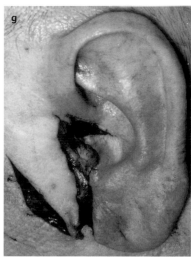

Fig. 10.20 Peripheral defects: helical defects
(see **Fig. 5.41**).

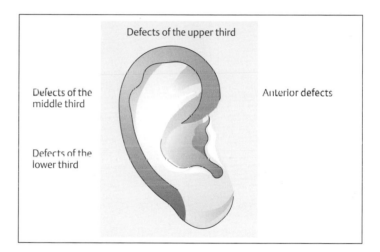

Defects of the upper third

Defects of the
middle third

Anterior defects

Defects of the
lower third

Peripheral Defects
(**Fig. 10.20**)

Peripheral defects refer in particular to defects
located on the helix (**Fig. 10.20**; see **Fig. 10.1**).

Helix Reconstruction with Auricular Reduction

The techniques described for reduction of the auricle
during correction of macrotia are very well suited for
treating defects of the helix secondary to tumor excision or trauma (see, for example, Di Martino 1856, as
cited in Joseph 1931; Trendelenburg 1886, as cited in
Joseph 1931; Cocheril 1894, as cited in Tanzer et al.
1977; Joseph 1896, 1931. If the age and general condition of the patient allow it, some of these operations can be performed under local anesthesia, on an
outpatient basis.

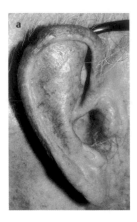
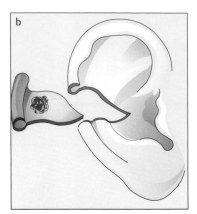
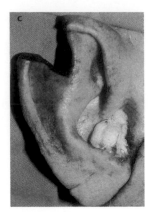
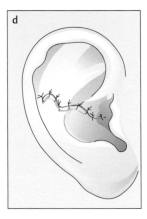
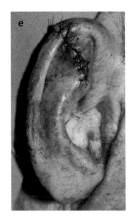
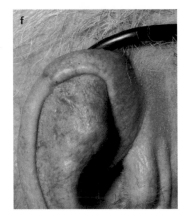

Fig. 10.21a–f Wedge-shaped excision without Burow's triangles (for defect sizes up to ~1 cm).
a Helical tumor.
b, c Wedge-shaped excision.
d, e Closure.
f Result.

Recommended Defect Reconstruction

Wedge excisions and reconstruction with advancement of the helix can be recommended.

Simple Wedge Excisions
(**Fig. 10.21**)
For small helical lesions or small defects, a simple extension of the wound in the form of a wedge excision is enough to achieve an adequately pleasing esthetic result (see **Fig. 5.41**; p. 55).

Wedge Excision and Burow's Triangles
(**Fig. 10.22a–j**)
Because irregularities in form and contour can result from simple wedge excision, Trendelenburg (1886, as cited in Joseph 1931) recommended the removal of Burow's triangles. This procedure has since been modified in many ways (see for example Trendelenburg 1886, as cited in Joseph 1931; Joseph 1896; Goldstein 1908; Lexer 1933). Whenever possible, we place the Burow's triangles in the scapha (**Fig. 10.22e**) or along the border between the concha and its transition to the antihelix (**Fig. 10.22a**; Converse and Brent 1977).

Gersuny's (1903) Technique of Defect Closure by Transposition of the Helix
(**Fig. 10.23**)
Gersuny performed a full-thickness crescent-shaped excision in the scapha of a female patient who had sustained a helical lesion, and transposed the helix into the resultant defect (**Fig. 10.23a, b**). This elegant method has been modified in several different ways (see **Figs. 10.24, 10.29, 10.30**).

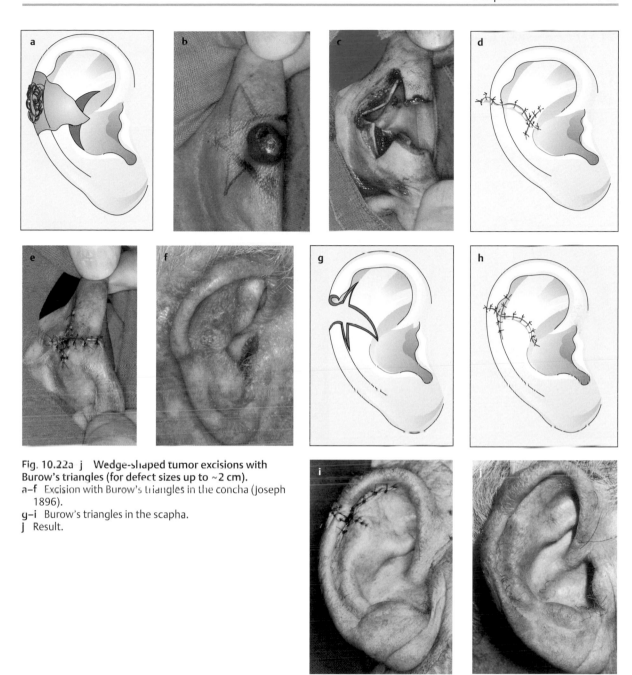

Fig. 10.22a–j   Wedge-shaped tumor excisions with Burow's triangles (for defect sizes up to ~2 cm).
a–f Excision with Burow's triangles in the concha (Joseph 1896).
g–i Burow's triangles in the scapha.
j Result.

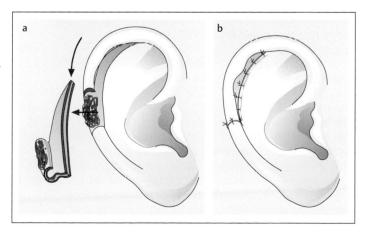

Fig. 10.23a, b   Gersuny's (1903) technique for full-thickness tumor excision.
a Tumor excision and full-thickness, crescent-shaped upper scaphal excision.
b Closure of the defect by rotating the helix downward (see **Figs. 10.23, 10.28, 10.29**).

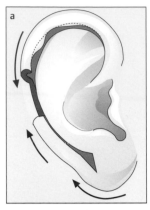
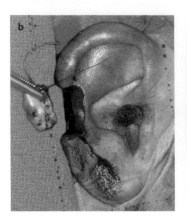
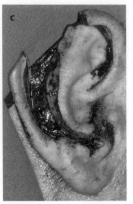
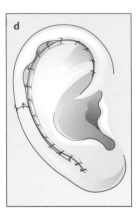

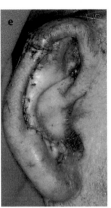
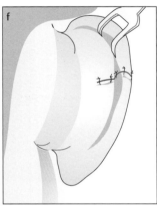
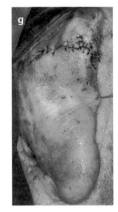
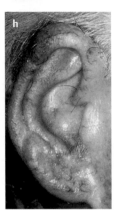

Fig. 10.24a–h   Excision of small defects in the helical region and closure using Gersuny's technique (1903), modified after Antia and Buch (1967), Antia (1974), and Weerda and Zöllner (1986).

a, b Tumor excision and two-layer, crescent-shaped excision in the scapha with a Burow's triangle in the earlobe.

c–e Mobilization of the entire helix on the postauricular skin and closure of the wounds.

f, g Excision of a dog ear on the postauricular surface and suture.

h Result.

Modification of the Gersuny Technique by Weerda and Zöllner (1986) (Fig. 10.24)

Similar to Antia and Buch (1967) and Antia (1974), and in contrast to Gersuny (1903; see **Fig. 10.23**), we made only a two-layer, crescent-shaped excision in the scapha after excision of the tumor and dissected the skin on the posterior auricular surface (**Fig. 10.24b, d, e**).

Antia and Buch's Modification with Mobilization of the Helical Crus

(**Fig. 10.25**; Antia and Buch 1967, Antia 1974)

In a modification for larger defects, the helical crus was additionally incised (it remains pedicled posteriorly and superiorly).

Lexer's (1933) Modification

(Fig. 10.26)

This modification is a full-thickness crescent-shaped excision from the scaphal and antihelical margin after excision of the tumor. The postauricular skin is excised slightly higher and then elevated. The defects are slid into each other, and the auricle is reduced by closing cartilage and skin (**Fig. 10.26b**; Ginestet et al. 1967).

Argamaso and Lewin's (1968) Technique of Ear Reduction and Defect Reconstruction

(Fig. 10.27)

For smaller defects, a Z-plasty is performed by transposing the inferior portion into the superior segment (**Fig. 10.27c**) in the form of a chondrocutaneous flap (**Fig. 10.27a, b**).

Meyer and Sieber's (1973) Modification of the Technique

(Fig. 10.28)

The concha or the preauricular defect can be treated together with tumors of the ascending helix (**Fig. 10.28a–d**; Argamaso 1989).

Tenta and Keyes' (1981) Excision of the Triangular Fossa with Reduction of the Auricle

(Fig. 10.29)

After full-thickness excision (**Fig. 10.29a**), the helix is used to cover the defect (**Fig. 10.29c**), as with Gersuny's technique (1903); **Fig. 10.29b**; see also **Figs. 10.30** and **10.42**).

Fig. 10.25a–d Helix reconstruction of a small defect (Antia and Buch 1967; Antia 1974).
a Debridement of the wound margins.
b Incisions around the helical crus and dissection of the postauricular skin pedicled on the entire helix extending from the scapha; incision within the scapha down to the earlobe, where a small Burow's triangle is excised.
c, d Closure of all defects with transposition of the helical crus and reduction of the auricle (see **Fig. 10.25**).

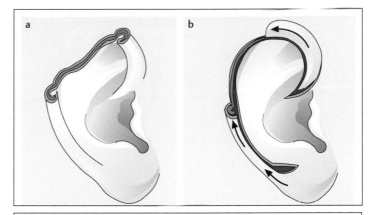

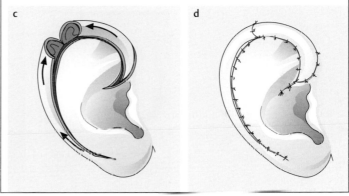

Fig. 10.26a, b Lexer's method for reconstruction of a helical defect with scaphal excisions (Lexer 1933; Ginestet et al. 1967).

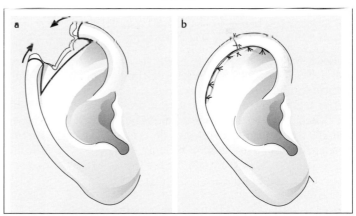

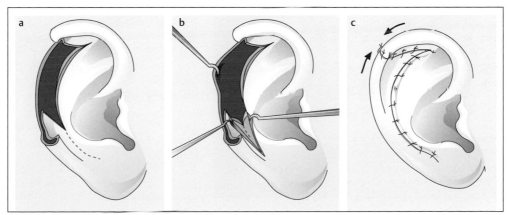

Fig. 10.27a–c Ear reduction (defect reconstruction), using the technique of Argamaso and Lewin (1968).
a Tumor excision, crescent-shaped, two-layer excision from the scapha (antihelix).
b Elevation of the postauricular skin and excision of the cartilage toward the earlobe.
c Closure of all defects; excision of a dog ear from the earlobe and the postauricular skin.

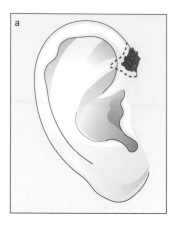
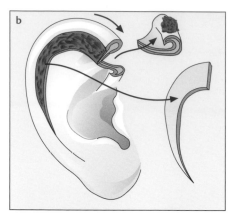
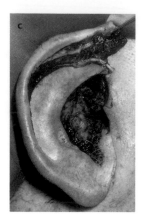

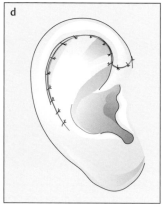
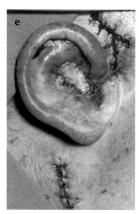
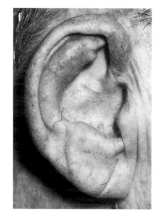

Fig. 10.28a–f Wedge excision of an anterior tumor of the helix and closure with auricular reduction, as described by Meyer and Sieber (1973).
a Tumor excision.
b, c Crescent-shaped, two-layer excision from the scapha. (Excision of an additional tumor of the concha).
d Closure.
e Closure, full-thickness skin graft covers the defect of the concha.
f Result (see **Figs. 10.24** and **10.25**).

Critique:
Here too, techniques that preserve the size of the auricle should usually take preference.

The techniques of reconstruction described here for conchal defects and defects of the antihelix can also be used for larger **combined defects of the concha and antihelix** (see also p. 137ff.).

Weerda and Zöllner's (1986) Technique for Defects of the Helical Crus and Preauricular Region
(**Fig. 10.30**; Weerda and Zöllner 1986; Weerda 1988d; see also **Fig. 10.43**)
The entire helix can be rotated anteriorly to treat tumors in the region of the anterior ascending helix, the helical crus, and the preauricular region, with the

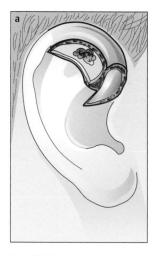
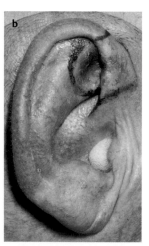
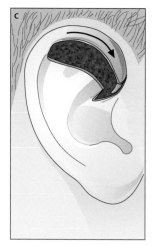
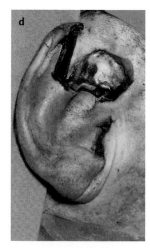

Fig. 10.29a–g Tumor excision in the triangular fossa with reduction of the auricle, as described by Tenta and Keyes (1981; see Figs. 10.30 and 10.42).
a, b Excision of a tumor in the triangular fossa.

c, d Excision of the skin behind the tumor, including part of the helical crus.

Fig. 10.29e–g ▶

Fig. 10.29e–g
e, f Closure of all defects.
g Result 1 year after reconstruction.

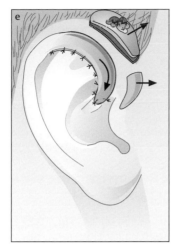
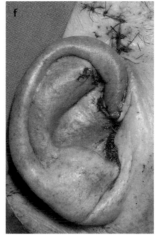
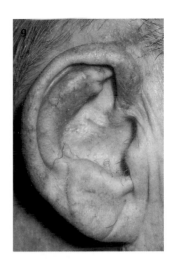

Fig. 10.30a–f Defect of the preauricular region and in the region of the helical crus and anterior helix.

a, b Elevation of a preauricular Dufourmentel flap and anterior transposition of the helix as a Gersuny plasty (see **Fig. 3.26**).
c–e Closure of all defects.
f Result (see also **Fig. 10.28**).

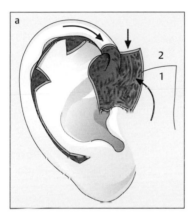
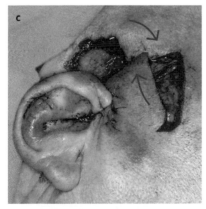
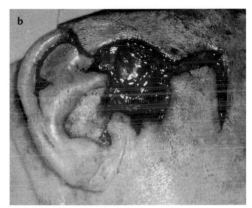
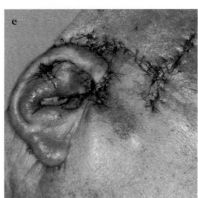
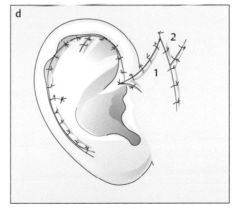
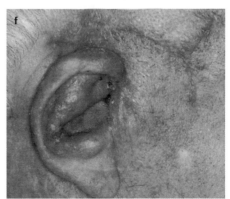

preauricular defect subsequently being covered by a Dufourmentel rhomboid flap (see also p. 26).

Nonrecommended Methods of Defect Reconstruction

Pegram and Peterson's (1956) Reconstruction with a Free Full-Thickness Composite Graft from the Contralateral Ear
(Pegram and Peterson 1956; see also the section "Middle third of the auricle", p. 168).

Even Körte (1905) and Lexer (1910) had previously used composite grafts for reconstruction of the ear. Similar techniques to reconstruct partial defects are described by Day (1921), Melchior-Breslau (1928 as cited in Joseph 1931), Wachsberger (1947), Pegram and Peterson (1956), Nagel (1972), Brent (1975), and Converse and Brent (1977). The margins of the defect are freshened, or the tumor excised; a wedge-shaped, full-thickness composite graft of half the defect size is removed from the contralateral ear and inset into the defect; the cartilage is adapted with a 5-0 braided suture; and the skin is closed with a 6-0 or 7-0 mono-filament suture. The wedge defect of the contralateral side is closed in a similar fashion.

Critique:
These techniques may be suitable, if at all, for smaller defects (see **Fig. 3.16**) because adequate nutrition of larger, freely transplanted composite grafts cannot be guaranteed. We see a high rate of graft loss, especially when this technique is performed by less experienced surgeons (see Weerda 2007, pp. 32–40, 57).

Helix Reconstruction without Auricular Reduction

Since the defects (see **Fig. 10.21**) frequently involve more than one region, reference will be made in the text and in the figure legends to similar reconstructions in other chapters.

Anterior Defects: Helical Crus and Ascending Helix (**Figs. 10.31** and **10.32**)

The ascending helix, as well as the helical crus, can be reconstructed with a small U-shaped advancement flap (**Fig. 10.31**), a rotation flap (**Fig. 10.32a, b**), or a preauricular, superiorly or inferiorly based transposition flap (**Fig. 10.32**).

Superior and Middle Thirds of the Helix

Superiorly Based Postauricular Transposition Flap
(**Fig. 10.33**; Weerda and Siegert 1999a; Weerda 2007)
A superiorly based posterior flap is raised in the sulcus, patterned from a template made from aluminum foil (Pennisi et al. 1965; Tebbetts 1982; Mellette 1991; Weerda and Siegert 1999a; Weerda 2001) and inserted over a cartilaginous support (**Fig. 10.33a–f**). After resection of the pedicle in a second stage, we can obtain a good result (**Fig. 10.33d, g, h**).

Preauricular Transposition Flap
(**Fig. 10.34a–c**)
As with the posterior flap, a patterned preauricular flap is used to reconstruct the superior helix.

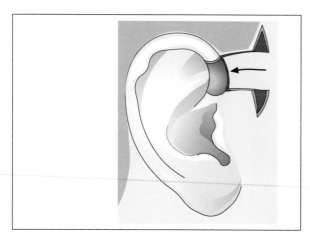

Fig. 10.31   U-shaped advancement flap to cover a defect of the ascending helix.

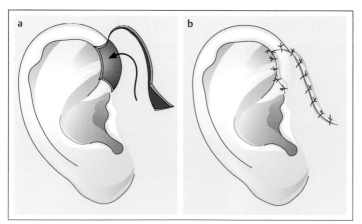

Fig. 10.32a, b   Coverage of the ascending helix with an inferiorly based rotation flap.

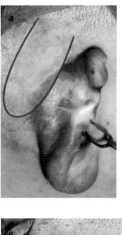
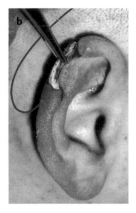
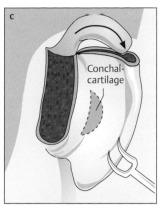
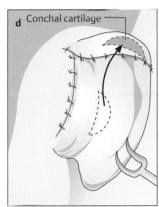

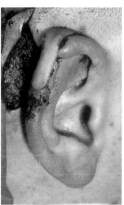
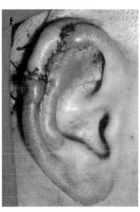
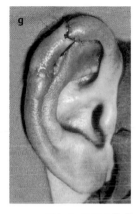
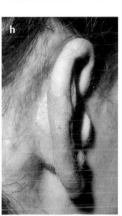

Fig. 10.33a–h Reconstruction of the superior helix with a posterosuperiorly based transposition flap.
Stage I:
a, b The superiorly based transposition flap is marked and the helix supported by a conchal cartilage strut.
c–f The flap is brought into position.

Stage II:
g After at least 3 weeks, the base of the flap is inset in a fish mouth manner (see **Figs. 10.38** and **10.39**).
h Result after 2 years.

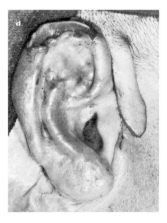
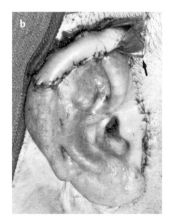
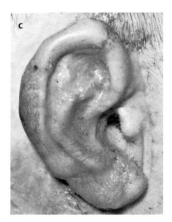

Fig. 10.34a–c Reconstruction of the superior helix with a preauricular flap secondary to necrosis of this region after total auricular reconstruction following an avulsion injury.
a Total reconstruction, necrosis of the superior helix: the superior helix has been reconstructed with cartilage from the contralateral concha and the preauricular tubed flap has been incised (it must be of adequate length; see **Figs. 10.38–10.40**).
b The flap is brought into position and attached in a fish-mouth fashion; the non-epithelialized end of the flap is protected with a small silicone plate (arrow).
c Result after the flap pedicle is inset, ~3 weeks later.

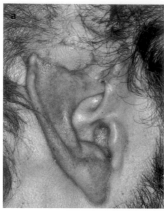
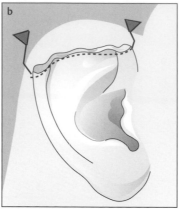
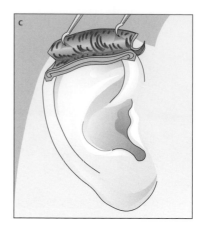
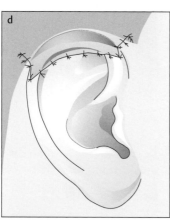
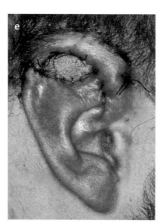
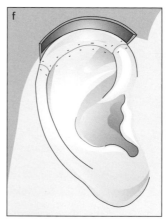
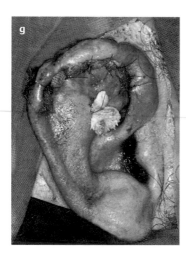
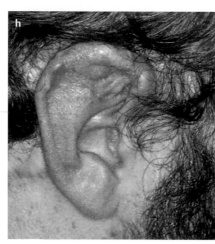

Fig. 10.35a–h Coverage of the superior, middle, and inferior helix with a broad-based superiorly pedicled retroauricular flap, as described by Smith (1917).

a Resorption of the cartilage after insertion of the denuded cartilage placed into a cutaneous pocket secondary to an avulsion injury.

Stage I:
b The flap is outlined.
c Incision and dissection.
d, e Inset with cartilage strut (pink) in a fish-mouth manner onto the helix (see **Fig. 10.38d**).

Stage II:
f, g After ~3 weeks, separation from the mastoid skin and posterior inset, coverage of the mastoid defect with thick split skin (Nagata 1994a–d).
h Result after 4 months.

Retroauricular Flap of Smith (1917)
(**Fig. 10.35a–h**)

The upper (middle) third of the auricular helix is reconstructed with a broad-based, superiorly pedicled retroauricular flap (see **Fig. 10.57**).

Tube-Pedicled Flap
(**Fig. 10.36**)
Pre-, post-, and retroauricular tube-pedicled flaps can be employed for all regions of the helix. Tube-

pedicled flaps of the neck (**Fig. 10.36a**; Pierce 1925; Hamblen-Thomas 1938; McNichol 1950; Converse 1958; Cosman and Crikelair 1966; Pitanguy and Flemming 1976; Davis 1987) can usually no longer be recommended, given that they produce conspicuous hypertrophic scars in the neck region (**Fig. 10.36b**). "Migrating" flaps of the supraclavicular region are better.

Defects of the upper, middle, or lower third of the helix can be reconstructed with a tunneled (bipedicle) or tubed pedicle flap that is raised in the sulcus

Fig. 10.36a, b Tube-pedicled flap from the neck, as described by McNichol (1950): **a technique no longer used**.
a Reconstruction of the helix with a tube-pedicled flap from the neck.
b Unsightly scar on the neck after a reconstruction by the author in the early 1970s.

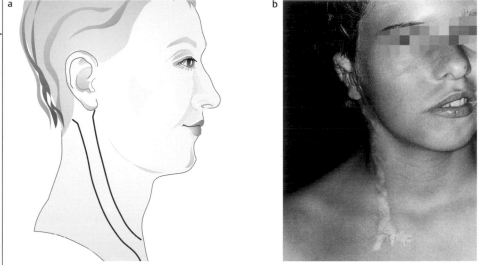

Fig. 10.37a–d Reconstruction of a longer helical defect with a tubed bipedicle, tunneled flap in three stages (see text; Steffanoff 1948; Weerda and Siegert 1999a; Weerda 2001).
Stage I:
a Cartilage harvested from the concha, access via the donor defect of the tunneled flap in the sulcus.
b After suturing in the cartilage strut, the wound margins are freshened before the tunneled flap is inset onto the defect.
Stage II:
c Three weeks after reconstruction, the flaps are separated and inset onto the helical defect at an acute angle. The remains of the tunneled flap are incorporated into the mastoid surface (see **Figs. 10.38** and **10.39**).
d Result at the end of the second stage.

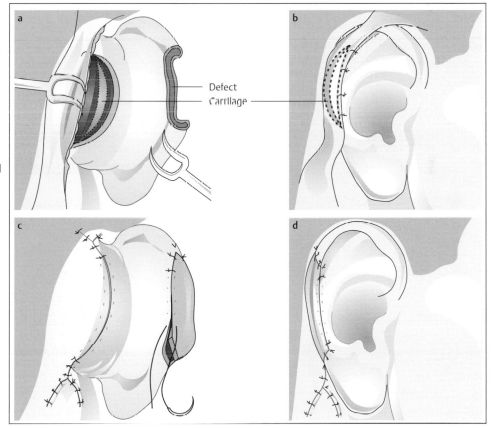

Defect
Cartilage

and initially based superiorly and inferiorly (see **Fig. 10.37;** Streit 1914; Troha et al. 1990; Dujon and Bowditch 1995).

Recommended Techniques for Defect Reconstruction

Tube-Pedicled Flap for the Superior Helix
(**Fig. 10.37;** see also, **Fig. 10.34**)
The tube-pedicled flap for the superior helix can also be used as a tubed bipedicle (tunneled) flap (see also **Fig. 10.38**).

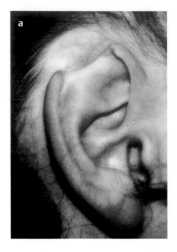

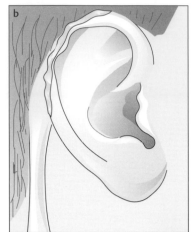

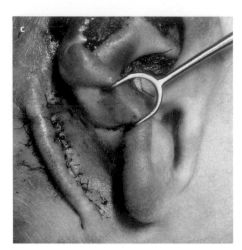

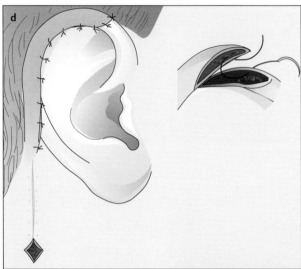

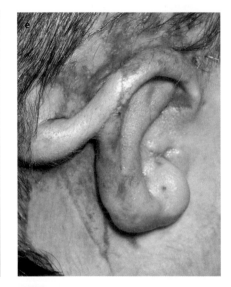

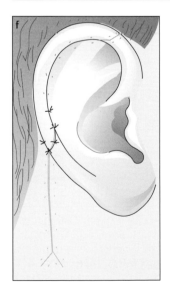

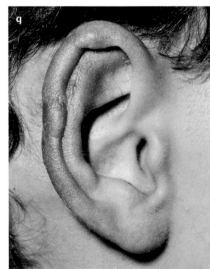

Fig. 10.38a–g Reconstruction of the helix with a tubed bipedicle flap in three stages, as described by Steffanoff (1948).

a Defect.

Stage I:

b, c The flap is incised and rolled up; if insufficient skin is available, the flap is enclosed in a silicone foil (0.2 mm thick).

Stage II:

d, e After 3 weeks; separation of the flap base inferiorly and incorporation into the defect in a fish-mouth manner. If necessary, a cartilage strut may be incorporated (see **Fig. 10.33**).

Stage III:

f After ~3 further weeks, incorporation of the remaining flap.

g Result.

Tubed Bipedicle Flap for Defects of the Superior and Middle Thirds
(Figs. 10.38 and 10.39)

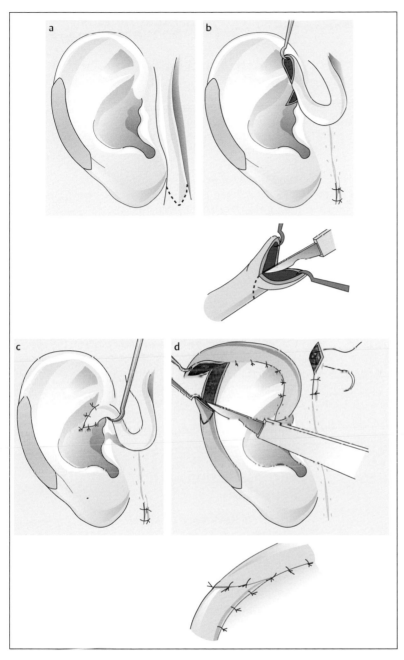

Fig. 10.39a–d Reconstruction of the entire helix with a tubed bipedicle flap, modified from the technique of Converse and Brent (1977).
Stage I:
a The posterior helix is reconstructed (see **Fig. 10.37**); a preauricular tubed bipedicle flap can be raised concurrently.
Stage II:
b, c Incorporation of the flap as a helical crus.
Stage III:
d After 3 weeks at the earliest, incorporation of the flap (see **Fig. 10.38d**) into the helix (for a similar technique of flap elevation in two stages, see **Fig. 10.34a, b**).

Three-stage Reconstruction of a Defect of the Middle Third with a Tube-Pedicled Flap

(**Fig. 10.39**; Steffanoff 1948; Converse and Brent 1977; Weerda and Siegert 1999a; Weerda 2001)

Unlike reconstruction with a tunneled flap (see **Fig. 10.37a**), the tube-pedicled flap is first raised and rolled into a tube (**Fig. 10.39b, c**). If there is not sufficient skin for closure, we use split skin for coverage, or wrap the exposed tube-pedicled flap with silicone foil (see also **Fig. 10.33b**).

Converse and Brent's (1977) Reconstruction with a Preauricular Tube-Pedicled Flap

(**Fig. 10.39**)

Similar to the flap previously described, a preauricular tube-pedicled flap can be raised for defects of the anterior and superior helix as well as for the helical crus (Berson 1948; Converse 1958; Converse and Brent 1977).

Reconstruction with a Superiorly Based Posterior Flap
(see **Fig. 10.33b**)

Inferior Helix

These reconstructions are similar to those of the superior and middle thirds of the helix; further reconstructions are discussed under "Lower partial reconstructions" (see p. 174).

Partial Reconstruction of the Auricle

Although a number of reconstructions are similar or identical for the upper and middle thirds of the auricle, and in part also for the lower auricle, as well as for subtotal and total defects, a distinction will be made between the upper, middle, and lower auricle, to make it easier for the surgeon to select options for reconstructions in particularly problematic cases. When necessary, reference is made to reconstructive procedures found in other chapters of this book.

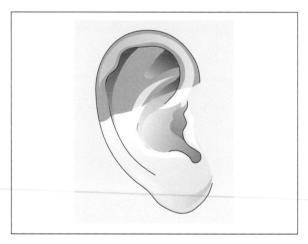

Fig. 10.40   Superior third of the auricle.

Upper-Third Auricular Defects (Fig. 10.40)

Reconstruction with Auricular Reduction

Reconstructions of the auricle with reduction of the ear are only appropriate in rare cases, for example, for auricular lesions in elderly patients, or for very large ears.

Wedge Excisions
(**Fig. 10.41**; see Helix Reconstruction with Auricular Reduction, **Figs. 10.21** and **10.22**).

Helical Sliding Flap of Antia and Buch (1967) (Figs. 10.42 and 10.43)
This technique lends itself for reconstructions with auricular reduction (see **Fig. 10.25**) as a modification of Gersuny's technique (1903; see **Figs. 10.23** and **10.24**).

Full-thickness Composite Grafts of the Contralateral Ear, as Described by Pegram and Peterson (1956)
This technique involves replacement of wedge-shaped defects with a full-thickness composite graft taken from the contralateral ear.

Critique:
There is a danger of losing the composite graft and deforming the other ear.

Reconstruction without Auricular Reduction

Historical Review

Although there are reports of attempts at auricular reconstruction, dating back to ancient and medieval times (Goedecke 1995), it was not until Tagliacozzi in 1597, Dieffenbach in 1845 and von Szymanowski in 1870 that reconstructive techniques were first

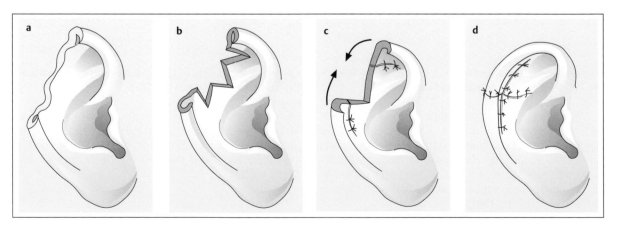

Fig. 10.41a–d   Reconstruction by auricular reduction with wedge resection and Burow's triangles (see also **Fig. 10.22**).
a Defect.
b Burow's triangles in the scapha.
c, d Closure of the defects (see **Fig. 10.23**).

Fig. 10.42a, b   Helical sliding flap and Dufourmentel rhomboid flap (see also **Figs. 3.24; 10.28–10.30**).
a Preauricular defect and defect of the superoanterior auricle.
b Coverage with a helical sliding flap and a rhomboid flap, with considerable reduction of the auricle (see **Figs. 10.28** and **10.29**).

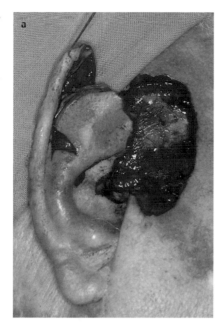
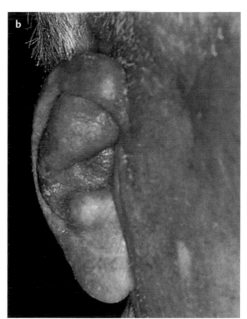

Fig. 10.43   Coverage of a superior defect with a posterior and anterior helical sliding flap (Gersuny technique), modified from the technique of Antia and Buch (1967). Two-layer incision in the scapha, continued around the helical crus with a Burow's triangle in the earlobe, and postauricular skin mobilization (explained in more detail in **Fig. 10.25**).

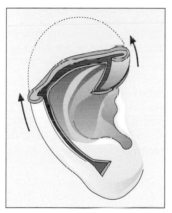

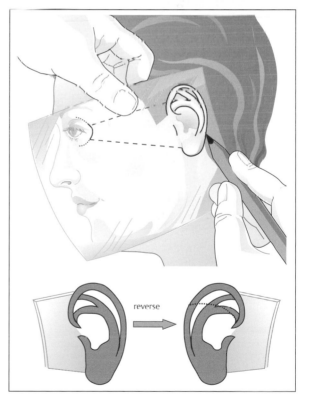

described; however, these almost certainly resulted in very contracted reconstructions.

Schmieden (1908) was the first to use autologous cartilage; he reconstructed part of the ear by suturing a square-shaped, pedicled flap from the ipsilateral arm to the margin of the defect. However, the results of such distant flaps are still poor in terms of color and texture match (Mündnich 1962; Toplak 1986; Goedecke 1995).

It was Gillies (1920) who first used a carved autologous costal cartilage framework for reconstruction.

Fig. 10.44   A template based on the healthy ear, made from transparent material (e. g. X-ray film). Place the film on the orbital margin, outline the auricle, and excise the scapha, the triangular fossa, and the concha (a template of the auricle alone will suffice for partial defects). The size of the defect is marked out on the template (dotted line). For template, see **Fig. 10.90**.

reverse

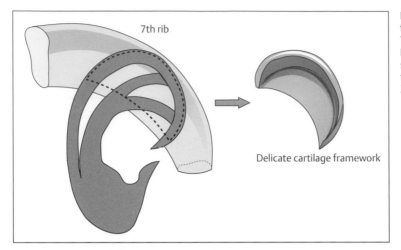

7th rib

Delicate cartilage framework

Fig. 10.45 Carving of a delicate cartilage framework patterned from a template (6th, 7th, or 8th rib). The template is reversed (see **Fig. 10.44**). The framework is 2 to 3 mm smaller (dotted) than the auricular segment to be reconstructed (see **Fig. 10.47a**; see p. 207ff.).

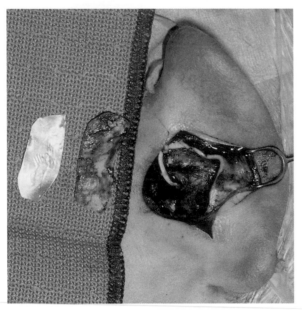

Fig. 10.46 Harvesting the support of the contralateral concha using a template (see **Figs. 10.44, 10.45, 11.3**).

Recommended Reconstruction

Reconstruction with a Costal or Conchal (see **Fig. 10.48**) Cartilage Framework and Skin Pocket

Informed consent:
Detailed and extensive informed consent should be obtained before the reconstruction.

Positioning:
The patient should be supine. The contralateral ear should also always be prepped; any possible harvesting of full-thickness skin and/or conchal cartilage (see **Fig. 10.46**) should also have been included in the informed consent.

Fabrication of a template:
Before the operation, a template of the healthy ear (**Fig. 10.44**) should be fashioned from transparent film

material (unexposed X-ray film or thick transparent foil). The contours are outlined with a marker pen and then cut out and reversed. The reversed template is placed over the injured ear and the margins of the defect are outlined. Usually, the position of the auricle can be determined exactly from the position of the residual ear, which is why the fabrication of a template the size of the healthy auricle with the defect outlined should suffice (see **Fig. 10.96**, p. 199).

Harvesting costal cartilage:
We have the harvesting performed by a second team (see p. 207ff.). **The cartilage framework is carved ~2 to 3 mm smaller than the part of the ear to be reconstructed** (**Fig. 10.45**; see also p. 208).

Fabrication of an auricular framework:
A second template, 2 to 3 mm smaller, is cut to make the framework. The framework, which should be as delicate as possible (see pp. 209, 210) and made entirely of costal cartilage (**Fig. 10.45**), is carved with the aid of appropriate instruments, and kept moist until the pocket over the mastoid surface has been developed and is ready to receive it.

Harvesting conchal cartilage:
(**Fig. 10.46**; see also **Figs. 2.23, 10.33b** and **10.49c**). The cartilage is prepared and excised using an incision in the retroauricular sulcus (**Fig. 10.46**).

Stage I: implantation of the cartilage framework:
The first stage of the operation is shown in **Fig. 10.47a–h** (see also **Fig. 10.57**).

Possible errors:
It is essential to reconstruct the auricular profile, that is, the cartilage framework must be attached to the stump in such a way as to ensure that it does not become folded during insertion into the pocket. The pocket must therefore be made sufficiently large, and the auricular stump may need to be set back and attached to the mastoid surface.

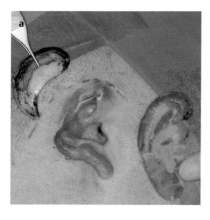
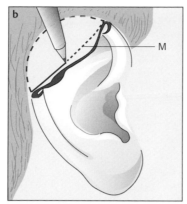
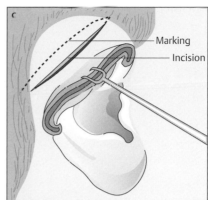
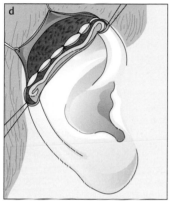
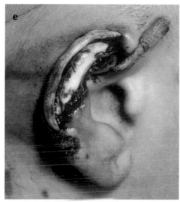
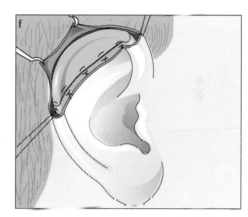
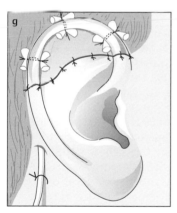
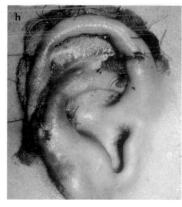

Fig. 10.47a–h   Reconstruction of the upper auricle with a subcutaneous pocket over the mastoid (Converse and Brent 1977). **Stage I:**

a Cartilaginous framework is carved (see **Fig. 10.45**); defect and template.

b The height of the stump (M) is marked on the skin of the mastoid surface, and the superior auricular rim is outlined according to the template (see **Figs. 10.44** and **10.45**).

c The skin is incised ~3 to 4 mm lower than the marked height of the stump.

d A subcutaneous pocket is developed, ~1 cm larger than the height of the superior helical margin, and the postauricular stump skin is sutured to the lower margin of the incision.

e, f The framework (amputated ear denuded of skin or carved cartilage framework, 2 to 3 mm smaller in size) is attached using a 5-0 braided suture and inserted into the pocket.

g, h Closure of the skin wound, vacuum drainage, and mattress sutures without pressure (see text, stage II: **Fig. 10.48**).

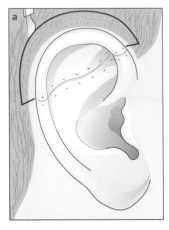

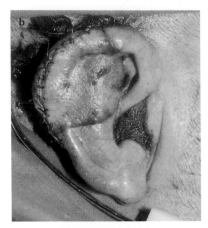

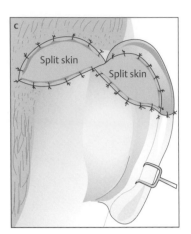

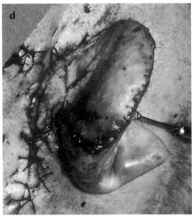

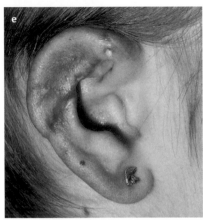

Fig. 10.48a–e   Second stage of the reconstruction of the upper auricle: elevation of the auricle as described by Nagata (1994b) (Fig.10.91; pp 192, 193).

a, b Incision of a full-thickness skin flap pedicled on the helix, above the level of the hair follicles. Fibrous tissue is left behind on the periosteum and on the posterior surface of the auricle.

c, d Coverage of the remaining defects with thick split skin, which is secured with sutures and fibrin glue; dressing (see **Fig. 10.91**).

e Result after 4 weeks (A contouring lateron is necessary; see p. 199).

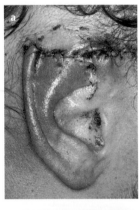

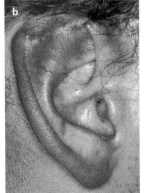

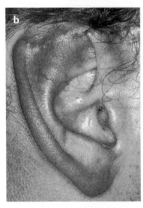

*Stage II: elevation of the auricle (*Fig. 10.48a–e*):*
The auricle is elevated after 6 to 8 weeks (some surgeons do it even later). For this purpose, according to the suggestions made by Nagata (1994; see **Fig. 10.59**), a thick split-thickness skin flap ~8 to 10 mm in width is elevated above the helix and above the hair follicles in the direction of the helix, leaving some fibrous tissue on the helical cartilage (**Fig. 10.48a**). Next, the entire postauricular surface is exposed in such a way that a good layer of fibrous and granulation tissue remains on the framework. The postauricular surface and the mastoid surface are covered with a thick split-thickness or full-thick-

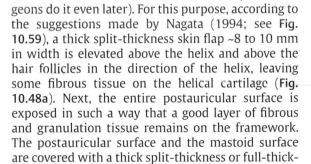

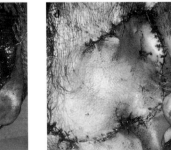

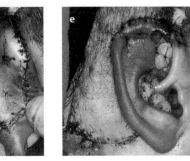

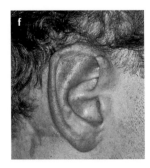

Fig. 10.49   Reconstruction of the upper auricle with a conchal cartilage (c) and a retro-postauricular rotation flap (see Fig. 10.81q).

Stage I:

a, b Resorption of the cartilage after the posttraumatic reconstruction (see **Figs. 10.45** and **10.46**).

c–e Reconstruction with cartilage of the same concha (c) and a retro-postauricular rotation flap (c–e).

f Result.

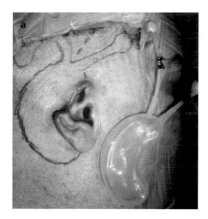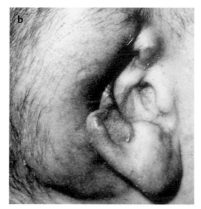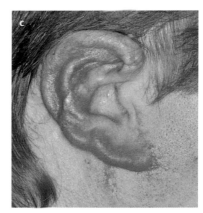

Fig. 10.50a–c Additional skin expansion before reconstruction.
a Outline of the 35 mL expander.
b Appearance after implantation (via an incision through hair-bearing skin) and expansion.
c Reconstructed ear (see **Fig. 10.51**).

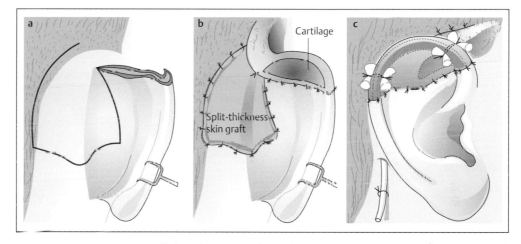

Fig. 10.51a–c Anterosuperiorly based retroauricular and postauricular transposition flap, as described by Crikelair (1956).
a Elevation of the flap.
b Incorporation of the patterned framework, coverage of the secondary defect with a thick split-thickness skin graft.
c Mattress sutures are used to form the contours, and a drain is inserted.

ness skin graft taken from the thorax donor site, the groin area, or the buttocks (**Figs. 10.48b–e** and **10.50**; Ombredanne 1931; Cronin 1952; Converse 1958; Musgrave and Garrett 1967; Converse and Brent 1977; Weerda 1984a, 2001; Weerda and Siegert 1999a).

Reconstruction by Insertion of an Expander
Where there is insufficient skin or after burn injuries, a 35-mL expander is implanted (**Figs. 10.50a, b**) and inflated continually twice a week over a period of ~8 weeks. The expanded skin is then used for reconstruction (**Fig. 10.50c**).

Crikelair's (1956) Reconstruction using an Anterosuperiorly Based Posterior Flap
(**Figs. 10.51; 10.52**)

The anterior and posterior auricular surfaces can be reconstructed with the flap described by Crikelair, which is superiorly based and includes the skin of the mastoid and postauricular regions (**Fig. 10.51a–c**). In cases with larger defects and insufficient skin, only the anterior surface of the ear need be reconstructed in a first stage, with the posterior surface then being raised in a second stage after 6 to 8 weeks, and covered with a free thick split-thickness skin graft (see **Fig. 4.66d–f**).

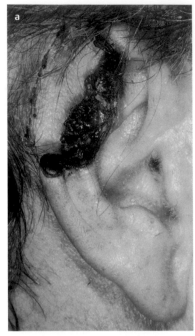

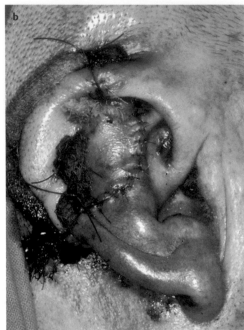

Fig. 10.52a–e
Stage I:
a Defect.
b A mastoidal flap is used for
coverage of the support
(see **Figs. 10.45, 10.47** and
Fig. 10.59b, c). With
mattress sutures, the contour is formed.
Stage II:
c The flap is divided after 3
weeks (see **Fig. 10.89**) and
the postauricular region is
covered with a thick split-
thickness skin graft (see
Figs. 10.13; 10.86).
Stage III:
d Contouring of the reconstructed area (see **Fig.
10.96**).
e Result after 3 weeks.

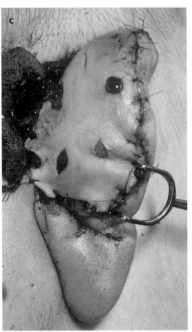

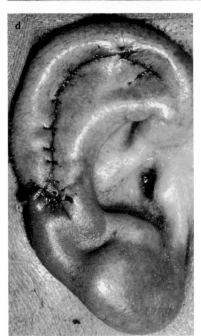

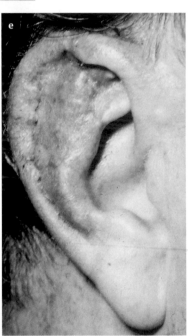

Methods of Reconstruction Described in the Literature

Primary management involves suturing the skin of the stump to the mastoid skin (see **Fig. 10.47**; see also "reconstruction of the middle third of the auricle").

Crikelair's Flap for Coverage of Large Defect
(**Fig. 10.52**)
This flap can also be used for reconstruction of a defect of the upper auricle (**Fig. 10.51a**), using a cartilaginous support (see **Figs. 10.33, 10.45, 10.47, 10.81**).

Harvesting a Skin Graft from the Thorax
(**Fig. 10.53**)
To use thick or full-thickness skin grafts in the retro-auricular or postauricular region (see **Fig. 10.51**), we harvest from the thorax (**Fig. 10.52a**), if rib cartilage has previously been harvested.

Secondary Reconstruction Using a Postauricular Flap Pedicled on the Helix (Ombredanne 1931)
(**Fig. 10.54**)

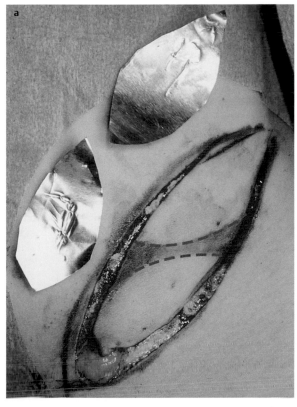
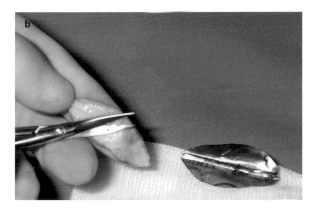
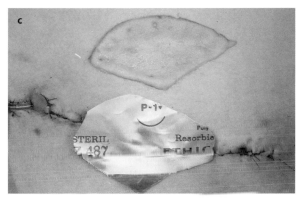

Fig. 10.53a–c   Full-thickness skin graft of the thorax (when cartilage was harvested in an earlier operation).
a Templates (aluminium foil) for two full-thickness skin grafts.   b Removing fat and connective tissue with delicate/curved sharp/sharp scissors.
c Result; the secondary defect is sutured.

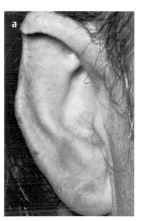
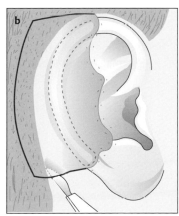
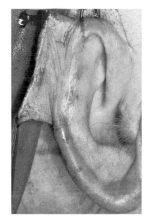
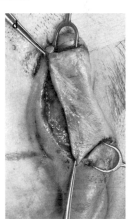

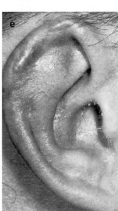

Fig. 10.54a–e   Secondary reconstruction with a postauricular flap pedicled on the helix (Ombredanne 1931).
a Defect.
b, c Posteriorly raised flap, pedicled on the scar. Placement of a strut fabricated from costal or conchal cartilage.
d The flap is sutured to cover the cartilage. Closure of the residual defect with a U-shaped advancement flap (see **Fig. 4.64b**) or thick split-thickness skin graft (see **Fig. 4.64f**).
e Outcome (surgeon: R. Katzbach).

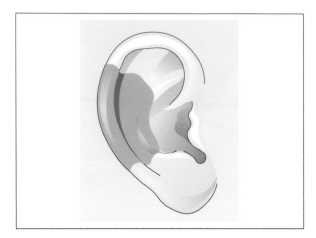

Fig. 10.55   Middle third of the auricle.

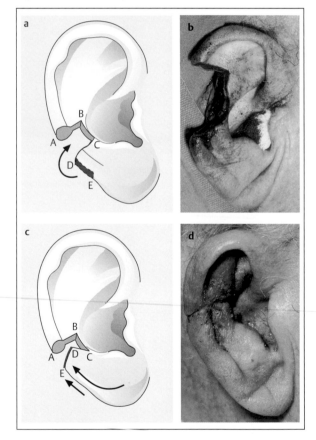

Fig. 10.56a–d   Reconstruction of the middle third of the auricle, as described by Templer et al. (1981).

a, b The margins of the defect and the lower helical region are freshened, D, E.

c The inferior auricle is rotated into the defect.

d Result.

Partial Reconstruction with a Temporoparietal Fascial Flap (Fan Flap)

(see **Figs. 10.62; 10.93**, p. 195, p. 196)

The use of a fascial flap for the reconstruction of the superior auricle is described in detail later. This flap is particularly suitable when the skin is exhausted, after burns, or after previous unsuccessful opera-

tions (Park and Suk Roh 2001), and it can also be used as a free flap from the opposite side.

Middle-Third Auricular Defects (Fig. 10.55)

Reconstruction with Auricular Reduction

The methods described for partial reconstruction of the upper auricle can also be employed in the region of the middle third of the ear.

Mention should be made of:

• Reconstruction of wedge-shaped defects with Burow's triangles (see **Fig. 10.41**)
• Techniques as described by Antia and Buch (1967) (see **Fig. 10.25**)
• Techniques as described by Day (1921) and Pegram and Peterson (1956), among others.

Reconstruction of the Middle and Lower Thirds, as Described by Templer et al. (1981)
(**Fig. 10.56**)

We freshen the wound margins and restore the contour of the ear by rotating the lower part into the defect (**Figs. 10.56a–d**). If required, the opposite ear can be reduced with the Gersuny technique (see **Fig. 10.24**).

Reconstruction without Auricular Reduction:

Recommended Methods of Reconstruction

Advancement and transposition flaps of the retroauricular region are the most frequently used, extending on occasion beyond the sulcus to include the postauricular region (**Fig. 10.57**).

Retroauricular U-shaped Burow Advancement Flap
(**Fig. 10.57**)

Stage I (**Figs. 10.57b–e**):

A wide, posteriorly based, retroauricular flap can be used for defects of the middle third of the helix. The hair should be generously shaved before the operation (**Fig. 10.57b**).

After suturing in the cartilage (C) (**Fig. 10.57c. d**), the height of which should be 2 to 2.5 mm lower than that of the defect, and which is sutured onto the cartilage stump with a 4-0 or 5-0 braided suture, the flap can be advanced into the defect and sutured to the anterior and posterior skin of the defect with 6-0 monofilament. The form of the helix can then be molded with two deep mattress sutures (**Figs. 10.57d–f**).

Stage II (**Fig. 10.57g**):

After ~3 weeks, the flap is divided from the posterior skin of the defect and its superior part incorporated. The residual defect is covered with a split-thickness

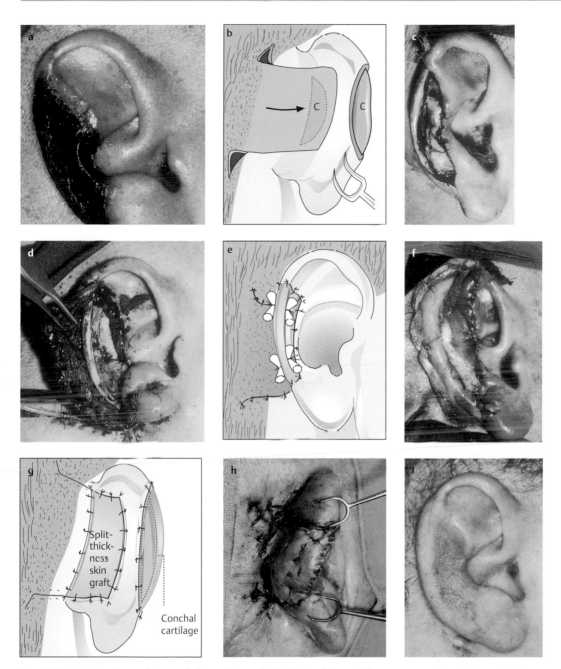

Fig. 10.57a–i   Smaller and larger defects of the middle third of the auricle; coverage with a U-shaped advancement flap (see **Fig. 10.78b**).

a Loss of the middle third of the ear after "classic replantation."

Stage I:

b–d The wound margins are freshened and a cartilage frame-work (C) is inserted. A postauricular U-shaped flap is incised and remains pedicled in the region of the scalp.

e, f This flap is sutured to the anterior skin of the stump and the contours molded with mattress sutures.

Stage II:

g, h The flap is divided after 3 weeks and incorporated into the postauricular region; if necessary, split-thickness graft is used to cover the residual defect (**Fig. 10.57**).

i Result (see also **Fig. 5.67**).

skin graft after freshening its margins and returning the U-shaped flap into its original position (**Fig. 10.57g, h**; Nelaton and Ombredanne 1907; Ombredanne 1931; Berson 1948; Musgrave and Garrett 1967; Converse and Brent 1977; Weerda 1981, 2001; Jackson 1985; Weerda and Siegert 1999a).

Avulsed auricular cartilage can also be denuded of skin and used as a strut, as can cartilage from the concha of the contralateral ear (see **Figs. 10.39a–d** and **10.40**; Musgrave and Garrett 1967).

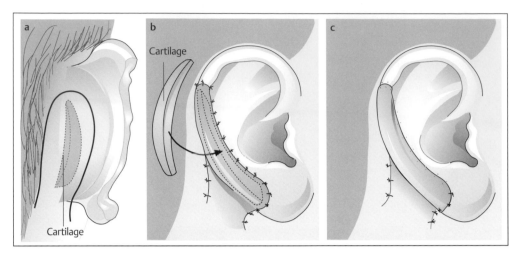

Fig. 10.58a–c   Retro-postauricular inferiorly or superiorly based transposition flap, as described by Scott and Klaasen (1992) (see **Fig. 10.66**).

a Elevation of the patterned flap, harvesting of a patterned strut fabricated from concha and anterior antihelix.

b The strut is placed in position and sutured with 4-0 or 5-0 braided resorbable suture material, and

the transposition flap is sutured to the trimmed wound margins.

c Separation and incorporation of the flap pedicle after 3 weeks.

Inferiorly and Superiorly Based Transposition Flap of Scott and Klaassen (1992)

(**Fig. 10.58**; see also **Figs. 10.59** and **10.78**)
A superiorly based transposition flap was described by Joseph (1931). It should have sufficient length when raised (see **Fig. 10.79c**).

Reconstruction with a Subcutaneous Pocket or a U-shaped Advancement Plasty

(**Fig. 10.59**; see also **Figs. 10.47** and **10.48**)
This procedure is used for larger defects of the upper and middle thirds of the auricle.

Stage I:
As previously described for smaller defects, here the retro- and postauricular skin is incised and dissected toward the hairline. An auricular template is patterned from the healthy ear, the defect is outlined (see pp. 161, 162), and, based on this template, a costal cartilage framework is carved to achieve a contour that is ~2 to 3 mm smaller than that of the expected reconstruction. A vacuum drain is secured with a suture for 6 days (**Fig. 10.59b, c**; see **Fig. 10.57c, d**).

Stage II:
Following suggestions made by Nagata, after 3 to 4 weeks, a thick split-thickness skin flap is raised ~1 cm above and parallel to the posterior margin of the frame, but not quite reaching it (see **Fig. 10.91f–k**).

The scapha can be formed in a further stage. Some later refinements can be made to improve overall form and contour (see **Figs. 10.96d–i** and **10.97c**).

Reconstruction with a Pocket as a Tunneled Flap

(**Figs. 10.60a–h**; Millard 1966; Converse and Brent 1977; Weerda 1980, 1991)

After trauma and partial avulsion, the stump was incised to the scalp (see **Fig. 10.49**).

Stage I:
Small incisions are made (**Fig. 10.60b–e**) and the scalp flap is tunneled. The support is pulled into the pocket; this operation dates back to the 1970s; nowadays we use a full-thickness support (see **Fig. 10.57c**). The incisions are closed and the helix is molded with mattress sutures (**Fig. 10.60f, g**).

Stage II (**Figs. 10.59d–f**):
After ~5 to 6 weeks, the reconstructed part can be divided, the posterior surface dissected using Nagata's technique, and the secondary defect reduced. The residual defects are then resurfaced with a thick split-thickness skin graft (**Fig. 10.60h**).

Caution:
Thin scar tissue and poor vascularity can result in necrosis.

Critique:
Excise the scar if it is hypertrophic, and proceed as shown in **Fig. 10.59b**. The transitions from stump cartilage to framework cartilage are not always satisfactory.

Reconstruction with a Rotation Flap

(see **Fig. 10.61**)
Likewise, a superiorly based rotation flap can be used if the hairline here does not allow reconstruction with a U-shaped advancement flap. **It is important to use a template to determine the form of the flap precisely, in advance of the reconstruction.**

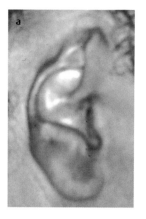
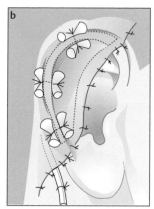
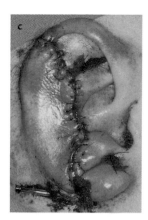

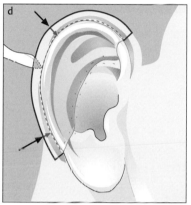
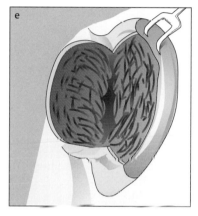
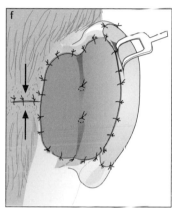

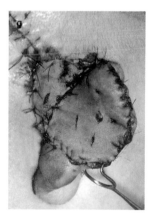
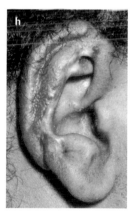
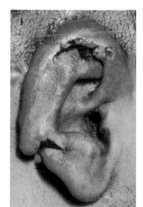
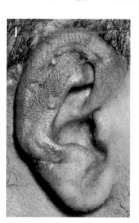

Fig. 10.59a–j Reconstruction of a large defect of the upper and middle thirds of the auricle with a subcutaneous pocket (or a U-shaped advancement flap).

Stage I:

a The wound margins of the defect are freshened. The delicate cartilaginous framework is put into place (see **Figs. 10.57c** and **10.66c**).

b, c The skin surrounding the defect is mobilized and sutured to the anterior skin of the auricular stump, a vacuum drain is inserted, and the auricle molded into shape (if necessary, large U-shaped advancement flap, see **Fig. 4.64b, d**).

Stage II:

d Incision placed 1 to 1.5 cm behind the cartilage margin and a thick split-thickness skin flap extending near to the helical margin is dissected with a size 15 blade (as described by Nagata 1994a–d, see **Fig. 10.90**).

e Careful dissection of the new postauricular surface, leaving behind a layer of fibrous tissue on the cartilaginous frame-

work. The dissected split-thickness flap is draped over the raw surface of the posterior helix.

f, g Reduction of the defect over the mastoid (arrows) and coverage of the residual defect with a split-thickness skin graft (taken from the scalp, groin, buttocks, or the old thoracic wound), which is glued with fibrin adhesive and sutured with 6-0 monofilament, while 5-0 sutures with a P3 needle are used for molding the sulcus (Weerda and Siegert 1999a; Weerda 2007).

Final refinements, if necessary:

h Small defects of contour are seen superiorly and at the transition to the earlobe.

i The defect is filled out with cartilage (above) and Z-plasty performed (below).

j Result 4 weeks later.

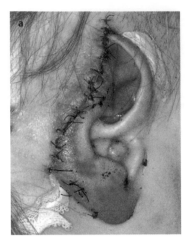

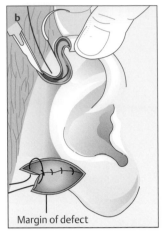

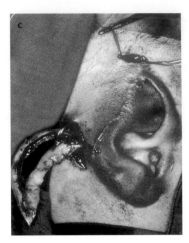

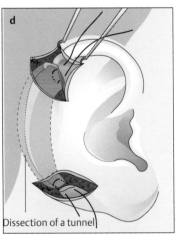

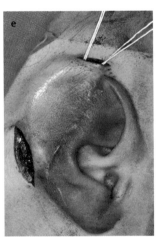

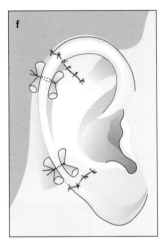

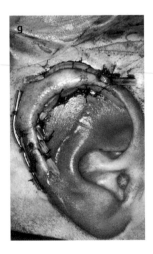

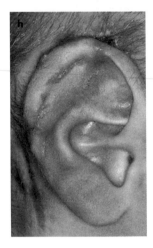

Fig. 10.60a–h **Secondary reconstruction after earlier simple debridement and closure** (after Converse and Brent 1977).
- **a** The stump was sutured to the scalp primarily.
- **b** After wound healing, incision slightly above and below the margins of the auricular defect. Dissection of a tunnel extending just beyond the hairline.
- **c–e** A delicate framework carved from costal cartilage (conchal cartilage) is drawn into the tunnel and attached to the stump with 4-0 or 5-0 braided suture material.
- **f, g** Closure of all wounds with 6-0 monofilament sutures and molding of the helix with mattress sutures.
- **h** Result after 6 weeks (see **Fig. 10.59d–j**).

Weerda's Rotation–Transposition Flap

With this flap, the defect can be closed in a single operation (**Fig. 10.61a–e**; Weerda 1980, 1984, 1991, 2007; Weerda and Siegert 1999a).

A second stage is not usually required, but if necessary some fine tailoring can be undertaken, 3 to 4 weeks after the operation (see **Fig. 10.61f**).

Critique:

This procedure involves more extensive skin mobilization and increased scar formation. We have therefore used it only on rare occasions in recent years, especially in oncosurgery (see **Fig. 10.103**).

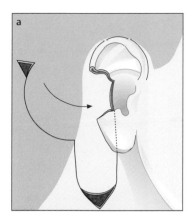
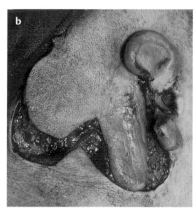
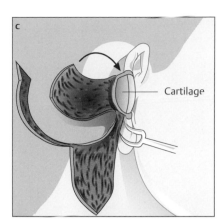
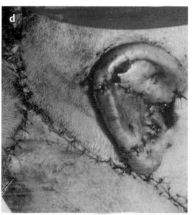
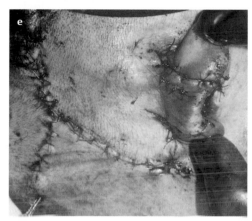
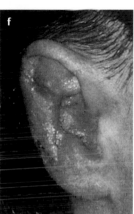

Fig. 10.61a–f   Reconstruction of a larger defect of the middle third of the auricle with the one-step Weerda rotation–transposition flap (1978, 1981).

a, b The rotation–transposition flap is outlined. The hairless retroauricular transposition flap (**reconstruction flap**) is transported into the correct retroauricular position by the hair-bearing rotation flap (**transport flap**).

c The transposition flap now lies behind the defect. The cartilaginous strut spans the defect and is 3 mm less in height. The area surrounding the secondary defect is mobilized.

d, e Appearance after reconstruction of the anterior and posterior surfaces in one stage (the suture line runs along the hairline).

f Result (slight edema; later contouring of the helix was recommended).

Other Types of Flaps Described in the Literature

Posterior Auricular Flap Based on Scar Tissue

(see also **Figs. 10.52** and **10.53**; Navabi 1964; Millard 1966; Davis 1987)

This is used for defects of the middle third of the auricle that have scar adhesions to the postauricular skin. A postauricular flap, pedicled on the scar, and extending into the sulcus, is raised according to the size of the defect, with dissection continued in a superior direction. The secondary defects are closed by mobilizing the surrounding skin.

Reconstruction with a Fan Flap (Temporoparietal Fascial Flap)

(Fig. 10.62)

These flaps and their use are described in detail in **Fig. 10.93**.

Reconstruction with Tubed Flaps

These flaps are described in detail under the discussion of reconstruction of the upper third of the auricle (see **Fig. 10.38**, pp. 155, 158 and 159).

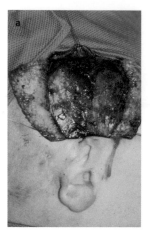
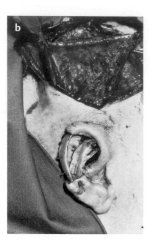
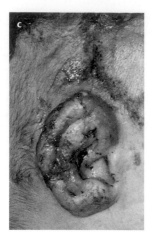
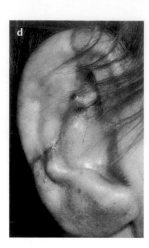

Fig. 10.62a–d   Reconstruction of the middle third of the auricle with a temporoparietal fascial flap (fan flap) (see **Fig. 10.93**).
a The fascia is exposed, the support embedded.
b Elevation of the vascular-pedicled fascia.

c The flap is inset and covered with a full-thickness skin graft harvested from the posterior region of the contralateral ear (coverage of the secondary defect with split-thickness skin graft).
d Appearance after healing (surgeon: R. Siegert; see also **Fig. 10.93**).

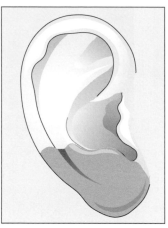

Fig. 10.63   Lower third of the auricle.

Lower-Third Auricular Defects
(Fig. 10.63)

Recommended Methods

Superiorly and Inferiorly Based Transposition Flap
(Fig. 10.64)

Stage I:
As with the reconstruction of central defects (see **Fig. 10.11**) or of the upper auricle (see **Fig. 10.51**), coverage can also be achieved in the region of the lower third in two stages, using a superiorly or inferiorly based transposition flap. Cartilage from the same or contralateral concha, or from a rib, is also used in the lower auricular region to prevent any significant contracture of the flap (**Fig. 10.64a–e**).

Stage II:
The flap is inset after 3 weeks at the earliest (**Fig. 10.64f–i**).

Reconstruction of the Entire Lower Auricle Using a Gavello Flap
(**Fig. 10.65**; Gavello 1907, as cited in Nelaton and Ombredanne 1907, Weerda 1989d)
A flap for reconstruction of the earlobe was originally devised by Gavello, and previously mentioned by von Szymanowsky in 1870. The situation after trauma avulsion. We have modified the Gavello flap

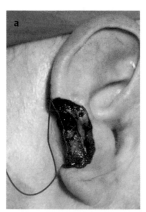
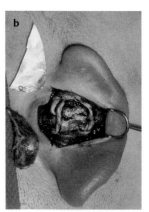
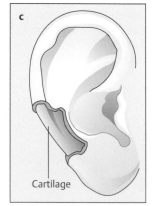

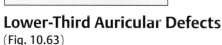
Cartilage

Fig. 10.64a–i Reconstruction of the lower third of the auricle with an (inferiorly or) superiorly based transposition flap (see also Figs. 10.13 and 10.33).
Stage I:
a Defect; flap outlined.
b Harvesting a cartilaginous support.
c Defect with incorporated cartilaginous strut from the ipsilateral or contralateral ear, harvested following a template; see i.

Fig. 10.64d–i   ▶

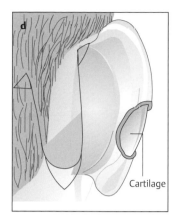

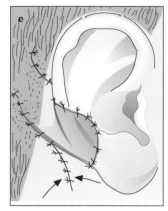

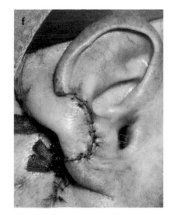

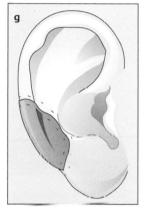

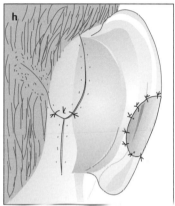

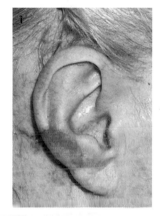

Fig. 10.64d–i

d Transposition flap.

e, f Flap inset over the cartilaginous framework.

Stage II:

g, h After ~3 weeks, division of the flap and incorporation into the postauricular surface and incorporation of the flap base.

i Result.

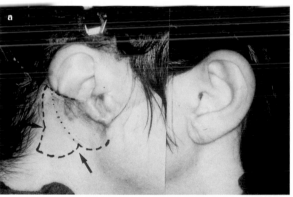

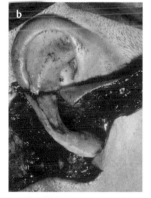

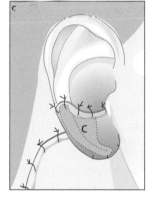

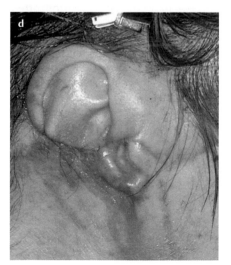

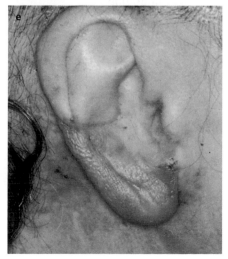

Fig. 10.65a–e Reconstruction of the lower auricular third (Weerda, 1989d) using a Gavello flap.

a Defect; the bilobed flap is planned and outlined with a Gavello flap technique.

b A large, anteriorly based, bilobed Gavello flap is elevated and, after preparation of the flap, the costal cartilage framework is sutured into place.

c The framework (C) is enveloped by the flap, and all defects are closed (see text).

d, e Result: before and after a single-stage reconstruction.

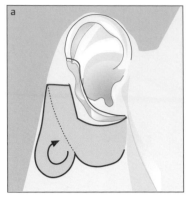
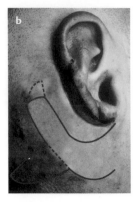
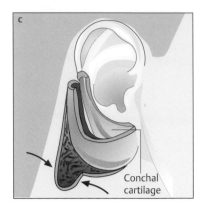
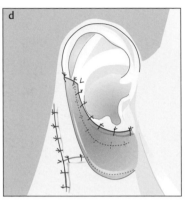
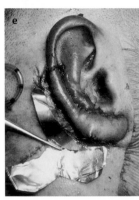
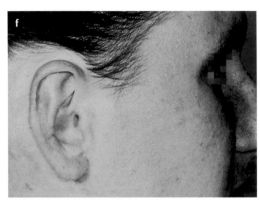

Conchal cartilage

Fig. 10.66a–f   Modification of the von Szymanowsky–Gavello flap (1870/1907) for a single-stage reconstruction of the helix and lower auricle after failure of primary reconstruction.

a, b Defect. The flap is outlined, designed from the previously prepared template (e; see **Fig. 10.73**: low insertion of the double flap due to the split-skin graft, which had previously been placed behind and below the auricle in another institution).

c The wound margins have been freshened, the flap is raised, and the patterned cartilage harvested from the contralateral

concha (or carefully carved from the costal cartilage) is sutured to the cartilage stump with a 4-0 or 5-0 braided resorbable suture.

d, e Closure of all defects, template.

f Result after 1 year.

slightly. To prevent contracture of the lower reconstructed auricle, a framework carved from costal cartilage is inserted into the lower auricle and earlobe. The costal cartilage is attached, with a 4-0 braided suture, to the cartilage stump of the auricle, after its wound margins have been freshened. The patterned flap is raised and sutured to the anterior and posterior skin of the auricular stump (**Fig. 10.65b, c**). The suture is placed slightly behind the earlobe, to achieve a good round curvature in the anterior region. A good round curvature of the earlobe is achieved if the earlobe curvature incised for coverage in the lower region is slightly larger than the earlobe curvature of the second flap. Good results can be obtained with this method (**Fig. 10.65e**).

Modified Gavello Flap

(**Fig. 10.66**; Weerda and Siegert 1999a; Weerda 2001) If, in addition to the earlobe, parts of the helix are also missing, the latter can be reconstructed with a modified Gavello flap (**Fig. 10.66a–e**). After carving a costal cartilage framework or harvesting conchal cartilage from the contralateral auricle patterned

from a template, it is attached to the cartilage stump with 4-0-braided sutures, after freshening the wound margins. The raised Gavello flap is then draped around the frame and sutured to the anterior and posterior wound surfaces, thus reconstructing the earlobe and helix. With the additional aid of a slightly larger anterior flap, the curvature of the earlobe can be given a somewhat better form. All the defects can be closed primarily by mobilizing the surrounding skin. This type of reconstruction was used for a female patient in whom the postauricular region had previously been resurfaced elsewhere with a split-thickness skin graft (**Fig. 10.66b**).

Reconstruction with a Modified Gavello Bipedicled Flap

(**Fig. 10.67**; Gavello flap 1907, first described by Szymanowski, 1870)

The posterior surface can also be covered with a thick split-thickness skin graft.

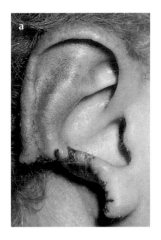
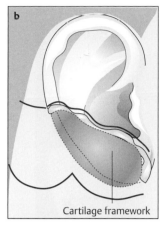
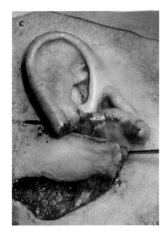

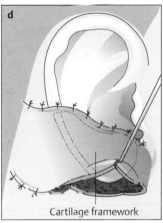
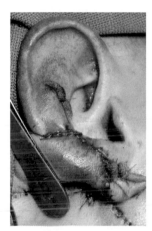
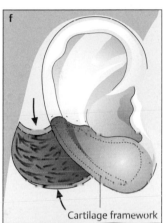

Fig. 10.67a–h   Modified Gavello bipedicled flap.

Stage I:

a Defect.

b The posteriorly and anteriorly based flap is raised, the margins of the stump are freshened, and the framework, carved from a template, is sutured on with 4-0 braided suture (see **Fig. 10.65b**).

c–e The flap is incised and the skin flap is sutured to the skin of the anterior surface of the stump.

Stage II:

f, g After ~3 weeks, division of the posterior flap and reconstruction of the posterior surface, suture to close the secondary wound (see also **Fig. 10.65**).

h Result some time after reconstruction.

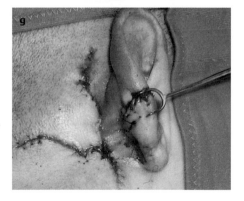
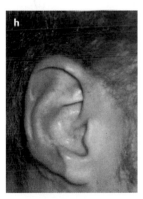

Fig. 10.68   Earlobe.

Reconstruction of the Earlobe
(Fig. 10.68)

Since the earlobe, unlike the lower third of the auricle, contains no cartilage, procedures can differ from those to reconstruct the lower auricle (see pp. 175, 176). Operations to repair tears, as well as procedures for reconstruction, will be presented.

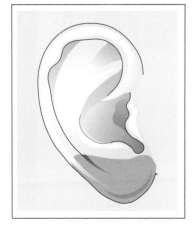

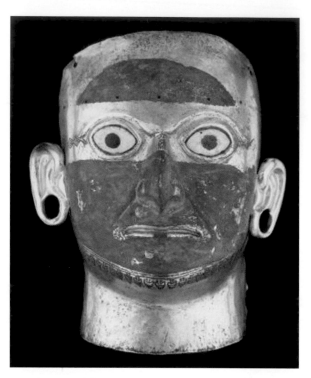

Fig. 10.69 **Earlobe defects in a mask of a king of the Moche culture, Northern Peru, 300–400 AD** (Linden Museum, Stuttgart, Germany; photograph by A. Dreyer).

Traumatic Earlobe Cleft

Example: earring avulsions.

Historical note:
In many cultures, it is customary to wear earrings, and sometimes extremely heavy or large pieces of jewelry are inserted into the earlobe (**Fig. 10.69**).

Thus, Celsus (25 BC to AD 30, in Zeis 1863) writes:

If the hole in the earlobe is large, as it tends to be in those who wear heavy ornaments in their ears, then the remaining bridge should be divided and the margins of the hole additionally freshened with a knife. The wound margins are then sutured and a medication to promote adhesion is applied (Goedecke 1995).

Reconstruction without Preservation of the Earring Perforation

Like Celsus ~2000 years ago, McLaren (1954) also freshens up the margins of the defect within the split earlobe and then closes the margins in layers.

Passow's Procedure
(**Fig. 10.70**; as cited in Mündnich 1962)
After avulsion injury, the wound margins are excised in a stepwise fashion (**Fig. 10.70b**) and the earlobe subsequently reconstructed.

Reconstruction with Preservation of the Earring Perforation

The perforation also requires reconstruction to allow further wearing of earrings.

Pardue's (1973) Method of Reconstruction
(**Fig. 10.71**)
A superiorly based epithelial flap is incised within the perforation (**Fig. 10.71g**), the opposite side is de-epithelialized, and the flap is folded in on itself (**Fig. 10.71h**). The defects are then closed (**Fig. 10.71i**).

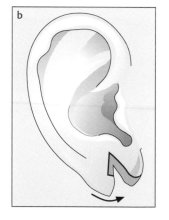

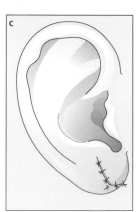

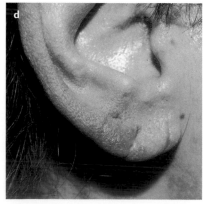

Fig. 10.70a–d **Passow's reconstruction of a cleft earlobe** (Mündnich 1962).
a Defect after avulsion injury.
b L-shaped freshening of the margins.
c Suture without reconstruction of the earring perforation.
d Delicate, L-shaped scar.

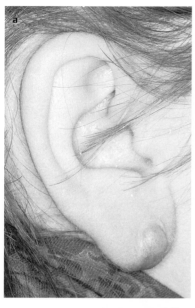

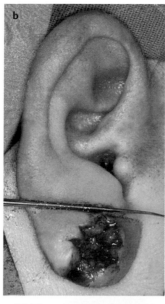

Fig. 10.71a–h   **Reconstruction of a torn earlobe without (a–e) and with f–h), preservation of the perforation for an earring,** as
described by Pardue (1973).
a Hypertrophic scarring of the earlobe.
b Excision and staggering of the scar with a
  W-plasty.
c Closure of the wound.
d Result after 14 days (steroid solution was
  infiltrated).
e Result after 1 year, with new perforations
  and ear studs.
f An epithelialized flap is prepared and the
  wound margins are freshened.
g, h The flap is rolled in upon itself and the
  wounds are closed with 6-0 or 7-0 monofilament sutures.

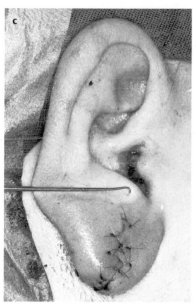

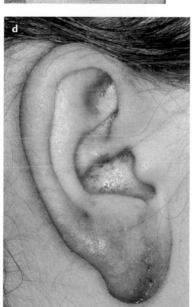

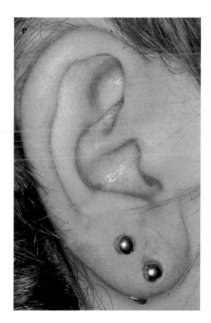

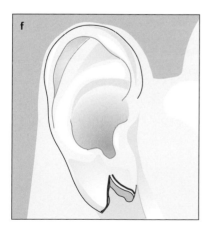

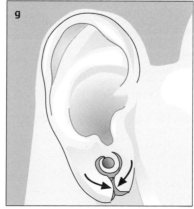

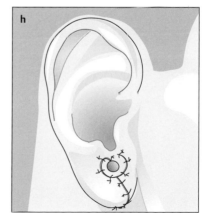

Defects of the Earlobe

These can be resurfaced with local flaps.

Loss of the Earlobe

Traumatic loss, keloids: hypoplasia or aplasia.

Historical note:
Sushruta (1000 AD, as cited in Zeis 1883; Meyer and Sieber 1973; Davis 1987) reports on the reconstruction of the earlobe, which had most likely been performed in this manner for hundreds of years:

"A surgeon can reconstruct the earlobe in a person devoid of them by slicing off a patch of living flesh from that person's cheek in a manner so as to have one of its ends attached to the cheek. Then the part where the artificial earlobe is to be made should be slightly scarified, and the living flesh should be made to adhere to it" (Celsus 25 AD).

The first description of a pedicled flap from the vicinity of the defect has, from that time on, been referred to as the "Indian method" (Goedecke 1995). In 1597, Tagliacozzi also described the reconstruction of the lower auricle (Mündnich 1962).

The reconstruction of the earlobe is described in a similar way by Dieffenbach (1845). After freshening the margins of the defect, the infra-auricular skin is incised, elevated, and sutured into position. After 3

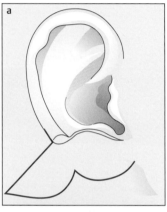
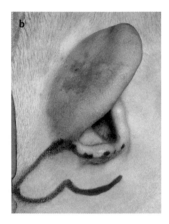
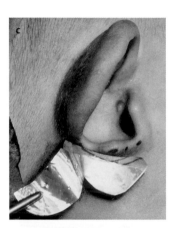
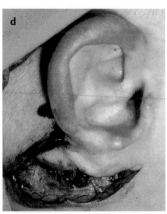
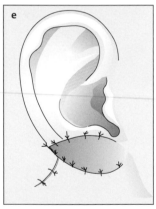
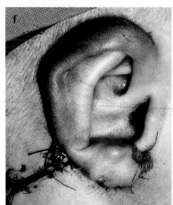
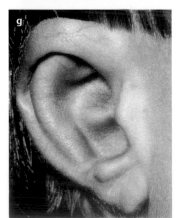

Fig. 10.72a–g Reconstruction of the lower auricle with a bilobed flap (corresponding to the Gavello flap (1907; see **Fig. 10.66 Aplasia of an ear lobe**; in von Szymanowski 1870).
a–c Outline and template.
d Incision.
e, f The flap is folded and the wound closed.
g Result (after additional otoplasty).

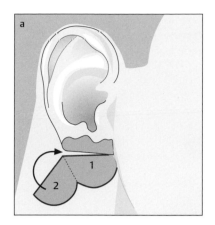
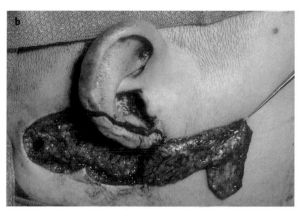
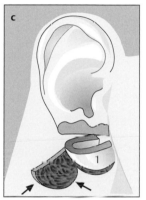
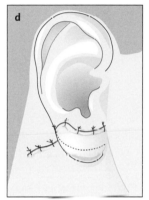
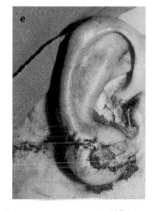
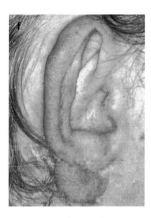

Fig. 10.73a–f Earlobe reconstruction using a Gavello flap (1907; in von Szymanowski 1870; see **Figs. 10.65** and **10.66**).

a, b Anteriorly based, bilobed flap (1, 2) is raised below the auricular defect after fashioning a template (see **Figs. 10.64e** and **10.71c**), as descibed earlier.

c The second flap (2) is folded over behind the first (1).

d, e Closure of the wounds (by mobilizing the inferior skin, the scar of the donor region comes to lie behind the auricle).

f One of the author's first Gavello flaps, from the early 1970s: result.

weeks, this flap is divided inferiorly and folded over to cover the posterior surface.

For his "total auricular reconstruction," von Szymanowski (1870) incised around the earlobe in a manner similar to a Gavello flap.

This flap is very suitable for reconstruction of the earlobe and the lower part of the auricle, and the author has used it in a lot of injuries (see **Figs. 10.65j, 10.66, 10.67, 10.72**)

Recommended Operations

Gavello's Method of Earlobe Reconstruction (1907; Figs. 10.65 and 10.66)

(**Fig. 10.73**; as cited in Nelaton and Ombredanne 1907; von Szymanowski 1870)

As previously described for the reconstruction of the lower auricle, we often use the double-flap method reported by Gavello for reconstruction of the earlobe (see also **Figs. 10.63–10.67**), previously described by von Szymanowski (1870). After freshening the margins of the defect, the flap is raised, patterned from a template made of aluminum foil or similar material, and folded over. For this purpose,

the anterior flap (**Fig. 10.73a, b, 1**) is chosen slightly larger than the second flap, bringing the lower suture line to lie on the posterior surface of the new earlobe.

The secondary defect is then closed by mobilizing the surrounding skin. Larger defects will require a cartilaginous framework, harvested from the ipsilateral or contralateral concha, which is sutured into the flap (see **Figs. 10.64** and **10.68**).

A **turnover flap** (**Fig. 10.74a**) was described by Bethmann and Zoltan in 1968.

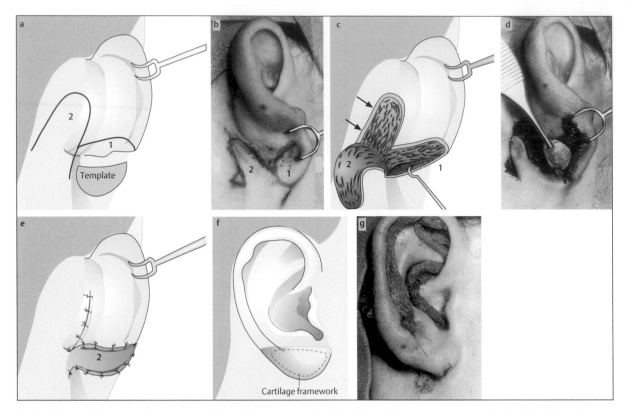

Fig. 10.74a–g   Reconstruction of the earlobe with a turnover flap (1) designed from a template, and an inferiorly based transposition flap (2), as described by Bethmann and Zoltan 1968 and by Converse and Brent (1977).

a, b Turnover flap (1) designed from a template, and an inferiorly based transposition flap (2).

c–e The flaps are dissected and inset and, in addition, a small conchal cartilage is inserted as a strut.

f, g Reconstructed earlobe at the end of the operation and otoplasty (surgeon: R. Katzbach).

Posterior Defects

The simplest method is to use thick split-thickness or full-thickness skin grafts if the periochondrium or periosteum is intact (see **Fig. 10.86**).

Postauricular defects
(**Fig. 10.75**)

Recommended Methods

Small Flaps
(**Figs. 10.76** and **10.77**)
Smaller, two-layer defects can be closed with an inferiorly or superiorly based rotation flap (**Fig. 10.76**), or with a transposition flap. An additional island flap can be used for small, full-thickness defects (**Fig. 10.77**).

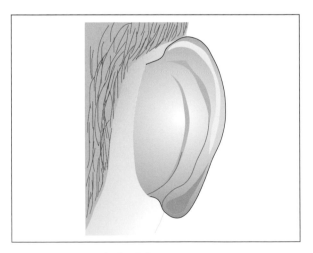

Fig. 10.75   Postauricular defects.

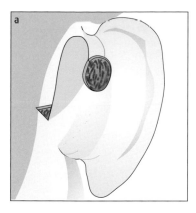
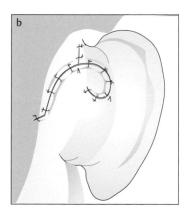
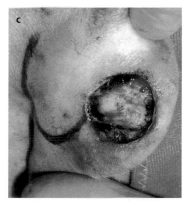

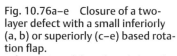

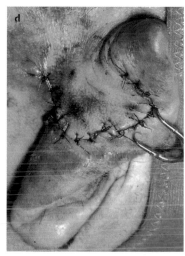
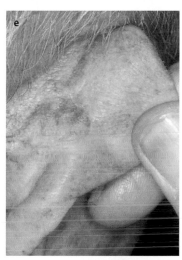

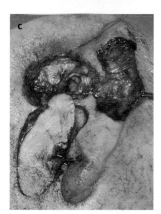
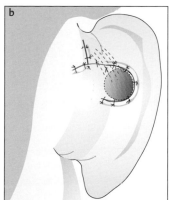

Fig. 10.76a–e Closure of a two-layer defect with a small inferiorly (a, b) or superiorly (c–e) based rotation flap.

a, b Incision of the inferiorly based rotation flap and coverage of the defect.

c Incision of the superiorly based rotation flap.

d Closure.

e Result.

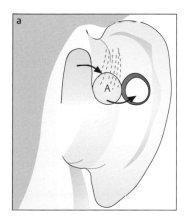
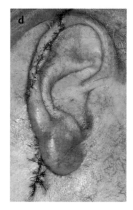
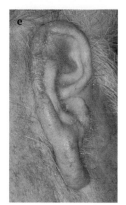

Fig. 10.77a–e Closure of a full-thickness defect with an island flap and a transposition flap.

a Elevation of an island flap (A) (see p. 138), which needs to be rotated, and the transposition flap.

b Closure of the defects (see also **Fig. 10.76**).

c Large, superiorly pedicled island flap (see **Fig. 10.5**) for reconstruction of the postauricular region and the helix).

d Closure of all defects.

e Result one year after reconstruction.

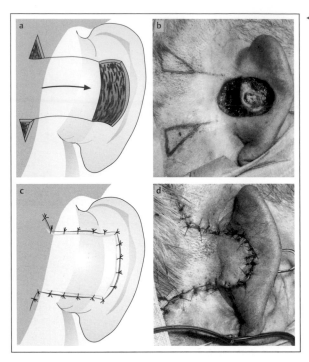

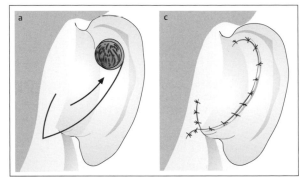

◄ **Fig. 10.78a–d   Closure of a two-layer defect with a U-shaped Burow advancement flap** (1853, as cited in Weerda 1991).
a, b Elevation of the flap with Burow's triangles in the hair.
c, d Closure of the defects.

Fig. 10.79a, b   V-Y advancement (Petres and Rompel 1996) for a two-layer defect.

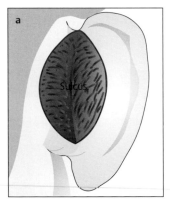

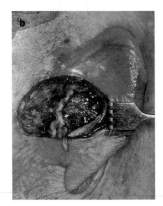

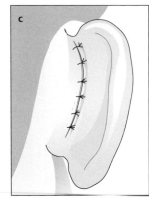

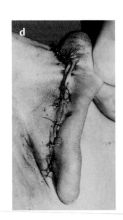

Fig. 10.80a–f   Tumor excision or skin harvest, and primary closure by coverage with the auricle.
a, b Defect after tumor excision or excision of a full thickness skingraft (see **Fig. 10.94b**).

c Closure using the entire auricular defect (and consequently reduction of the sulcus). The posterior helix should remain free.
d Result (the sulcus is diminished the helix remains free).

U-Formed Advancement Flap
(**Fig. 10.78**)
Advancement flaps are also suitable for covering a large number of two-layer defects (**Fig. 10.78a–d**), as we have already previously encountered with the reconstruction of partial auricular defects (see **Fig. 10.57**).

V-Y advancement
(**Fig. 10.79a, b**)

Closure of Defects Caused by Skin Harvesting
(**Fig. 10.80**)
Wounds caused by tumor excision, skin harvesting (**Fig. 10.80a, b**), island flap elevation, or similar procedures can be closed primarily, particularly in the

sulcus. After excision of the entire post- and retroauricular skin, especially in the sulcus, the defect can be resurfaced with split-thickness skin (see **Fig. 10.86**), or the auricle can be sutured to the mastoid surface (**Fig. 10.80c, d**). The helix should remain free (**Fig. 10.80d**).

Weerda's Bilobed Flaps
The hair-bearing **transport flap** transports the **reconstruction flap** that is raised behind the defect (**Fig. 10.81**, see **Figs. 10.87, 10.88, 10.103**).

Weerda's Rotation–Transposition Flap
(Weerda and Münker 1981; Weerda 1983a; Weerda and Siegert 1999a; **Fig. 10.81a–f**).

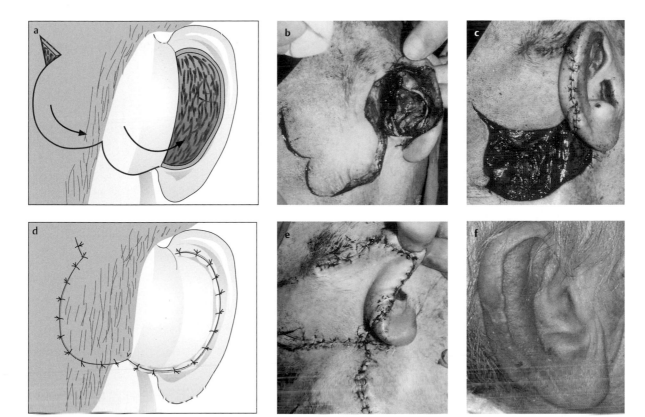

Fig. 10.81a–f   Single-stage reconstruction of a posterior auricular defect using Weerda's double rotation flap (1983a).
a, b Defect; the hairless reconstruction flap and the hair-bearing transport flap are outlined.
c, d, e Mobilization and closure of the defects.
f Result with partial reconstruction of the helix (see c, e).

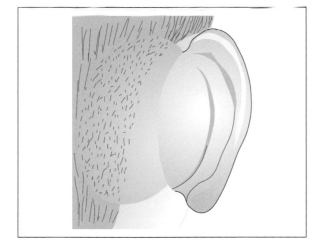

Fig. 10.82   Retroauricular (mastoid) defects.

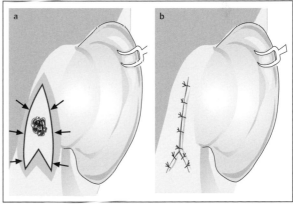

Fig. 10.83a, b   Elliptical or W-shaped excision and primary closure (Petres and Rompel 1996).

If sufficient skin is not available for a transposition or rotation flap, then a transposition flap based on a hair-bearing rotation flap can be used as a bilobed flap.

Weerda's Double Rotation Flap
(Fig. 10.81; Weerda 1983a)
As with the flap described above, a double rotation flap can be employed for large posterior defects (**Fig. 10.81a–d**).

Retroauricular Defects (Fig. 10.82)

If primary closure is not possible for defects of the mastoid region, a split-thickness or full-thickness skin graft can be used in the "ear's shadow" (see **Fig. 10.86**). Smaller and medium-sized defects can be closed by a number of flaps.

Elliptical or W-shaped Excisions and Primary Closure
(Fig. 10.83)

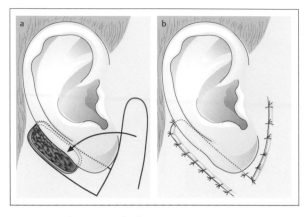

Fig. 10.84a, b Preauricular flap.
a Preauricular, inferiorly based transposition flap.
b Appearance after closure (Pennisi et al. 1965).

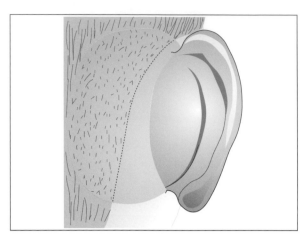

Fig. 10.85 Combined post- and retroauricular defects.

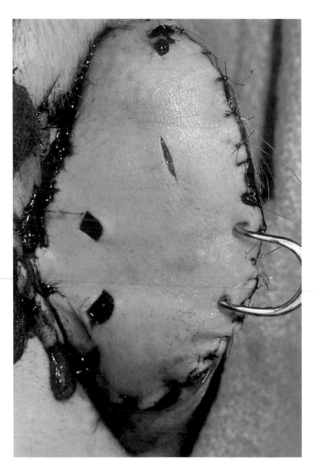

Fig. 10.86 Coverage of a post- and retroauricular defect with a free full-thickness skin graft, sutured and glued with fibrin adhesive (see Fig. 5.52c).

Preauricular Transposition Flap
(Fig. 10.84)

Coverage with Skin of the Postauricular Surface and Rotation of the Cavum
(see Fig. 10.80)

Combined Post- and Retroauricular Defects (Fig. 10.85)

Here we use free split-thickness or full-thickness skin grafts (**Fig. 10.86**) and the same flaps as described for coverage.

More extensive defects are dealt with in the following section on "Subtotal Defects."

Free Skin Grafts
(Fig. 10.86)

For larger defects, or for harvesting skin to cover defects of the face, we use split-thickness or full-thickness skin grafts from the thorax, abdominal, groin, or thigh regions, for coverage.

Subtotal Defects

Depending on their site, subtotal auricular defects can be managed in the same way as reconstructions of the upper segment, the middle third of the auricle, or the lower auricle.

Special Reconstructive Techniques

These special techniques may be useful for cases where the helix and earlobe have been preserved.

Single-stage Reconstruction with Weerda's Bilobed Flap as a Transposition–Rotation Flap
(**Fig. 10.87**; see also **Fig. 10.61**; Weerda and Münker 1982; Weerda and Siegert 1999a; Weerda 2001)

After a full-thickness, subtotal defect with loss of the mastoid skin and preservation of the helix and earlobe (**Fig. 10.87a–e**), a framework is first fashioned in the usual manner (see pp. 207–211). Next, using a rotation–transposition flap, the part of the **reconstruction flap** beneath the helix is de-epithelialized, and this flap is then transported into the

Fig. 10.87a–g Single-stage reconstruction of a subtotal auricular defect and a defect of the mastoid surface with a Weerda bilobed or trilobed flap (Weerda and Münker 1982).

a, b The flaps are outlined.

c The flaps are incised and mobilized.
The two hairless transposition flaps (1, 2 = reconstruction flaps) are used for reconstruction of the auricle (1) over a cartilage framework (d) and for coverage of the secondary defect. The rotation flap (3 = transport flap) transports the flaps into the correct position (see a).

d The flaps are sutured in situ, the transposition flap (1) is de-epithelialized at the site that comes to lie beneath the tunnel when passed anteriorly (broken line in a). The cartilaginous support is put in situ, and the flap 1 pulled through the defect.

e Closure of the defect: posterior region. Excision and closure of a Burow's triangle above the retroauricular defect.

f, g Reconstructed ear and resurfaced adjacent region.

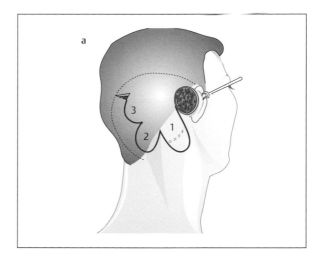

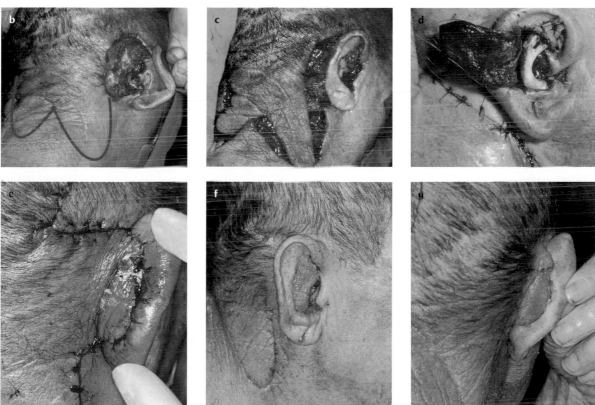

defect via the rotation flap (**transport flap**). It is thus possible to close all the defects in a single stage.

Two hairless transposition flaps (**Fig. 10.87a**1 and 2) are raised as reconstruction flaps, to close the secondary defect. These flaps are transported into the defects by the hair-bearing rotation flap (**Fig. 10.87a–e**). The flap 1 has to be de-epithelialized.

Single-stage Reconstruction of the Anterior Surface with a Bilobed Flap
(**Fig. 10.88**)

A carcinoma invading the auricular soft tissue, the petrous bone, and the surrounding skin was removed. The patient was left with only the auricular frame comprising the helix, earlobe, and tragus (**Fig. 10.88b, c**). This huge defect was covered with a double rotation flap, over which the auricular frame was placed (**Fig. 10.88d, e**). The outcome was a good esthetic result (**Fig. 10.88f, g**).

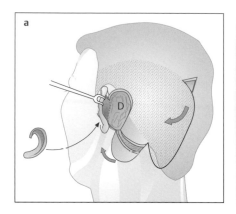

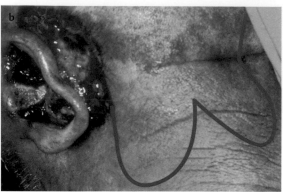

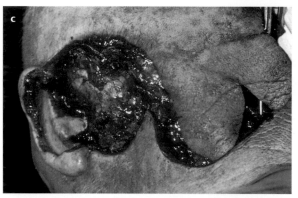

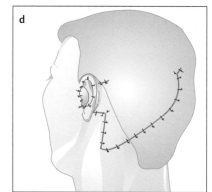

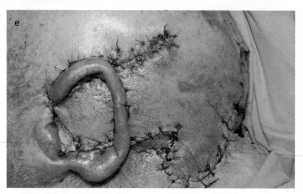

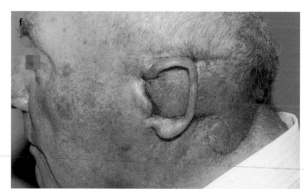

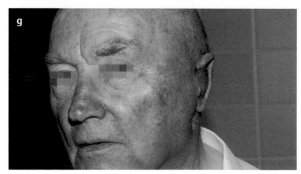

Fig. 10.88a–g Subtotal auricular defect. Single-stage reconstruction of the anterior auricular surface with a bilobed flap in a case with preservation of the auricular frame and a large defect of the periauricular region.

a–c Defects of the mastoid region and the central auricle after tumor excision. The helix, tragus, and earlobe are still intact, outline (**a, b**). Elevation of a bilobed flap (**c**).

d, e Flap in situ and appearance after placing the "frame" over the flap, which has been de-epithelialized along the corresponding margin.

f, g Good cosmetic result in profile and in half-profile in a patient over 80 years of age.

Loss of the Auricle

Fresh Avulsion Injuries

Microvascular Replantation
Microvascular replantation of the avulsed ear should be attempted whenever possible (Pennington et al. 1980). The success rate is 23% (Weerda and Siegert 1998; Weerda 2007, pp. 40–42).

Replantation of the Auricular Cartilage
Analogous to auricular reconstruction with rib cartilage, the skin of the avulsed ear can be removed and the auricular cartilage implanted into a pocket developed in the area above and behind the defect (see **Figs. 10.47** and **10.52**; Weerda 2007, pp. 35–38). The cartilage is sutured to the auricular cartilage stump and inserted into the pocket, and the skin of the pocket is sutured to the skin of the stump (see **Fig. 10.89**).

Replantation by the Technique of Mladick et al. (1971)
In this technique, the amputated ear part is dermabraded with a large diamond or corundum wheel, then inserted into a retroauricular skin pocket and sutured to the stump, as in the replantation of auricular cartilage. Four weeks later, the skin pocket is opened, the largely epithelialized segment is taken from the pocket, and the skin of the pocket is fixed in the retroauricular sulcus. The replantation of small auricular segments by the Mladick technique has a success rate of ~65% (Weerda and Siegert 1998).

Auricular Replantation by the Technique of Baudet (1972) and Arfai (in Spira 1974) (Weerda 1980) (Fig. 10.89)
The replantation of ear parts is doomed to failure in most cases (Weerda et al. 1986). The overall success rate reported in the literature is ~40% (Weerda 2007; p. 42).

Stage I:
Avulsed ear parts should be kept cool and clean by placing them in a moist paper towel or special box, for delivery to the operating room. Small auricular composite grafts can be successfully replanted even after 24 hours, but necrosis increases with the size of the replanted part and the duration of exposure to room temperature. The procedure described by Baudet (1972) and later by Arfai (in Spira 1974; **Fig. 10.89**) increases the raw surface in the mastoid area and promotes anterior revascularization by fenestrating the salvaged cartilage (**Fig. 10.89a–c**)

Fig. 10.89a–l Replantation of an avulsed auricle by the technique of Baudet (1972) as modified by Arfai (in Spira 1974).
a A total avulsion.
b, c Preparation of the posterior side of the avulsed auricle. The skin is dissected back to the helical rim as a full-thickness skin flap (A). The auricular cartilage is fenestrated by excising segments down to the perichondrium on the anterior side of the auricle.
d, e Preparation of the **recipient bed** on the mastoid. The flap (B) is developed toward the scalp, creating a large raw surface.

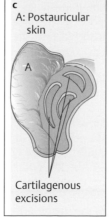

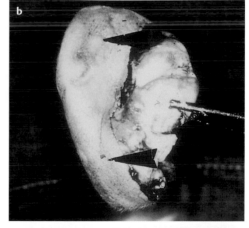

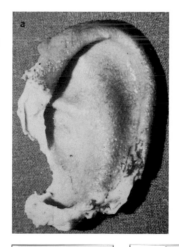

c
A: Postauricular skin

A

Cartilagenous excisions

d
B: Mastoid flap

B

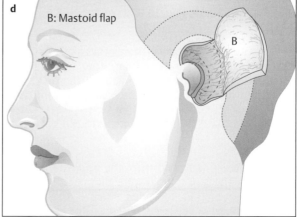

Fig. 10.89e–l ▶

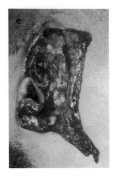
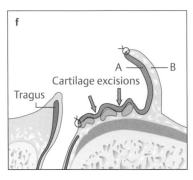
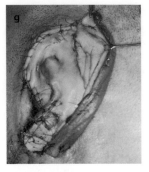
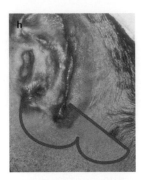
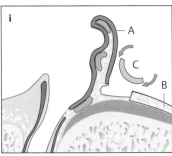
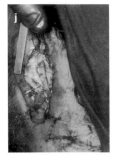
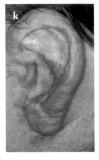
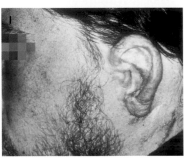

Fig. 10.89f–l Replantation of an avulsed auricle.

f, g Stage I: the fenestrated cartilage is sutured and glued to the recipient bed. The postauricular skin flap (A) is attached to the mastoid flap (B) with sutures and glue (g).

h–j Stage II: 5 weeks later, (Fig 10.89h). The postauricular flap (A) is separated from the mastoid flap (B), and both

flaps are returned to their original positions. Residual defects are grafted with split-thickness skin (C). The lobule is reconstructed with a Gavello flap (see **Fig. 10.73**): outline in **h**.

k, l Result after 1 year (see p. 196).

Stage II (Fig. 10.89d):

After 4 to 8 weeks, the auricular skin flap (**Fig. 10.89a**, A) can be separated from the mastoid flap (**Fig. 10.89b, c**; B). The auricle is raised from the mastoid plane as in a total ear reconstruction, and the flaps are returned. Residual defects are covered with a thick split-thickness or full-thickness skin graft (**Fig. 10.89d**). The reported success rate is ~40% (Weerda and Siegert 1998). If the earlobe is missing, it is reconstructed by the Gavello technique (**Fig. 10.89h**; see also **Figs. 10.72, 10.73**).

Auricular Reconstruction Following Total Amputation

(**Figs. 10.90, 10.91, and 10.92;** Weerda 1983c, 1987, 1997; Weerda and Siegert 1998)

When the entire auricle has been lost as a result of accidental trauma or tumor surgery, there is generally enough skin left to proceed with reconstruction. Otherwise, the available skin should be expanded by implanting a 20- to 35-mL tissue expander for ~8 weeks (Siegert and Weerda 1994; see **Figs. 4.4** and **5.50**).

Stage I:

First, a pattern is traced from the opposite, normal ear, onto a sheet of radiographic film or other transparent material (**Fig. 10.90d**; see **Figs. 3.8** and **11.1d, f**). The pattern is reversed, the position of the new

auricle is precisely determined (**Fig. 10.90a**), and a skin pocket is developed past the hairline (**Fig. 10.90b**). The skin should be dissected thin enough to conform well to the underlying framework but thick enough to preserve an adequate blood supply. After the rib cartilage has been harvested (see **Fig. 11.1**), a cartilage framework is carved from the synchondrosis of the ipsilateral or contralateral sixth and seventh ribs. The framework should be ~3 mm smaller in all dimensions than the proposed auricle (see **Fig. 11.3** and **Fig. 10.90c, d**).

Generally, the eighth rib is used to reconstruct the helix; it should be at least 8 to 10 cm long (see **Fig. 11.3**). Remnants of rib cartilage are reimplanted subcutaneously in the thoracic wound for the second stage of the operation. The cartilage framework is inserted into the pocket (**Fig. 10.90e–g**), and one or two continuous-suction drains and bolster sutures coapt the skin to the frame. The bolster sutures are left in place for ~8 days (**Fig. 10.90g**). The suction drains are not removed before the sixth or seventh day.

Stage II (Brent 1992; Weerda 1996; Weerda et al. 1996; Weerda 2007; Fig. 10.91):

About 12 to 24 weeks later, a curved incision is made ~1 to 1.5 cm above and behind the rim of the implanted framework, and a thick split-thickness skin flap is sharply dissected to the rim on a shallow plane, using a no. 15 blade (**Fig. 10.89**). The frame-

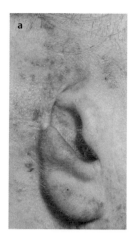

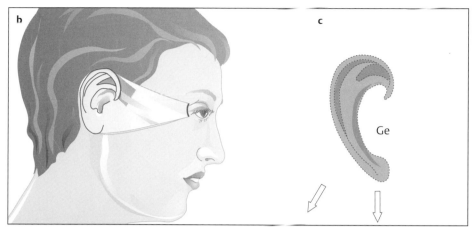

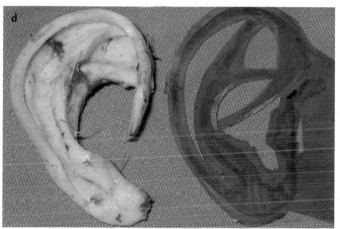

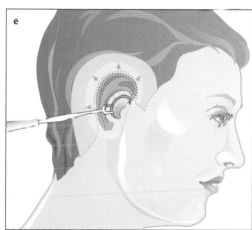

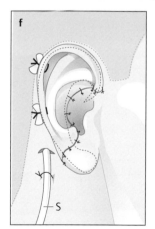

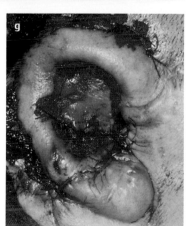

Fig. 10.90a–g Auricular reconstruction after total amputation.
Stage I:

a Total avulsion, the lobule and tragus are preserved.

b The film pattern traced from the opposite ear is reversed to determine the precise position of the reconstructed ear (see **Fig. 10.14**). Its position is also determined by the auricular remnants.

c In case of residual lobule, the template designed from the contralateral side (template 1; see **Fig. 11.3**) is placed over the stump remnants, and the future position of the ear is outlined, which is usually well defined by the stump remnants. A slightly smaller cartilaginous framework is carved using template 2 (see **Fig. 10.44**).

d, e The old wound is opened, the scars are carefully excised, and the skin is undermined. The old wound edges are freshened, and the cartilage framework (d) is implanted (see **Fig. 11.3**).

f, g The wound is closed. The earlobe remnant is placed at the anatomically correct site, and the skin is coapted to the framework by a suction drain (S) and several bolster sutures (g: see patient in Fig. 2.8h, the ear here is turned to the right side).

(Stage II: see **Fig. 10.91**)

work itself is not exposed, and care is taken to leave ample connective tissue on the back of the framework to ensure cartilage nutrition (**Fig. 10.91a, b, f, i**; see also **Fig. 10.89d, e**).

A crescent-shaped cartilage graft 35 to 40 mm long, 10 to 12 mm high, and ~8 mm thick is carved from the rib cartilage that was banked in the thoracic pocket during the first operation (**Fig. 10.91e, f**). The cartilage graft is mobilized until it can be separated from the

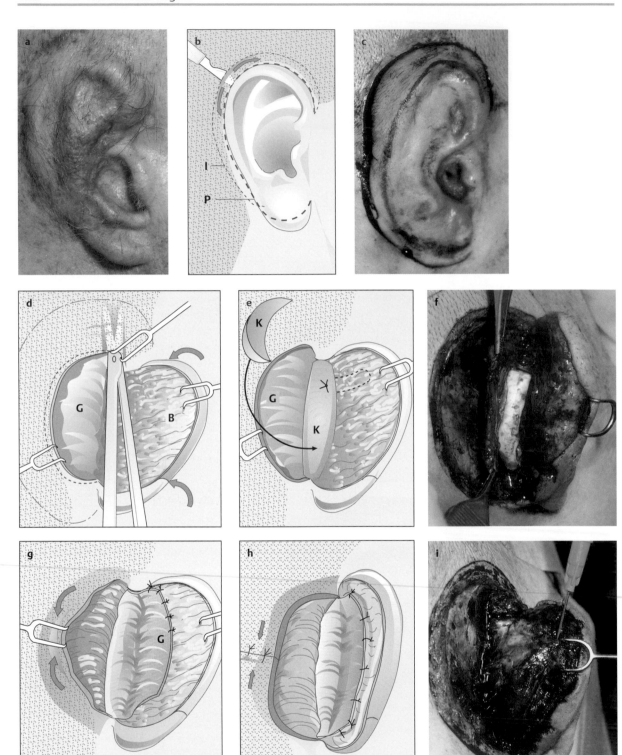

Fig. 10.91a–o Second stage of auricular reconstruction ~4 to 6 months later (Nagata 1999; Weerda 1999; Weerda 2007).

a Result 4 months after the first stage (**Fig. 10.90**).

b, c An incision (I) is made 1 to 1.5 cm above and behind the rim of the framework. A full-thickness skin flap is dissected with a no. 15 scalpel above the level of the hair bulbs, developing to flap close to the framework; P = limit of the dissection. The framework itself should not be exposed.

d The cartilage framework is dissected from its bed, preserving the layer of granulation and connective tissue (B) over the frame. A galea–fascia–muscle flap (G) of adequate size is then outlined and raised on the mastoid.

e, f A crescent-shaped cartilage graft (K) measuring ~35 to 40 mm × 10 mm × 12 mm (height) is inserted and sutured into place. The graft functions as a spacer to maintain the auriculocephalic angle. The flap is held by forceps.

g–i The cartilage graft is covered with the galea–fascia–muscle flap (G), which is secured with sutures and fibrin glue. The raw surface on the mastoid is reduced in size. (h)

Fig. 10.91j–o ▶

Fig. 10.91j–o

j, k One or two split-thickness skin grafts (Sp) are glued and sutured into the defects. A tie-over Vaseline gauze bolster is secured with adhesive tape to create a light pressure dressing (see **Fig. 10.95; see text**).

l Sectional view of the individual layers.

m Result.

n Before reconstruction.

o After reconstruction.

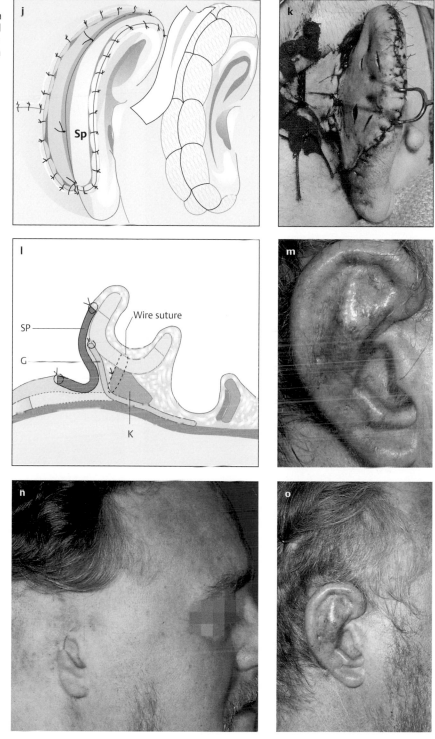

head by ~25 mm (distance from superior helical rim to mastoid) without tension. The crescent-shaped cartilage graft (K) is positioned under the new antihelix to function as a spacer (**Fig. 10.91e**) and is fixed to the antihelix with two sutures. An anteriorly based galea–fascia–muscle flap (G) is folded over the cartilage graft (**Fig. 10.91e–g**) and secured to the connective tissue with absorbable sutures and fibrin glue (Immuno, Vienna, Austria) (**Fig. 10.91l, G**). Perichondrium is left attached to the mastoid plane. The surrounding skin is mobilized and advanced behind the auricle. A Burow's triangle is excised, and the wound is closed in two layers (**Fig. 10.91g, h**). If there is adequate separation of the auricle from the mastoid (ideally ~2.0 cm to the upper helical rim), the remaining defects can be grafted with split-thickness skin from the groin or

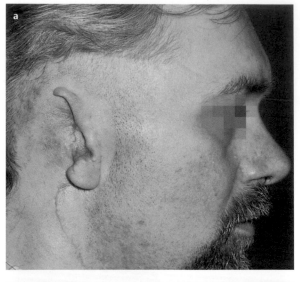

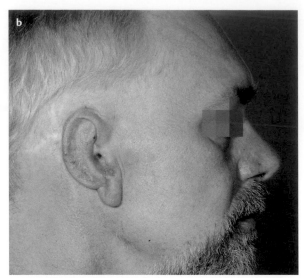

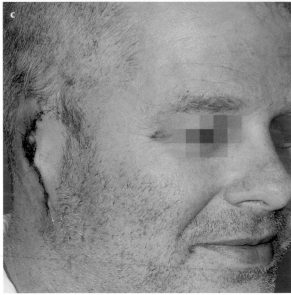

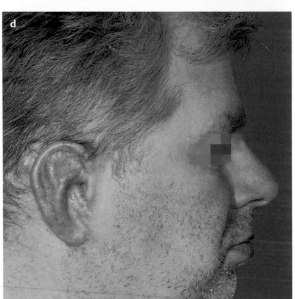

Fig. 10.92a–d   Examples of reconstruction.
a, b Defect of residual crus helicis tragus and lobule and result (b).

c, d Reconstruction after total avulsion.

buttock (**Fig. 10.91g, k, l**). This graft is covered with a light pressure dressing (**Fig. 10.91e**), and the first ear bandage is not applied before day 6. The split-thickness skin graft can also be obtained from the head, keeping above the plane of the hair follicles in the scalp to permit rapid re-epithelialization and normal hair growth that will conceal the donor site. Additional touch-ups can be performed later. **Fig. 10.91l** shows the individual layers in cross-section. It is possible to obtain a graft from the thoracic scar (see **Figs. 10.59** and p. 167).

Some results of reconstruction of the auricle after loss are shown in **Fig. 10.92a–d**.

Reconstruction of the Ear or Auricular Region in Patients with Skin Loss or Burns
(**Fig. 10.93**)

If the skin around the ear cannot be used, the parietotemporal fascia (**Fig. 10.93**) on the ipsilateral side can be transferred as a "fan flap," to cover the auricular framework. Split-thickness skin is then used to cover the fascia. The preferred donor site for this skin is the posterior surface of the opposite auricle, as this will provide the best color and texture match. The entire postauricular surface and mastoid area can be utilized, while leaving the perichondrium on the auricle. A large split-thickness skin graft from the

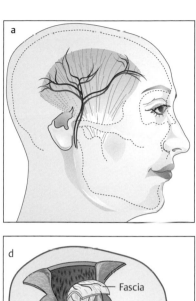

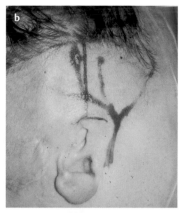

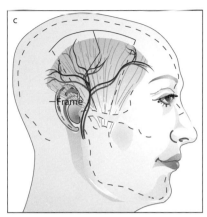

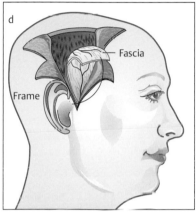

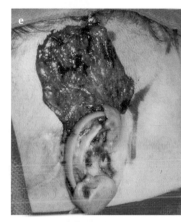

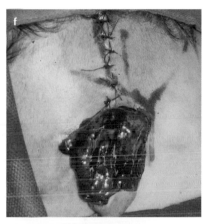

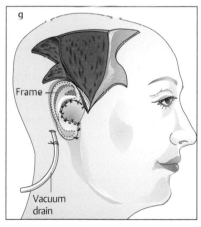

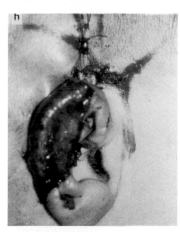

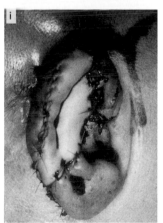

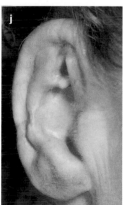

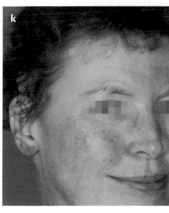

Fig. 10.93a–k Partial reconstruction with a parietotemporal fascial flap (fan flap) pedicled on the superficial temporal artery and vein above the thicker temporal fascia, as described by Weerda 2007 (see **Fig. 10.62**).

a, b Ear loss. The superficial temporal artery and vein are identified using Doppler ultrasound.

c The parietotemporal fascia and vessels are exposed through a zigzag incision.

d, e The fascia is raised together with its vascular pedicle, and the cartilaginous support is inserted (e).

f–h The cartilage frame is covered with vascularized fascia.

i Coverage with a thick split-thickness or full-thickness skin graft harvested from the retroauricular and postauricular region of the contralateral side, or from a similar site (see text, Abul-Hassan et al. 1986), and closure of all wounds.

j, k Result (surgeon: R. Siegert).

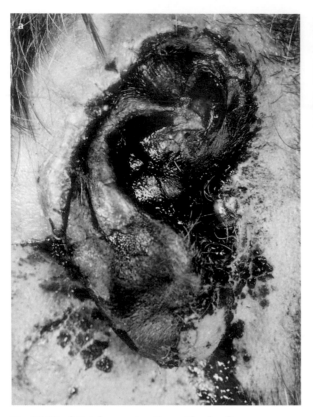

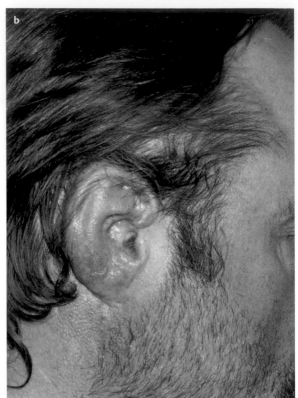

Fig. 10.94a, b Total reconstruction with a fan flap.

a Loss of an ear following avulsion and replantation performed in another institution using Baudet's technique (1972) (see **Fig. 10.89**; p. 190).

b Appearance after reconstruction with a fan flap and a full-thickness skinflaps of the contralateral post auricular region (see **Fig. 10.80a, Fig. 10.93**).

groin or buttock is then used to cover the postauricular surface and mastoid area on the normal side, and, if necessary, it can be used for the reconstructed postauricular surface as well. Split skin from the nearby scalp can also be used in a thickness of approximately 0.3 mm. If an ipsilateral parietotemporal fascial flap (**Fig. 10.93**) cannot be used because of an inadequate blood supply (evaluate by Doppler, see **Fig. 10.93b**) or a severe burn, the surgeon may try to obtain a fan flap from the opposite side. This would require a free transfer and thus a surgical team trained and equipped to perform microvascular anastomosis. Another option is a **forearm fascial flap** with **microvascular anastomosis**.

Fan Flap of Parietotemporal Fascia
(**Fig. 10.93**)

The head is shaved on the designated side. A Doppler probe is used to locate and mark the course of the superficial temporal artery (**Fig. 10.93a, b**), and the skin over the fascia is opened with a zigzag incision (**Fig. 10.93d, e**). The skin should not be incised too deeply, because the parietotemporal fascia directly overlies the deep temporal fascia and is just below the hair bulbs and fat. The scalp is dissected to the left and right, directly below the plane of the hair bulbs. At this point, the blood vessels can be clearly

traced upward from the preauricular area. A fascial flap is outlined, based on the size and shape of the auricular framework that has already been fabricated. The flap is dissected from the deep temporal fascia and turned downward on its vascular pedicle (**Fig. 10.93e–f**). The cutaneous wound is closed in layers, over a vacuum suction drain, and the auricular framework is covered with the fascia (**Fig. 10.93e, f**). Next, a split-thickness or full-thickness skin graft is obtained and attached to the fascia, with fibrin glue and a few interrupted sutures. The suction drain will coapt the fan flap to the auricular framework (**Fig. 10.93g**). A Vaseline pack is applied and secured with tape (for 1 week), to help shape and protect the reconstruction. Further touch-ups are added later as required (see Stage II, p. 197; **Fig. 10.95**).

Transient flap edema is normal initially, but the flap should assume the desired shape and thickness over a period of weeks. (**Fig. 10.93j, k**). A total reconstruction with a fan flap is also shown in **Fig. 10.94**. Free fascia harvested from the radial forearm can be used if temporalis fascia is not available (see **Fig. 14.1i, j**).

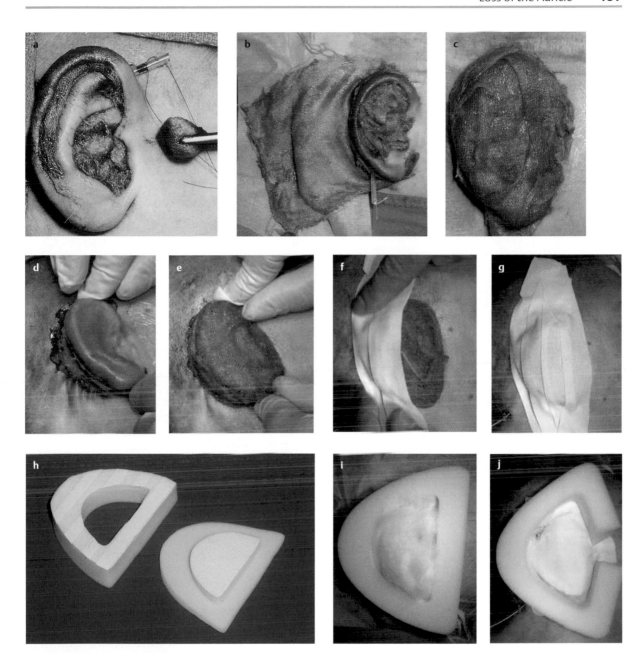

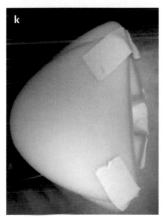

Fig. 10.95a–m   Dressing after auricular surgery.

a Dressing after **set-back otoplasty** and after individual operative stages. The concha is supported by packing with small swabs of ointment-soaked gauze.

b, c Dressing material is placed over the posterior and anterior surface.

d–g Dressing for the **second stage of microtia grades II** and III, subtotal oder total reconstruction.

d A free graft is inserted after reconstruction of grade III microtia.

e, f Dressing using split thickness skin grafts: The graft is bandaged under mild compression for 1 week. Coverage of the surrounding area. The skin is prepped with rubbing alcohol, and the first strips of adhesive plaster (2 cm) are applied to provide mild compression on the posterior (see b,c) padding and skin.

g Application of the adhesive plaster dressing .

h, i, j **Fenestrated sponge dressing which is also used without the adhesive-plaster dressing for the first stage, as for all other operations.**

k Fenestrated sponge dressing is used at **the end** of all auricular operations.

Fig. 10.95l–m   ▶

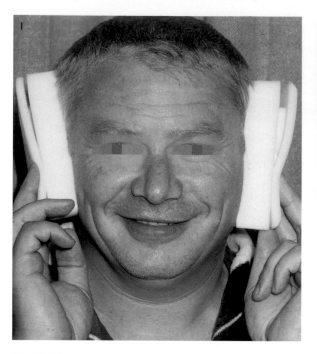

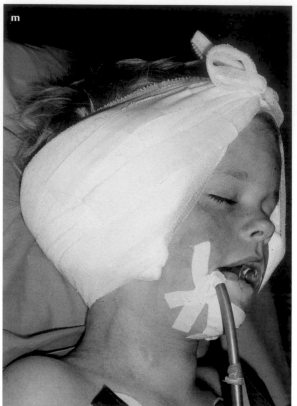

Fig. 10.95l–m
l Fenestrated sponge dressing.
m A large bandage or a Stulpa tubular bandage are wrapped around the head to secure the windowed foam pad that shields the ear from pressure.

Spiggle & Theis, Dieburg, Germany

Dressing the Ear
(Fig. 10.95)
We use ointment dressings soaked in a mixture of povidone–iodine and petroleum jelly for all of our dressings, and supplement with additional steroid ointments for otoplasty, and after individual operative stages. The auricle is covered with a fenestrated sponge dressing developed especially for this purpose, to avoid pressure on the external ear. We also apply additional cotton wool cushioning. Then, a circular dressing is put on, secured with a tubular dressing. (Fig. 10.95h–m)

At the second operative stage (coverage of the posterior region with a free graft), the cavity behind the ear is sealed off with the ointment dressing described above (see Fig. 10.95d–g) and the auricle is bandaged under mild compression for 1 week (Fig. 10.95l–m). Fibrin adhesive is used to glue the thick split-thickness or full-thickness graft over the postauricular surface, so partial or total loss of the split-thickness grafts has become very rare. With problem cases and for secondary interventions, we administer perioperative antibiotics, extended over at least 5 days.

A fenestrated sponge and a circular bandage covered by a tubular bandage, particularly at night, secures the entire dressing (Fig. 10.95h–m).

Removal of Sutures
This is done 6 to 8 days after surgery, preferably on the 8th day. The same applies for the chest wound, because of the intracutaneous suture used there. We then recommend short-term use of adhesive tape for 3 to 4 days, to secure the wound.

Fine-Tailoring After Operations
Occasionally, we find that the contours of the scapha are not readily apparent, or there is a lack of depth to the concha, a poorly defined tragus, or distortions from scar formation. We have to wait at least 6 months to get better results. If not, we have to deepen the scapha and triangular fossa, to model the cartilage (Fig. 10.96) or to construct the concha and/or tragus (Fig. 10.97).

An incision is made in the scapha, directed somewhat more toward the antihelix (Fig. 10.96c–f). If necessary, the skin is dissected as far as the upper concha and the scapha is deepened (Peer and Walker 1957; Fig. 10.96e–g). Deepening of the scapha, triangular fossa and depilation. In addition, refinements may also be made to the antihelical framework, the triangular fossa excavated, and the concha slightly enlarged (Fig. 10.96e, f–i). When hair is present on the helix, it is dissected off the framework, and the hair follicles are removed with fine pointed scissors.

Fig. 10.96a–j   Corrective surgery: deepening of the scapha, fossa and epilation.

a Total loss.

b Bad contour after reconstruction.

c, d Incision in the scapha, near the antihelix, dissection of the skin.

e, f Deepening of the scapha and scar excision.

g If required, deepening of the triangular fossa and widening of the concha. Lowering of the antihelix. Dissection around the superior helix and removal of the hair follicles (sharp/sharp fine scissors; see **Fig. 2.74**, p. 7 and **Fig. 2.7, d7**, p. 8).

h, i The skin incision is sutured with 6-0 (1) polydioxanone mattress sutures, knotted over a long cotton bolster soaked in petroleum jelly (2, 3), and also, if necessary, glued with fibrin adhesive.

j Result 2 years after reconstruction.

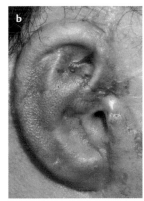

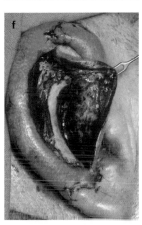

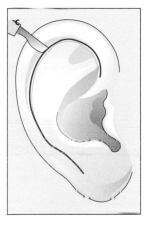

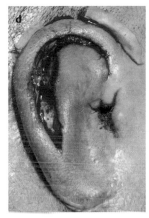

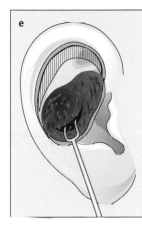

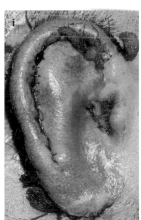

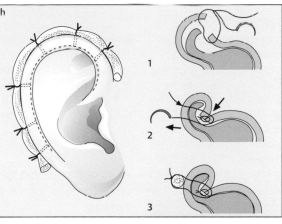

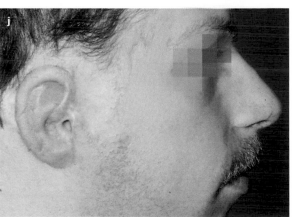

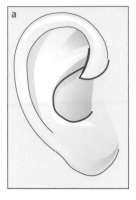
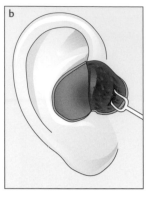
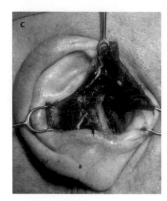

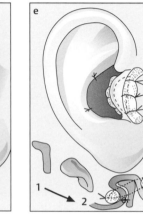
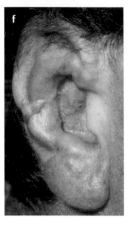

Fig. 10.97a–f Deepening of the concha, formation of the helical crus and the tragus, as described by Tanzer (1974), modified, and coverage of the concha with a full-thickness skin graft.

a   Incision around the helical crus and in the transition from concha to antihelix.

b, c   Elevation of the skin anteriorly by dissection. The concha is deepened down to the mastoid and anteriorly. If necessary, parts of the antihelical cartilage is excised.

d   A full-thickness skin graft, fashioned from a template and harvested from the sulcus of the contralateral ear, is sutured to the tragal skin.

e   An L-shaped segment of cartilage can be inserted as a tragal strut, the full-thickness skin graft is glued into place with fibrin adhesive, and the shape of the tragus is formed using mattress sutures tied over cotton bolsters; 1 and 2: schematic illustration.

f   Result.

The incision is closed with 6-0 monofilament sutures. Placing the incision close to the antihelix now allows the skin to reach down into the base of the scapha. By removing the scar tissue and lowering the antihelix and the crura, the skin of the antihelix also suffices to lend a good form to the scapha. The skin incision is closed (**Fig. 10.96b, i**). Mattress sutures (5–0 monofilament sutures, P3 or PS-3 needle), knotted behind the helix over long, thin bolsters soaked in a mixture of petroleum jelly and povidone–iodine, draw the skin into the scapha (**Fig. 10.96h, i**, 2, 3).

Tanzer (1974) suggests making only three to four incisions in the scapha, 7 to 8 mm in length, instead of a long incision, and deepening the scapha via these.

Deepening of the Concha Formation of the Concha and the Tragus (Fig. 10.97):
Because we usually fix the skin onto the concha using fibrin glue, suturing is often unnecessary.

Forming the shape of the Helical Crus, Concha, Antitragus, and Intertragic Notch
Figure 10.97a, b demonstrates Weerda's method.

Davis' (1987) method of forming the helical crus is shown in **Fig. 10.98c, d**.

In the absence of the helical crus, or if it is poorly defined, transposition of tissue from the preauricular region in the form of a Z-plasty can create a helical crus (**Fig. 10.98c, d**; **Fig. 10.17**, p. 145).

Reconstruction of Defects of the Auricular Region after Partial or Total Amputation

(**Fig. 10.99**)

(**Figs. 10.100** and **10.101**; see also p. 120ff.)
If, after amputation or any other loss of the auricle and skin of the auricular region (**Fig. 10.99**), the intention is merely to reconstruct the defect, then, depending on the size of the defect, free skin grafts (**Fig. 2.22a, b**), local skin (**Figs. 10.87** and **10.88**), myocutaneous island flaps (**Figs. 12.1, 12.2**) or, **nowadays, flaps anastomosed using a microvascular technique** (see Chapter 15) can be used for coverage.

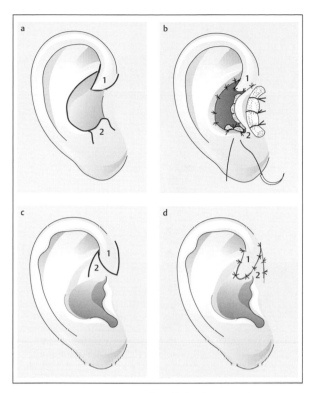

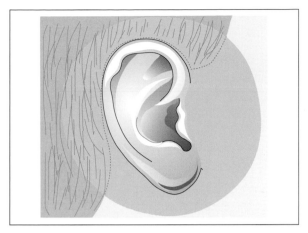

Fig. 10.99 Auricular region.

Fig. 10.98a–d Formation of the helical crus and intertragic notch and deepening of the concha (see also **Fig. 10.97**).
a Pattern of the incisions for formation of the helical crus (1) and intertragic notch (2).
b After elevation of the skin flaps, scar tissue, and, if necessary, cartilage (including the antihelix) are excised. A mattress suture is also used to form the notch (2). Epithelialization of the concha: see **Fig. 10.97**.
c Z-plasty forming the helical crus, using a preauricular flap (1; Davis 1987). Z-shaped incision (1, 2).
d Z-plasty and suture; if necessary, the crus can be underlaid with some fibrous tissue or cartilage (see **Fig. 10.17**; p. 145).

Free Skin Graft
(See **Fig. 2.22**, p. 16)

When the skin is exhausted, in multimorbid or very old patients, we still occasionally use free, thick split-thickness skin grafts after conditioning the wound bed for the graft. (**Fig. 10.100**, see also **Fig. 2.22**). Conditioning of granulation tissue is necessary if the color match is poor (see **Fig. 5.52j, l**).

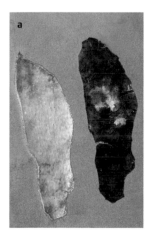
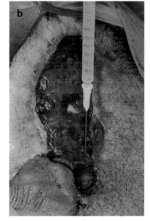
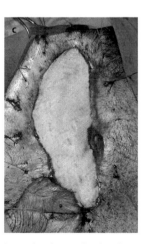
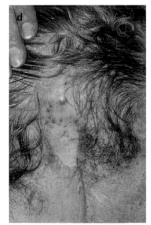

Fig. 10.100a–d Free split-thickness skin graft (from the upper leg or buttock).
a Pattern of the defect of the auricular region after tumor resection.

b, c The skin is glued and sutured to the defect (if there is bare bone, holes are drilled and granulation tissue should be conditioned). The graft fixation sutures are left long for light pressure dressing (see **Fig. 2.22b, c**, p. 16).
d Result years later.

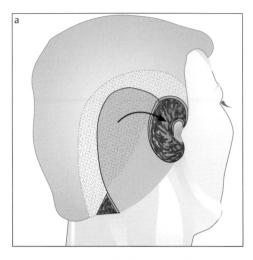

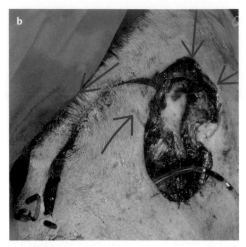

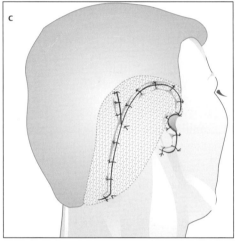

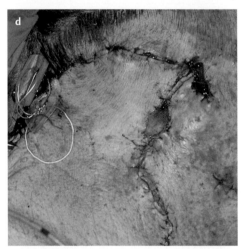

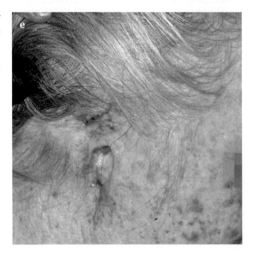

Fig. 10.101a–e   Reconstruction with an inferiorly and posteriorly based transposition or rotation flap.
a, b Incision of the flap.
c, d Closure of the defects (submandibular incision for neck dissection).
e Result.

Rotation Flap of the Neck
(**Fig. 10.101**)

Reconstruction with Rotation Flaps (Fig. 10.101) and Double (Bilobed) Flaps (Figs. 10.102 and 10.103)
Using recently introduced free microvascular flap transfer (see Chapter 14), we finally show some double flaps (bilobed flaps, see p. 187ff.) that we have used for auricular region repair, sometimes with neck dissection (**Figs. 10.102** and **10.103**). (Reconstruction with a free flap see pp. 213, 214).

Bone-Anchored Defect Protheses
In all these cases we offer bone-anchored retention elements and silicone defect prostheses (**Fig. 10.104**; see Weerda, 2007, pp. 269, 270)

Fig. 10.102a–c Reconstruction with posteriorly based neck rotation flaps.

a Neck flaps after tumor re-excision and neck dissection.

b The defects are closed.

c Result nearly 2 years after reconstruction.

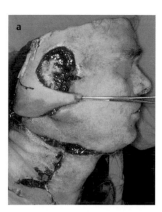
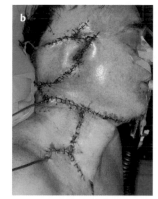
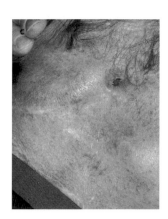

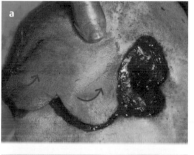
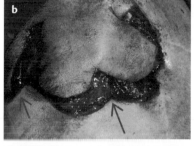
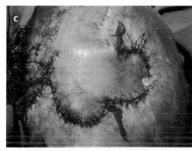

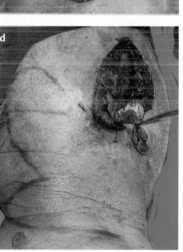
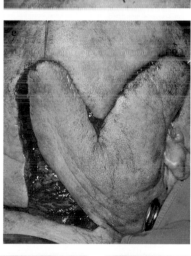
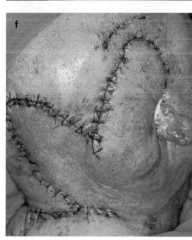

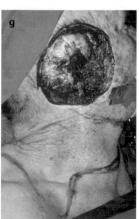
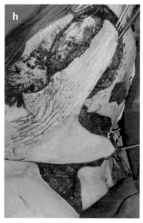
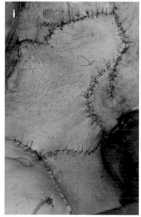
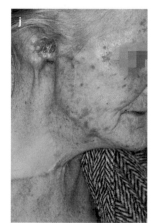

Fig. 10.103a–j   Different bilobed flaps for reconstruction of the auricular region.

a Petrosectomy, a superiorly, posteriorly based flap is incised.

b, c The defects are closed.

d–f Anteriorly, inferiorly based flap.

g–i Inferiorly posteriorly based flap.

j Result 2 years after operation.

(d–j with neck dissection)

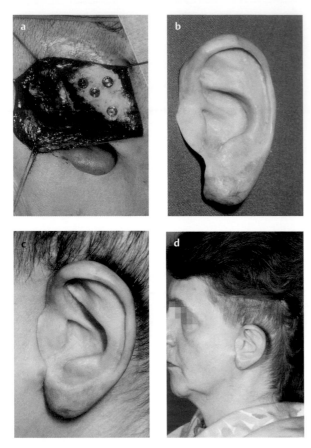

Fig. 10.104a–d Bone-anchored retention elements for fastening a silicone defect prosthesis.
a Retention elements.
b Silicone defect prosthesis.
c, d The prosthesis is fixed to the retention elements (Greiner and Weerda in Weerda, 2007, p. 268ff.).

III Rib Cartilage, Myocutaneous and Free Flaps, and Microvascular Surgery

11 Rib Cartilage

Cartilage is a bradytrophic tissue (scant blood supply) and, as such, is excellent for reconstruction and augmentation of the trachea, nose, cheek, skin, and ear (Weerda 1985a).

Obtaining Rib Cartilage for Ear Reconstruction
(Fig. 11.1)

Rib cartilage is generally obtained from the same side of the thorax, under general anesthesia. Small

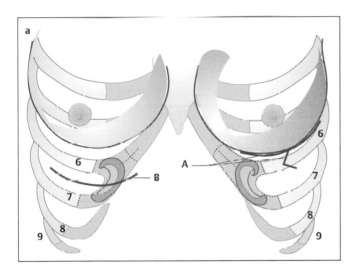

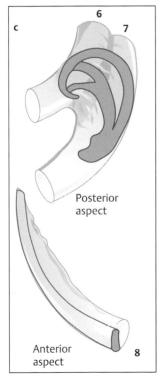

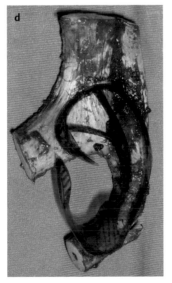

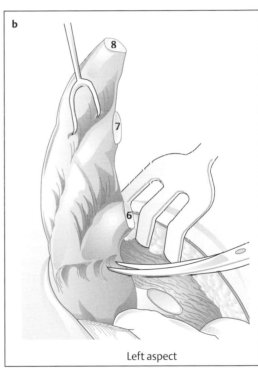

Left aspect

Fig. 11.1a, b Harvesting rib cartilage (generally we use the same side).
a In women, the incision is placed in the inframammary fold (A), aided if necessary by a small Z-shaped extension. In men, the incision is made between the sixth and seventh ribs (B). The synchondrotic region of ribs 6 and 7 will supply a sufficient block for carving the auricular framework.
b The incision is deepened through all layers to the sixth, seventh, and eighth ribs, which are sectioned at the chondro-osseous junction. The surgeon carefully dissects close to the rib surface or between the cartilage and perichondrium (risk of pleural injury; may use a cautery knife).
c, d Ribs 6, 7, and 8 (or 7, 8, and 9) are removed for the auricular reconstruction.
(c: preparing of the helix of the 8th rib.)

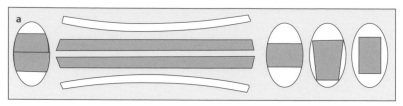
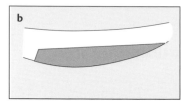
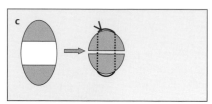
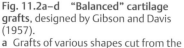

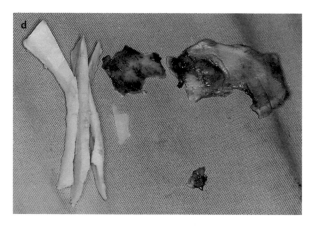

Fig. 11.2a–d "Balanced" cartilage grafts, designed by Gibson and Davis (1957).
a Grafts of various shapes cut from the center of a rib.
b Nasal dorsal onlay graft from the ninth rib.
c The graft shape can be stabilized by sewing together two pieces of cartilage that have opposite warping tendencies.
d Thin warped parts of the rib or preserved cartilage of the septum, as well as conchal cartilage (see **Figs. 2.24** and **10.46**; p. 162) can be used for partial or total nose reconstruction (see **Figs. 5.52–5.54**).

etal pleura, and an airtight layered closure, there should be no further difficulties. The fascial and subcutaneous layers should be closed separately. We generally use 4-0 (or 3-0) intracutaneous monofilament sutures for skin closure (see **Fig. 2.5**).

Preparation of Cartilage Grafts
(Fig. 11.2; Nagata 1994)

Some types of cartilage graft, such as nasal onlay grafts, can warp after implantation. This has led to the use of "balanced" grafts, as suggested by Gibson and Davis (1958) (**Fig. 11.2**). The graft should be cut from the center of the cartilage to minimize its warping tendency (**Fig. 11.2a, d**). Various techniques of graft preparation are illustrated in the figure. Cartilage segments with different warping tendencies can be assembled to produce a more stable graft (**Fig. 11.2c**). Generally, the perichondrium is removed, or at least scored, since the graft tends to warp in the direction of the perichondrium. Parts of the preserved nasal septum or the thin warped parts of the rib cartilage, as well as conchal cartilage (see **Fig. 2.24**), can be used for reconstruction after partial or total loss of the nose (**Fig. 11.2d**; see also **Figs. 5.52–5.54**).

amounts of cartilage can be taken from the fourth, fifth, or sixth rib, close to the sternum. We usually incise along the inframammary fold in women (**Fig. 11.1a, A**) and parallel to the donor site in men (**Fig. 11.1a, B**). The seventh rib is the longest cartilaginous rib and the last rib that extends to the sternum. The eighth rib is somewhat shorter and is often connected to the seventh rib by a synchondrosis. The sixth and seventh ribs generally supply a sufficient block to carve the body of the auricular framework (**Figs. 11.1** and **11.3**). The eighth rib can be used to make the **helical rim**, if it is at least 8 cm long (preferably 9–10 cm).

Operative Technique
We usually anesthetize the incision site with a local anesthetic solution containing epinephrine (diluted 1:200,000). The skin is incised parallel to the rib, or over the costal arch (eighth rib), and all layers are divided down to the rib. Attention is given to the pleura, which should remain intact if at all possible. When whole cartilaginous ribs are removed, the muscle is cut close to the cartilage with an electrocautery device, or the perichondrium is dissected from the cartilage surface. If pleural injury occurs (under general anesthesia), a small piece of fascia (free or pedicled) should be glued over the defect and the wound closed over a suction drain while ventilation is maintained. With a small wound in the pari-

Carving an Auricular Framework
(Fig. 11.3)

The framework should be as delicate as possible and **~3 mm smaller than the film pattern** in all dimensions (see **Fig. 10.44**, p. 161). The block from which the main framework is carved may be obtained from the ipsilateral side (Weerda, Nagata: operative side, easier access) or from the contralateral side (Brent 1976; Siegert) (**Figs. 11.1** and **11.3a, b**).

Instruments
The instruments for framework fabrication consist of no. 11 and no. 15 scalpel blades, special sharp gouges (see **Fig. 2.7a, 7**) 2 to 5 mm in width, 5-0 wire suture material, and 5-0 braided absorbable sutures

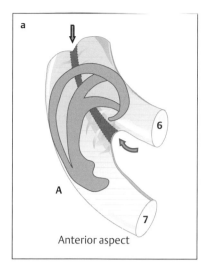

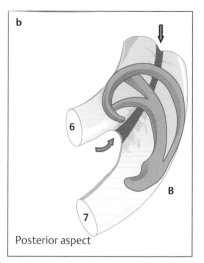

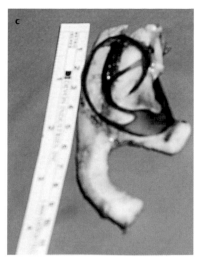

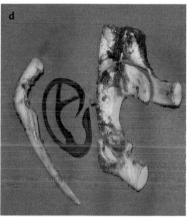

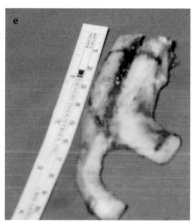

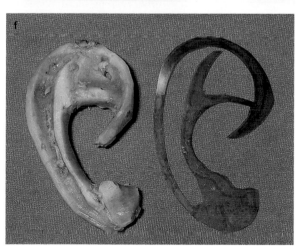

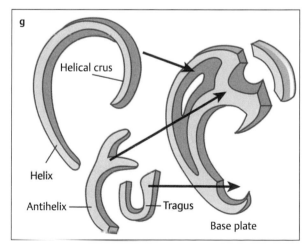

Fig. 11.3a–l Fabricating a **cartilage framework for total auricular reconstruction** (generally right-side thorax for a right auricle).

a, b The pattern is placed on the exposed cartilage: A, the **posterior side** of the cartilage for an **ipsilateral** reconstruction (A); the **anterior side** for a **contralateral** reconstruction (B; see **Fig. 11.1c**). Synchondrosis between the sixth and seventh ribs (arrow).

c–f Different possibilities of carving a cartilaginous support out of different rib blocks (the pattern is 2–3 mm smaller than the intact auricle).

g The main framework for a right ear (~3 mm smaller than the proposed auricle). Arrow: synchondrosis (see **Fig. 10.89d**). Helical rim carved normally from the eighth (or ninth) rib, 9 to 10 cm long (technique of Nagata, 1994, modification).

Fig. 11.3 h–m ▶

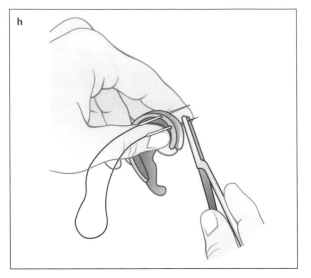

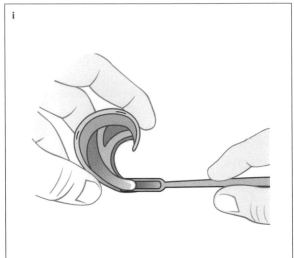

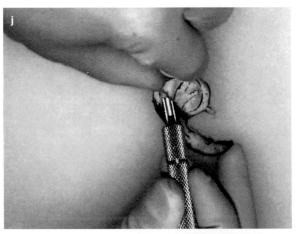

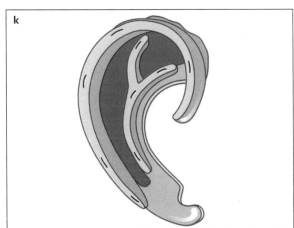

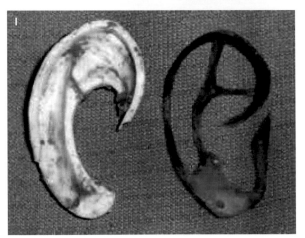

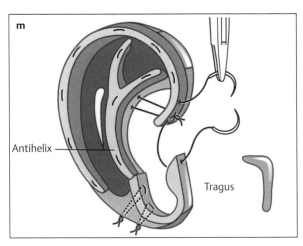

Antihelix

Tragus

Fig. 11.3h–m

h The helical rim is attached to the main framework with 5-0 wire sutures and/or 4-0 Vicryl (Ethicon, Germany) sutures (doubly armed, straight needles). Arrow: synchrosis.

i Carving a support, using 6th and 7th rib in this way, and the 8th rib is carved and sutured to the helical rim (see **Fig. 11.3h, i**).

k, l, m Supports for a right ear.

(e.g., Vicryl; Instruments see **Fig. 2.7a,7; g, 13**, see appendix p ...) on a P3 (Ethicon, Germany) needle. The framework is carved 3 mm smaller than the pattern. In most cases, all of the main framework can be fabricated from the sixth and seventh ribs (**Fig. 11.3a–c**); otherwise it must be assembled from smaller segments. The helical rim is carved separately from the eighth (or ninth) rib, which should be at least 8 to 9 cm long (see **Figs. 11.1c, 11.3d** and **g, k** and **m**). The rim should be 8 to 10 mm wide and is affixed to the main framework with doubly armed wire or absorbable suture material (4-0 or 5-0 on straight needles) (**Fig. 11.3e** in l pattern, 3 mm smaller than the contralateral ear). (The wire knots should be burried in the cartilage).

12 Myocutaneous Island Flaps

K. Sommer, S. Remmert, H. Weerda

Pectoralis Major Island Flap
(**Fig. 12.1**)

Flap type:
Myocutaneous island flap of the axial pattern type (see **Figs. 1.3** and **1.4**).

Flap components:
Skin, subcutaneous fat, fascia, muscle (pectoralis major, vessels).

Use:
Myocutaneous island flap for reconstructing major defects in the neck and face (microvascular free transfer is possible).

Vascular pedicle:
The skin and muscle are supplied by the **thoraco-acromial artery**, which is the second branch of the axillary artery past the scalene interval. The flap is supplied by the pectoral branches of the artery and their venae comitantes.

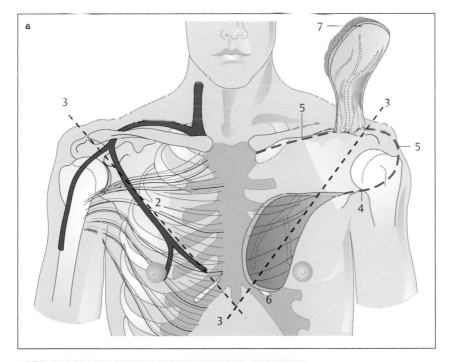
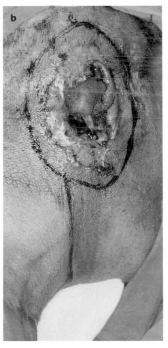
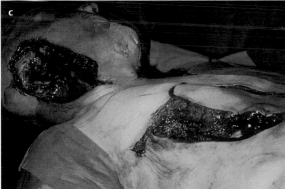

Fig. 12.1a–g
a **Myocutaneous pectoralis major island flap.**
1   Axillary artery.
2   Thoracoacromial artery.
3   Ariyan's line.
4   Incision for raising the flap (deltopectoral flap design).
5   Incision for a deltopectoral flap (see **Fig. 13.1**).
6   Incision outlining the myocutaneous flap.
7   Length of the flap.
b Tumor of the auricular region.
c Reconstruction of the auricular region after tumor resection and petrosectomia.

Fig. 12.1d–g   ▶

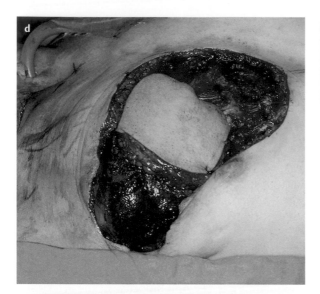

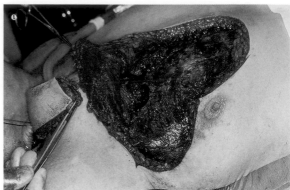

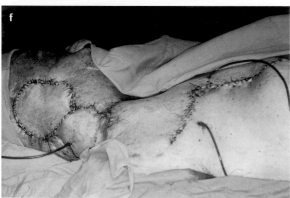

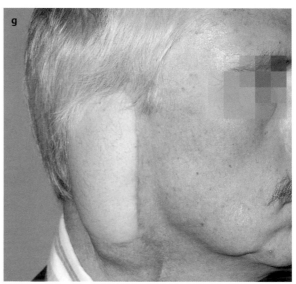

Fig. 12.1d–g
d, e The island flap is prepared and pulled through the skin bridge (**a** 5).

f The defect is covered and the wounds closed.
g Result.

Position:
Supine.

Flap size:
Maximum 10 × 20 cm.

Flap elevation:
An imaginary line from the acromion of the scapula to the xiphoid process of the sternum marks the axis of the nutrient pectoral branches (**Fig. 12.1**, 3). The pivot point of the pectoralis major island flap is located just below the middle third of the clavicle. The pedicle must be long enough to reach from the pivot point at the clavicle to the recipient site in the head and neck region (**Fig. 12.1**, 7). The skin paddle should be placed medial to the nipple whenever possible. The incision is carried across the thorax (**Fig. 12.1**, 4), the skin is undermined to the lower incision for the subsequent transfer (**Fig. 12.1**, 4), and the skin, muscle, and underlying fascia are incised to outline the flap (**Fig. 12.1**, 6). The muscular portion of the flap should be slightly larger than the skin pad-

dle. Next, the skin is sutured to the subcutaneous fat on the muscular fascia, to prevent shearing of the myocutaneous perforators. Proceeding from below upward, the pectoralis major muscle is elevated from the chest wall on its nutrient vascular pedicle, along with the deep muscular fascia. The arc of rotation can be increased by releasing the humeral and clavicular muscle attachments, leaving about a 4-cm-wide muscle pedicle to protect the nutrient vessels. **The skin outline of a deltopectoral flap should be preserved** (**Fig. 12.1**, 5) so that this flap will also be available if needed. When the island flap has been elevated to the clavicle, it is rotated 180° and carefully tunneled under the skin and over the clavicle to reach the defect (**Fig. 12.1**, 7).

Indications and advantages:
The pectoralis major island flap can be used in reconstructions of the pharynx, tongue, face, and neck, and especially to cover the carotid artery when this vessel is at risk because of prior irradiation. Tumor excision and reconstruction can be completed in one

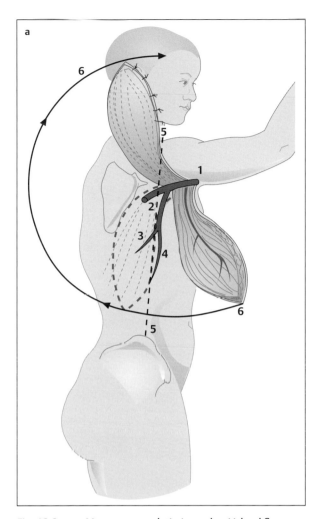

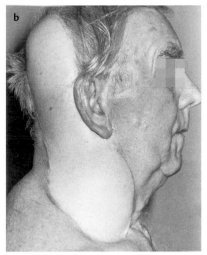

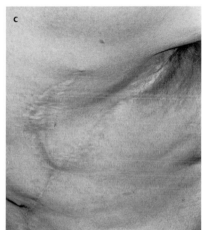

Fig. 12.2a–c   Myocutaneous latissimus dorsi island flap.

a
1   Axillary artery.
2   Subscapular artery.
3   Circumflex scapular artery.
4   Thoracodorsal artery.

The flap is raised behind a line from the center of the iliac crest to the anterior axillary fold (5). The flap is based on the thoracodorsal artery (4). The initial incision is made over the anterior border of the latissimus dorsi muscle, following the line shown (5). The very large flap has a long arc of rotation (6) that can reach all head and neck defects (see text).

b   Coverage of the scalp, postauricular region, and neck, with a latissimus dorsi island muscle flap following melanoma resection.

c   Donor site after completion of healing (surgeon S. Remmert).

operation (**Fig. 12.1b–g**). We find that the vascular pedicle has a consistent anatomic course. Direct closure is possible in most patients. There is no need to reposition the patient when raising the flap. The pectoralis major flap can be combined with a deltopectoral flap (**Fig. 12.1, 5**) or a latissimus dorsi island flap (see **Fig. 12.2**). It can also be used as a purely muscular flap or myofascial flap without a skin paddle.

Disadvantages and complications:
A large donor defect will require skin grafting. Esthetic objections are most common in women, owing to breast distortion, and the incision should be placed in the inframammary fold whenever possible. Thick subcutaneous fat and muscle bulk make it difficult to model the flap. Long-term results can be marred by volume reduction due to shrinkage and scarification.

Heavy body hair in male patients limits the indications for this flap in reconstructions of the oral cavity and pharynx.

Latissimus Dorsi Island Flap
(**Fig. 12.2**)

Flap type:
Myocutaneous island flap of the axial pattern type (see **Figs. 1.3** and **1.4**).

Flap components:
Skin, subcutaneous fat, fascia, muscle (latissimus dorsi).

Use:
Myocutaneous island flap, microvascular anastomosis (see **Fig. 14.3**).

Vascular pedicle:
The vascular bundle supplying the muscle consists of the thoracodorsal artery and vein (**Fig. 12.2**), which are a continuation of the subscapular artery and vein and give rise to the circumflex scapular artery and vein ~2 to 4 cm below their origin from the axillary artery and vein (**Fig. 12.2**). Several millimeters below the origin of the circumflex scapular artery, a vessel springs from the thoracodorsal artery to supply the serratus anterior muscle. The caliber of the vessel increases toward the axillary artery and is ~2 to 4 mm at its origin. The vascular pedicle is ~10 to 15 cm long. The venae comitantes are often paired but have a common termination in the axillary vein.

Flap size:
The latissimus dorsi flap is the largest myocutaneous flap used in plastic reconstructive surgery. It has a maximum useful size of 20 × 35 cm ("tennis racket" flap; **Fig. 12.2a**, 6).

Position:
Lateral decubitus.

Flap elevation:
A line is drawn (**Fig. 12.2a**, 5) from the center of the iliac crest to the posterior axillary line. The vascular bundle enters the muscle on that line ~10 to 12 cm below the axilla, and this point is marked on the skin. The connecting line runs ~2 cm behind the anterior border of the latissimus dorsi muscle and also represents the rotational axis of the flap. The skin paddle should be designed over the anterior border of the muscle, as this area has the greatest density of perforator vessels. The initial incision is made along the line to the level of the proposed flap, and the anterior border of the latissimus dorsi is exposed. The vascular pedicle is identified medial to the anterior border, and traced to the site where it enters the muscle. The vascular pedicle is dissected superiorly to its origin from the maxillary artery. The perimeter of the skin paddle is incised, and the latissimus dorsi muscle is bluntly separated from the serratus anterior muscle from the anterior side, using some sharp dissection

inferiorly. The skin is sutured to the subcutaneous fat on the muscle, to prevent shearing of the perforator vessels. A myocutaneous island flap is created by rotating the tissue 180° on the myovascular pedicle at the level of the axillary artery (**Fig. 12.2a**, 6). The flap is carefully passed through a prepared subcutaneous tunnel to its destination, and sutured into place. If the flap cannot reach the defect, it can be transferred as a microvascular free flap.

Indications and advantages:
- The long vascular pedicle can reach any site in the head and neck region.
- There is a constant, large-caliber vascular pedicle.
- It is the largest flap in reconstructive surgery.
- In most cases, the donor site can be closed primarily with an acceptable cosmetic result.
- We have seen no significant functional deficits at the donor site, and the flap can be used in conjunction with other flaps.
- The peripheral vascular pattern allows multiple flaps to be based on one pedicle.
- We have had no breast mutilation.

Disadvantages and complications:
- The patient must be repositioned during the operation.
- When a very large flap is raised, the donor site requires partial coverage with split skin grafts.
- The large wound area often leads to seroma formation.
- The transferred tissue tends to shrink and scarify over time.

The latissimus dorsi island flap can also be used as free flap (see **Fig. 14.3**).

Neurovascular Infrahyoid Myofascial Flap of Remmert et al. (1994)
(**Fig. 12.3**)

Flap type:
Neurovascular myofascial flap of the axial pattern type (see **Figs. 1.3** and **1.4**).

Flap components:
Muscle (infrahyoid muscle group), fascia.

Use:
As a neurovascular myofascial island flap or microvascular free flap with a neural pedicle (**Fig. 12.3a, b**).

Vascular pedicle:
The superior thyroid artery (**Fig. 12.3a, b**, 4) usually arises from the external carotid artery but may also arise from the bifurcation of the common carotid artery. The thyroid vein drains chiefly into the facial vein and internal jugular vein. A segmental drainage

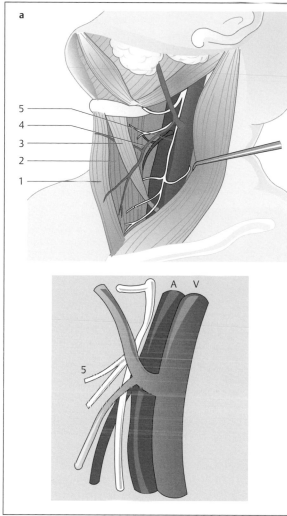

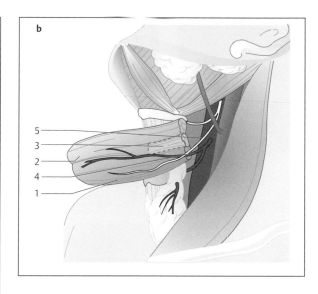

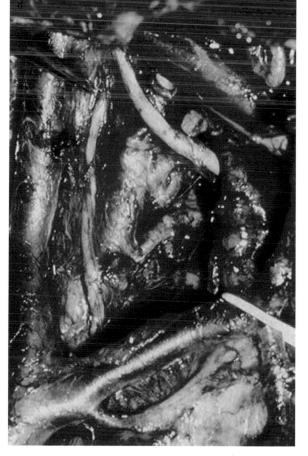

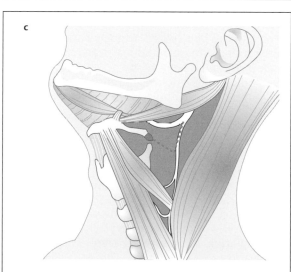

Fig. 12.3a–d Neurovascular infrahyoid myofascial flap of Remmert (1994).

a The infrahyoid muscles (1, 2, 3) are based on the superior thyroid artery and vein (4) and on the superior root of the ansa cervicalis (5).

b The myofascial flap is divided, and the nutrient vessels (4) and ansa cervicalis (5) are dissected.

c, d Junction of the hypoglossal nerve and the superior root of the deep ansa cervicalis, located 1 cm above and lateral to the posterior crus of the hyoid bone.

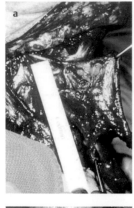

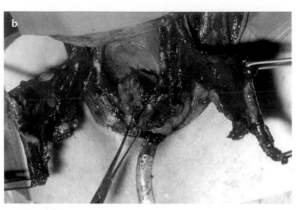

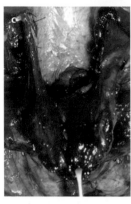

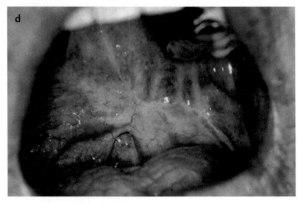

Fig. 12.4a–d Tongue reconstruction with the neurovascular bilateral infrahyoid myofascial flaps of Remmert (Fig. 12.3; see also Fig. 14.1; Remmert et al. 1994, 1997, Remmert 2001).

a The muscles are prepared and dissected.

b The upper part of the omohyoid muscle is separated, and the muscles of both sides are sutured together.

c The neo-tongue is pulled through into the oral cavity, and the upper parts of the omohyoid muscles are anchored in the tonsilar areas of both sides.

d The neo-tongue is covered with a radial forearm flap, and sensation is restored by anastomosing the lateral antebrachial cutaneous nerve to the lingual nerve. Situation 1 year after reconstruction.

pattern exists in 20% of cases. The dissected vascular pedicle is 2 cm long, with an arterial caliber of 1.5 mm and a venous diameter of 2 mm. The superior root of the deep ansa cervicalis, which supplies motor innervation to the infrahyoid muscles, is found just lateral and superior to the posterior cornu of the hyoid bone (**Fig. 12.3c, d**).

Flap size:
Up to 3.5 × 11.5 cm.

Position:
Supine.

Flap elevation:
The infrahyoid muscle group is reached through the approach for a standard neck dissection. The superior root of the ansa cervicalis is identified above and lateral to the posterior cornu of the hyoid bone (**Fig. 12.3c, d**), and must be preserved along with the superior thyroid artery and vein (**Fig. 12.3b**). The musculature is divided cranial to the hyoid bone and along the linea alba, whereupon the flap is elevated from the larynx and thyroid gland, in a medial to lateral direction (**Fig. 12.4a, b**). The thyrohyoid muscle should be left in place to protect the superior vascular bundles of the larynx. The rest of the dissection proceeds from below upward along the large vessels, including the ansa cervicalis of the hypoglossal nerve in the dissection. Based only on the neurovascular

bundle, the flap can now be rotated into the area of the defect (**Fig. 12.4c, d**).

Indications and advantages:
• The flap can be used unilaterally or bilaterally; it is particularly useful for reconstructing the tongue and pharynx, since it can actively contract, owing to voluntary innervation from the superior root of the ansa cervicalis.
• The flap can be exposed through a standard neck dissection, with no additional scars or cutaneous defects (**Figs. 12.3 and 12.4b**).
• Voluntary innervation via the ansa cervicalis tends to reduce shrinkage and scarring of the muscle tissue.
• The myofascial flap is relatively thin and pliable (Remmert et al. 1994, 1995, 1998).

Disadvantages and complications:
• The flap cannot be used in patients with extensive cervical metastasis.
• If the vascular pedicle has a low origin, the arc of rotation will be insufficient to reach the oral cavity, necessitating microsurgical transplantation and elongation.

13 Deltopectoral Flap

S. Remmert, K. Sommer, H. Weerda

Although this flap (see **Fig. 12.1a**, 5) is credited to Bakamjian (1965), it was first mentioned in the German literature during the 1900s, and in the American literature in the early 2000s. Once commonly used, the deltopectoral flap has now been largely superseded by the pectoralis major island flap and free flaps.

Flap type:
Fasciocutaneous flap of the random pattern type (see **Fig. 1.2**).

Flap components:
Skin, subcutaneous fat, muscular fascia.

Use:
As a regional transposition flap.

Vascular supply:
First through fourth perforating branches of the internal thoracic artery (internal mammary artery) (**Fig. 13.1a**).

Position:
Supine.

Flap size:
Width 8 to 12 cm, length 18 to 22 cm (the flap can be extended to the shoulder) (**Fig. 13.1a, b**).

Flap elevation:
The flap is designed larger than the size of the ablative defect. When the flap is raised, the fascial layers of the pectoralis major and deltoid muscles should be taken with the flap because they transmit the perforating branches. Care is taken not to kink the flap or rotate it excessively when suturing it into the defect. As much of the donor defect as possible is closed directly, and the rest is split-skin grafted. No pressure should be placed on the flap during the first few postoperative days, and the chest, shoulder, and neck should be immobilized. Adequate wound drainage should also be maintained, and any hematomas under the flap should be evacuated without delay.

Fig. 13.1a–c Deltopectoral flap for neck defect reconstruction after radiation treatment.
a The flap is incised (see **Fig. 12.1a**, 5) and extended to the shoulder.
b The cervical defect is covered.
c Result after weeks.

Indications and advantages:
- The deltopectoral flap is most commonly transferred upward to close postirradiation fistulas and resurface large cutaneous defects in the neck (**Fig. 13.1a, c**), especially in cases where the myocutaneous pectoralis major island flap is no longer available.

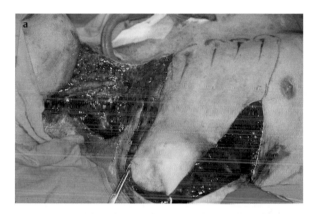

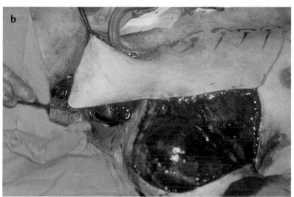

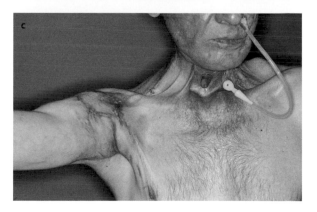

- The vascular supply is constant.
- The flap is easy to expose and dissect.
- The flap provides ~250 cm^2 of skin.
- The flap has an arc of ~45° to 135°.

Disadvantages and complications:
- When a large flap is raised, split-skin grafting of the donor site is required.
- There may be an unfavorable cosmetic result, owing to exposed scars.
- The flap has a significantly lower survival rate in patients who are emaciated, have undergone radiation therapy, or have severe cardiovascular problems. In these cases, there should be a delay before the transfer.

14 Free Flaps

S. Remmert, K. Sommer, H. Weerda

Radial Forearm Flap

(**Fig. 14.1**)

Flap type:
Fasciocutaneous (neurovascular) flap or pure fascial flap of the axial pattern type (see **Figs. 1.3** and **1.4**).

Flap components:
Skin, subcutaneous fat, and fascia (may include the sensory nerve).

Use:
Microvascular flap.

Vascular pedicle:
The flap is based on the radial artery, which is a continuation of the brachial artery. Its caliber is ~1 to 2 mm. The radial artery is accompanied in its distal portion by two venae comitantes (**Fig. 14.1a, b**, 2), which unite at the elbow to form one vein ~2 mm in diameter. The flap is innervated by the lateral antebrachial cutaneous nerve (**Fig. 14.1b**, 9), which runs parallel to the superficial cephalic vein.

Flap size:
Maximum 5 × 15 cm.

Position:
Supine.

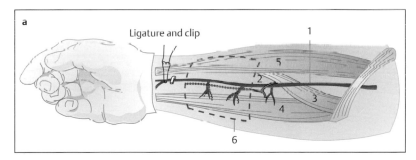

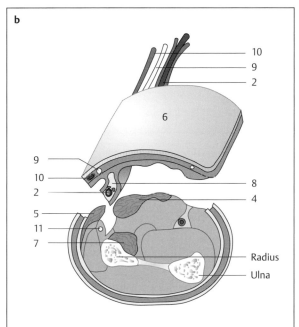

Fig. 14.1a–j
a Design of the radial forearm flap, a free flap based on the radial artery and two venae comitantes (2) (see text).
1 Brachial artery.
2 Radial artery.
3 Pronator teres muscle.
4 Flexor carpi radialis muscle.
5 Brachioradialis muscle.
6 Flap.
7 Flexor pollicis longus muscle.
8 Deep fascia.
9 Lateral antebrachial cutaneous nerve.
10 Cephalic vein.
11 Radial nerve.
b Cross-section of the forearm (viewed from above; from Walter 1997).

Fig. 14.1 c–j   ▶

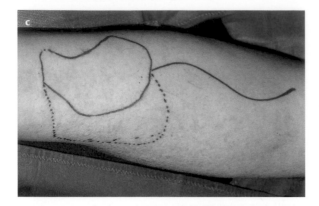

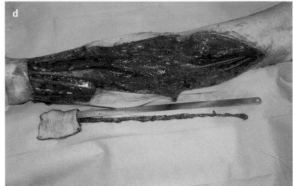

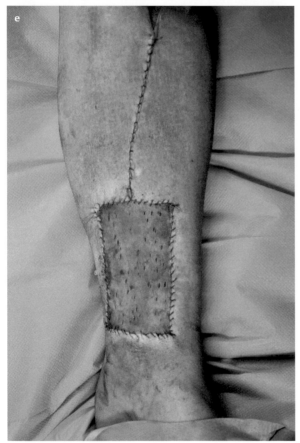

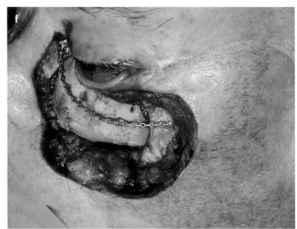

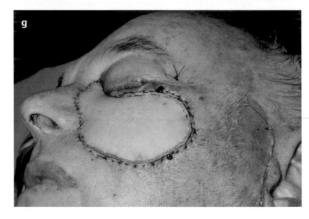

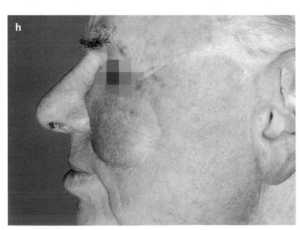

Fig. 14.1c–h
c The radialis flap is outlined (right arm).
d The flap is harvested with a long pedicle.
e The donor defect was closed by direct closure and a split-skin graft.
f Defect of the cheek after tumor excision, the orbital rim is reconstructed with rib and a miniplate.
g The flap is sutured to the defect.
h Result after 1 year. (The vessels were anastomosed to the facial vessels).

Fig. 14.1 i–j   ▶

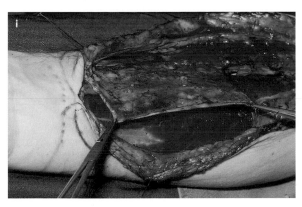
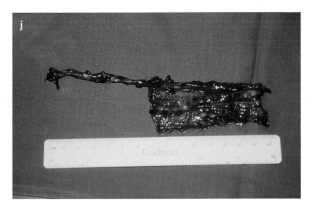

Fig. 14.1i–j
i, j   A fascial flap is harvested.

Flap elevation:
Before the operation, it is determined whether the hand will survive without radial arterial input. This is done by performing an Allen test or using Doppler ultrasound or angiography to check for adequate collateral flow via the ulnar artery. The flap size is marked on the skin (**Fig. 14.1c**), and an S-shaped incision is made from the elbow to the proximal margin of the flap, dividing the forearm fascia. Next, the muscle bellies of the flexor carpi radialis and brachioradialis are identified (**Fig. 14.1a, 4 and 5**) and separated from their intermuscular septum. The radial artery and its two venae comitantes lie between these muscle bellies on the fascia of the flexor digitorum superficialis. Next, the perimeter of the flap is incised, dividing the fascia of the flexor digitorum superficialis at the ulnar border. The dissection of the flap and muscular fascia (**Fig. 14.1b, 8**) proceeds from the ulnar to the radial side, avoiding injury to the peritendinous tissue. The flap should not be developed too far distally, to preserve the extensor retinaculum. Next the radial artery and its accompanying veins are ligated at the distal margin of the flap. The next step is to dissect the fasciocutaneous tissue from the radial side, as far as the abductor pollicis longus and brachioradialis muscles, preserving the superficial branch of the radial nerve. The vascular pedicle is raised with the fascia of the flexor digitorum superficialis in a distal to proximal direction, and finally the radial artery and venae comitantes (or one deep vein draining into the accompanying veins) are ligated (**Fig. 14.1d**). The donor site is closed by a combination of direct closure and split-skin grafting (Remmert 1995; **Fig. 14.1e**).

Indications and advantages:
- The radial forearm flap is very good for reconstructions of the oral cavity, tongue, pharynx, and neck, as well as for defects in the face (**Fig. 14.1f–h**) and ear region.
- The vascular pedicle has a consistent length (**Fig. 14.1d**).
- The flap is pliable.

- There is no need to reposition the patient intraoperatively.
- Tumor resection and reconstruction can be performed in one operation.
- Two teams can work concurrently: one removes the tumor, while the other harvests the flap.
- When a radial forearm flap is used for tongue reconstruction, for example, sensation is restored by anastomosing the lateral antebrachial cutaneous nerve to the lingual nerve. A radial forearm flap can be used for reconstructing the cheek (**Fig. 14.1f–h**). A facial forearm flap can be harvested for ear reconstruction (**Fig. 14.1i, j**).

Disadvantages and complications:
- The donor forearm must be immobilized for 10 days.
- Split-skin grafting of the defect may lead to wound-healing problems in the flexor tendon area, and cosmetic morbidity.
- The flap may shrink by up to 25%.

Allen Test

The Allen test is used to determine whether the ulnar artery will adequately supply the hand following ligation of the radial artery. The patient is told to make a tight fist with the affected hand. Then the examiner simultaneously compresses the radial artery and ulnar artery, the patient slowly opens the hand, and pressure on the ulnar artery is released. In an abnormal test, the fingers do not show significant capillary fill (blush) within 5 seconds after ulnar artery release, and a radial forearm flap is contraindicated. A similar test is used intraoperatively. Following the usual dissection of the radial forearm flap and exposure of the axial vascular bundle, the radial artery is clipped at the distal margin of the flap. If oxygen saturation measured on the thumb does not fall below 97%, it is assumed that the ulnar artery is providing an adequate collateral supply, and the radial forearm flap can be raised (Remmert and Sommer 1993).

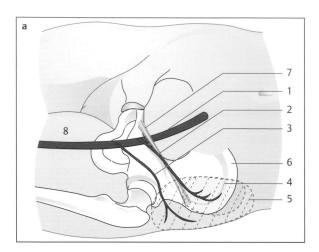

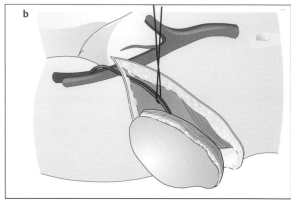

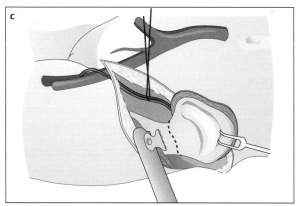

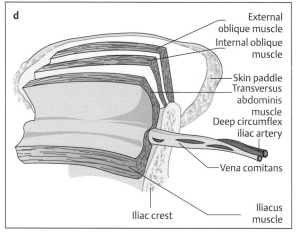

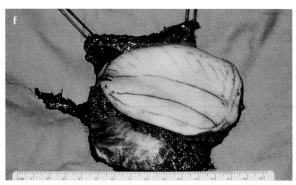

External oblique muscle
Internal oblique muscle
Skin paddle
Transversus abdominis muscle
Deep circumflex iliac artery
Vena comitans
Iliac crest
Iliacus muscle

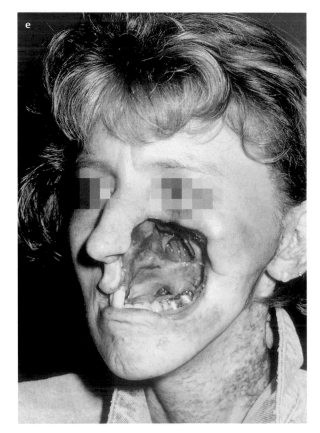

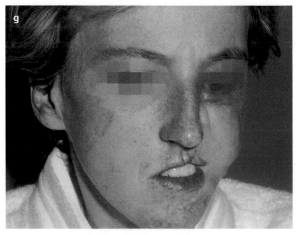

Groin Flap
(Fig. 14.2)

Flap type:
Osteomyocutaneous flap (composite or compound) of the axial pattern type.

Flap components:
Skin, subcutaneous, muscle (internal oblique), bone (ilium). The groin flap can be transferred as a bone graft only (iliac crest bone graft), as a bone graft with muscle, or as a bone graft with muscle and skin (osteomyocutaneous flap).

Use:
Microvascular transfer.

Vascular pedicle:
The osteomyocutaneous flap is supplied by the superficial and deep circumflex iliac arteries. The deep circumflex iliac artery is the more important of the two, arising from the external iliac artery posterior to the inguinal ligament (**Fig. 14.2a**, 1). Its vascular pedicle has a length of 80 to 120 mm and a caliber of 3 mm, and chiefly supplies the ilium. In 75% of cases, there is an ascending branch with perforators, which supplies the internal oblique muscle, along with a 2.5 × 8-cm skin area over the iliac crest (**Fig. 14.2a**, 4). The superficial circumflex iliac artery (**Fig. 14.2a**, 3) arises from the femoral artery 30 mm below the inguinal ligament. Its vascular pedicle has a length of 5 to 20 mm and a caliber of 1.5 mm. The vessel mainly supplies a 12 × 23 cm skin area over the iliac crest (**Fig. 14.2a**, 5). If only a small skin paddle is required, the deep circumflex iliac artery (**Fig. 14.2a**, 2) is the only vessel that needs to be anastomosed at the recipient site. If a larger skin paddle is needed, the superficial circumflex iliac artery (**Fig. 14.2a**, 3) should also be anastomosed (Remmert et al. 1998).

Position:
Supine.

Flap elevation:
First the inguinal ligament, femoral artery, and iliac crest are marked out on the skin (**Fig. 14.2a**, 6 and 7). The skin paddle is outlined and its perimeter incised, dividing the skin and subcutaneous tissue down to the abdominal wall musculature. When the skin paddle is raised from the external oblique muscle, an area of muscle ~3 × 8 cm is left on the upper iliac crest. The muscle and skin in this area should not be divided, to preserve the perforator vessels to the skin paddle. After the external oblique muscle has been divided, leaving a flap ~2 to 4 cm wide on the iliac crest, an adjacent internal oblique muscle flap based on the iliac crest is cut to match the size of the defect. The underlying transversus abdominis muscle is divided in the same way as the external oblique muscle, leaving a strip of muscle ~2 to 4 cm wide on the iliac crest. This muscular cuff transmits the deep circumflex iliac artery (**Fig. 14.2a**, 2) with its perforators. After the tensor fasciae latae and gluteus medius are separated from the lateral aspect of the ilium, the vascular pedicle is exposed by detaching all abdominal wall layers at the level of the anterior superior iliac spine. The deep circumflex iliac artery arises from the external iliac artery posterior to the inguinal ligament. The vascular pedicle is dissected free, proceeding in a medial to lateral direction as far as the anterior superior iliac spine. Finally, the iliacus muscle is released from the medial surface of the ilium, fully exposing both the medial and lateral aspects of the bone. A bone fragment of the necessary size and shape (determined from a pattern) is cut from the ilium, with an oscillating saw; the vascular pedicle is divided; and the osteomyocutaneous flap is transferred to the recipient site. The donor site is carefully closed in layers, to prevent hernia formation (Remmert et al. 1998).

Indications and advantages:
- This flap is used for reconstructions of the mandible, maxilla, cheek, and occasionally the forehead (**Fig. 14.2e–g**).
- There is consistent vascular anatomy.
- Skin, muscle, and bone can all be reconstructed with one flap.
- Bone from the iliac crest provides a good bed for dental implants.
- Tumor resection and reconstruction can be performed in one operation.
- There is no need to reposition the patient intraoperatively.

Fig. 14.2a–g
a The **groin flap** can be designed as a myocutaneous or osteomyocutaneous transfer (compound flap, see text).
1   External iliac artery.
2   Deep circumflex iliac artery.
3   Superficial circumflex iliac artery.
4   Size of the skin area supplied by the deep circumflex iliac artery.
5   Size of the skin area supplied by the superficial circumflex iliac artery.
6   Iliac crest.
7   Inguinal ligament.
8   Femoral artery.
b The skin paddle and muscle are elevated on the deep circumflex iliac artery and its venae comitantes (after Bootz and Müller 1992).
c The iliacus muscle is detached medially, the tensor fasciae latae and gluteus medius laterally, and the sartorius anteriorly. The bone fragment (outlined from a pattern) is removed with a saw.
d The composite (compound) iliac crest flap has been harvested with its skin paddle (viewed from the medial side).
e Defect after tumor resection.
f Compound iliaccrest flap (see **d**).
g Result 1 year after reconstruction, a lip refinement is planned (The vessels were anastomosed to the temporal vessels).

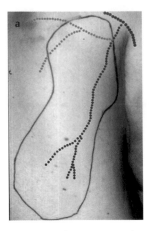
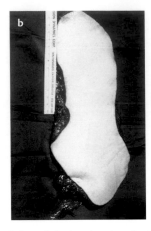
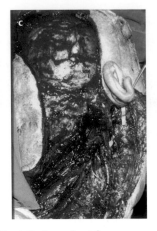
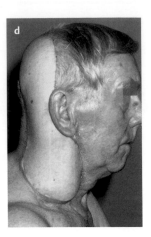

Fig. 14.3a–d   Covering a large defect of the head and neck with a latissimus dorsi flap.
a The flap is outlined and the vessels are marked.   c, d Defect and result after inset with microvascular anastomo-
b The flap is harvested.   sis.

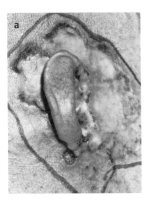
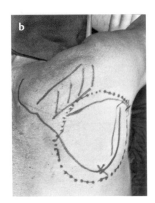
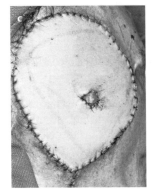
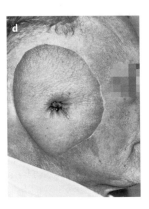

Fig. 14.4a–d   Coverage of the auricular region with a free parascapula flap anastomosed using a microvascular technique.
a Tumor recurrence of the auricular region after repeated   d Result after 4 weeks (the edema will settle with time) (sur-
  radiotherapy.   geon: S. Remmert).
b Parascapula flap, size (dotted line) and scapula outlined.
c Flap anatomosed on the temporal vessels and inset.

Disadvantages and complications:
- There is a risk of hernia formation.
- With a large skin paddle, both the deep and superficial circumflex iliac arteries must be anastomosed at the recipient site.
- Primary closure of the donor site is not possible when a large skin paddle is taken.
- Severe pain may occur.

The latissimus dorsi island (see **Figs. 12.2** and **12.3**) and the scapula and parascapula flap (see **Fig. 14.4**) can also be used as a free flap, using the microvascular anastomosing technique.

Transplants Anastomosed Using a Microvascular Technique
(**Figs. 14.3** and **14.4**)

These are, for example, the free latissimus dorsi flap, the radial artery forearm flap (see **Fig. 14.3**), the parascapular flap (**Fig. 14.4**), or the lateral upper arm flap.

Free transplants anastomosed on the superficial temporal artery and vein, the facial artery and vein, or other vessels are well suited to cover defects of the auricular region (**Fig. 14.4**) and are now the techniques of first choice (Weerda 2001).

Microvascular Surgery

Instrumentation
(Fig. 14.5)

The instruments required for microvascular surgery are relatively few in number: straight and curved microforceps (**Fig. 14.5a**), microscissors (**Fig. 14.5b**), and vascular clips and clip appliers (**Fig. 14.5c**). Microforceps or special spring-handled needle holders are excellent for suturing. Round-handled instruments are advantageous, as they can be rotated between the fingers and supported on the metacarpus. Vascular clips are needed to occlude the blood flow and keep the vessel ends from retracting into the soft tissues. Approximators (**Fig. 14.5d**) make it easier to hold the vessels in position and rotate them as needed to access the back wall. This special instrument set for microvascular suturing is complemented by various syringes, cotton swabs, and the suture material itself. Syringes are used to flush out the vessel ends with heparinized sodium chloride solution and to irrigate the vessels with lidocaine. Cotton swabs are used to soak up blood and irrigation fluid, and for hemostasis. The suture material of choice is monofilament Ethilon. Monofilament material does not have the wick action of multifilament material and does not cause tissue friction. Suture size is determined by the diameter of the vessels to be anastomosed. Sizes 9-0 and 10-0 are recommended for vessel diameters of ~1 mm, and 8-0 for diameters of 2 to 3 mm. We generally use ⅜ round-body needles such as MV-10, BV-4, and BV-2 (Ethicon).

Practicing for Microvascular Surgery

Cobbett coined the term "microvessel" for very small vessels that have an outer diameter of 3 mm or less. As the vessel diameter becomes smaller, there is greater potential for errors and complications associated with microvascular manipulations. For example, while 1 or 2 mm of narrowing in a large vessel like the femoral artery has virtually no functional significance, even a tiny reduction in cross-section can have major consequences when it occurs at the microvascular level. For this reason, microvascular anastomosis is a technically challenging procedure that requires a high degree of manual dexterity. In addition, a knowledge of coagulation processes, hemodynamics, the micromorphology of small vessels, and the terminal vascular branches in various tissues is essential for successful microvascular suturing and for the survival of transplanted or replanted tissues. These essential skills and knowledge are only acquired through experimental practice and study. A good way to learn the microvascular suturing technique is through a staged approach that starts with practice on experimental animals. White

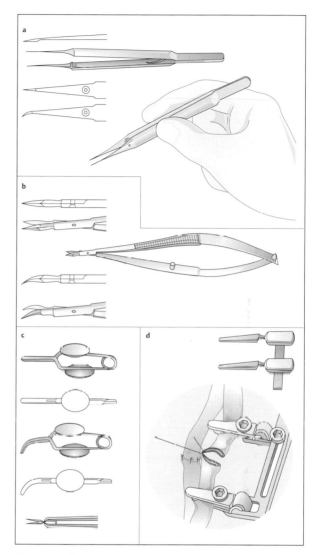

Fig. 14.5a–d Instruments for microvascular surgery.
a Straight and curved microforceps.
b Spring-handled microscissors, straight and curved (also: spring-handled needle holder with fine jaws).
c Vascular clips and clip applier.
d Approximators (double microclamps).

male rats with a body weight of 250 to 350 g are optimal. They have less fatty tissue than females, and the vessel diameters are larger.

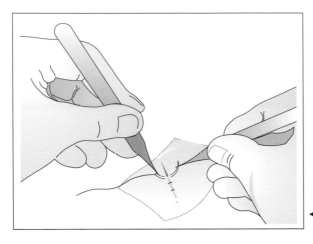

Knot-Tying Practice Under a Microscope or Binocular Loupe
(Figs. 14.6–14.9)

Microvascular Anastomosis in an Experimental Animal: Vascular Dissection in the Rat
(Fig. 14.10)

End-to-End Anastomosis of the Abdominal Aorta and Femoral Artery, Diameter 1 to 1.5 mm
(Figs. 14.11 and 14.12)

◀ **Fig. 14.6** **Knot tying** for microvascular anastomoses can be practiced on thin silicone film or surgical glove material.

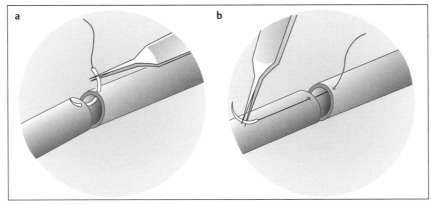

Fig. 14.7a, b
a End-to-end anastomosis, practiced in a thin silicone tube. The needle should enter and exit perpendicular to the vessel plane. Note the curved needle path.
b The needle (not the suture itself) is grasped with the needle holder and pulled. The suture is pulled through until the short end appears in the magnified field of view.

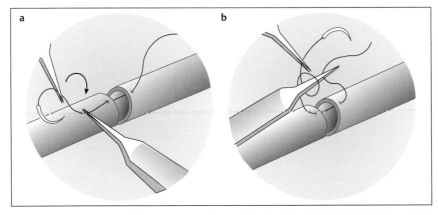

Fig. 14.8a, b Tying a right-handed knot.
a Held in the left forceps or micro-needle holder, the suture is passed once clockwise around the right forceps for an ordinary knot, or twice for a surgical knot.
b The suture is pulled through for the initial knot. A second knot can be added in the opposing direction (see **Fig. 14.9**).

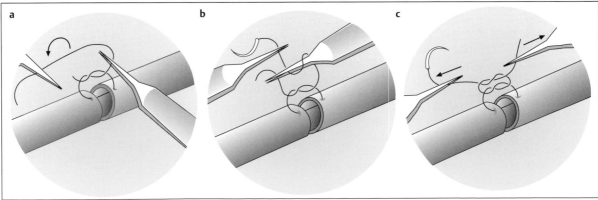

Fig. 14.9a–c Tying a **left-handed knot**.
a Held in the left forceps, the suture is passed counterclockwise around the right forceps.

b The other end of the suture is grasped with the right forceps.
c The knot is pulled tight.

Fig. 14.10a–c   Dissection in a rat, with exposure of major blood vessels.

a Supine dissection exposing the abdominal aorta, vena cava, and femoral vessels.

b The surrounding connective tissue is dissected off the vessels, grasping only the adventitia.

c The scissor dissection is directed parallel to the vessel axis.

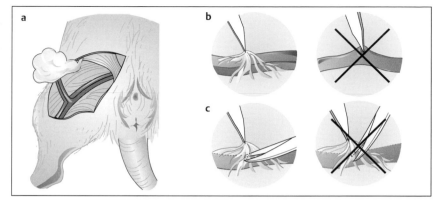

Fig. 14.11a–d   Preparing the **skeletonized vessel** for anastomosis.

a With the approximator in place, the vessel is divided perpendicular to the vessel axis.

b The cut ends are flushed out with heparinized Ringer solution, and/or milked with the forceps.

c, d Projecting adventitia is removed along with any remaining connective tissue, completely opening up the circumference of the vessel. The tissue is pulled past the vessel end with forceps, and cut flush with the edge of the media (visible through the transparent tissue).

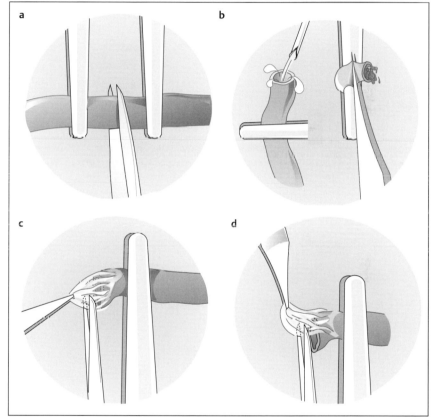

Fig. 14.12a–c   The approximated vessel ends are sewn together with interrupted sutures: placement of the **key sutures**.

a The first two sutures are the most important and most difficult. They are placed 120° apart in the line of the anastomosis (asymmetric biangulation). The left forceps are inserted into the vessel lumen and opened slightly to provide counterpressure for needle insertion (the forceps do not grasp the vessel ends).

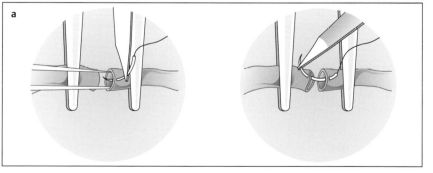

Fig. 14.12 b–c   ▶

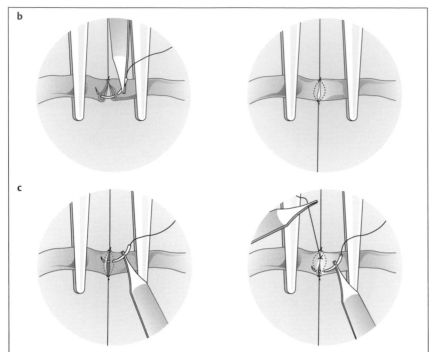

Fig. 14.12b–c
b The **second key suture** is placed 120° from the first. This causes the back walls of the vessel ends to retract slightly, clearing the way for placing intermediate sutures in the front wall.
c Placing the **intermediate sutures** in the front wall.

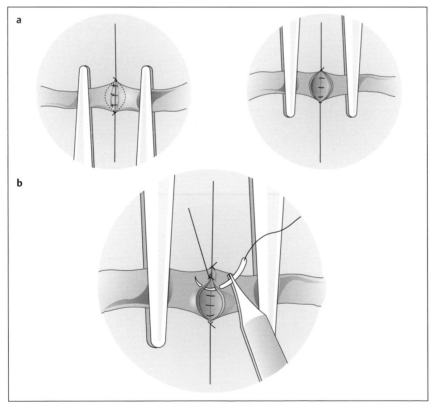

Fig. 14.13a–c   After the front wall sutures have been placed, the approximator is inverted, **rotating the vessels 180°**.
a The vessel ends at this stage show a typical diamond pattern.
b The intermediate sutures are placed as they were in the front wall. Gentle traction on the final suture opens up the lumen slightly and reduces the danger of grasping the front wall.

Fig. 14.13 c   ▶

End-to-End Anastomosis of the Inferior Vena Cava, Diameter 1 to 1.5 mm
(Fig. 14.13a)

End-to-Side Anastomosis
(Figs. 14.14 and 14.15)

Fig. 14.13a–c

c The end-to-end anastomosis is also used for veins. Traction perpendicular to the vessel axis places tension on the thinner-walled veins, opening up the collapsed lumen.

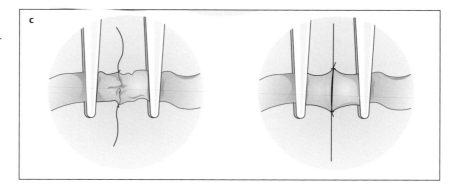

Fig. 14.14a, b End-to-side anastomosis.

a This technique is used to anastomose vessels of markedly different sizes, such as joining the typically small veins of a free flap to a large venous trunk at the recipient site. The suction effect provides for good venous return.

b The double clamps exert tension on the recipient vessel wall, which is incised longitudinally. The opening must match the lumen of the flap vessel. The elastic fibers in the vessel wall cause the opening to assume a rounded shape

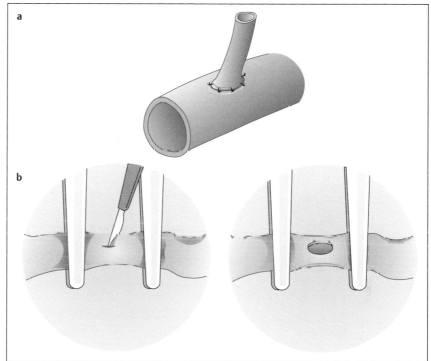

Fig. 14.15a–d Acland's technique of creating an **oval opening** for end-to-side anastomosis.

a The vessel wall is pierced with a microneedle. The wall tissue is elevated on the needle, and the raised area is excised with scissors.

b The **key sutures** are inserted. The first two sutures are placed **180° apart**.

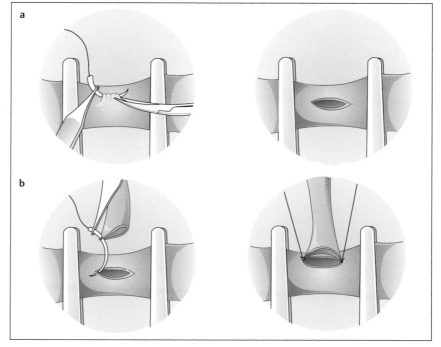

Fig. 14.15 c–d ▶

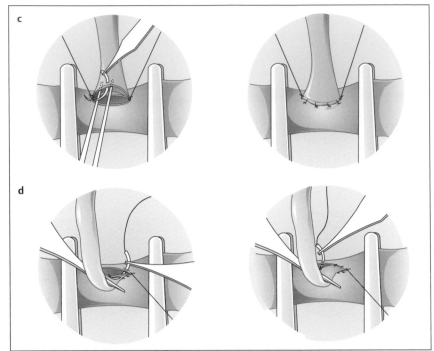

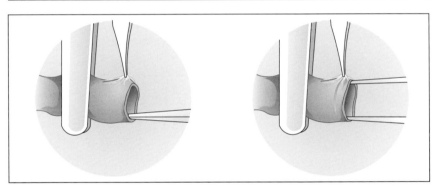

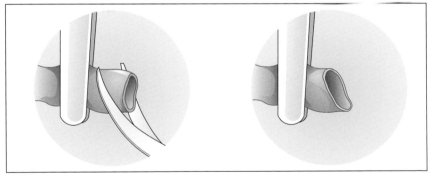

Fig. 14.15c–d
c The intermediate sutures are placed in the front wall.
d The flap vessel is lateralized with forceps or a heavy suture, and the **back wall is sutured**.

Fig. 14.16 If the **vessel calibers are nearly equal**, the smaller lumen can be gently dilated with forceps or a retractor.

Fig. 14.17 Vessel calibers can also be matched by **cutting** the smaller vessel end at an **oblique angle**.

Problems and Complications
(**Figs. 14.16–14.20**)

- Inequality of vessel diameters (**Figs. 14.16–14.18**).
- Gaps between the vessel ends (**Fig. 14.19**).
- Early or delayed thrombosis at the anastomotic site (**Fig. 14.20**).

Test for Patency
(**Fig. 14.21**)

Fig. 14.18   Fish-mouth technique.
The front and back walls of the donor vein are incised to enlarge the anastomotic lumen. This technique is particularly useful in an end-to-side anastomosis where the incision in the recipient vein has been made too large (Remmert 1995).

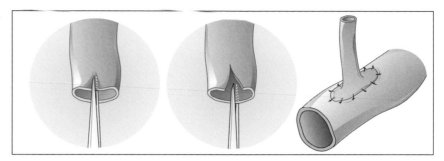

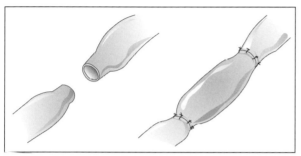

Fig. 14.19   Gaps between the vessel ends. The vessel ends must be apposed without tension, since traction on the anastomosis leads to thrombosis. Larger gaps should be spanned with an interpositional graft of equal diameter.

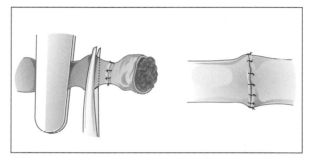

Fig. 14.20   Thrombosis. The most dreaded complication is anastomotic thrombosis. A clot that forms during suturing is flushed out with heparinized sodium chloride solution. If the anastomosis has already been closed, the segment is excised and a new anastomosis is performed.

Fig. 14.21a–c   Test for patency.
The patency of arterial and venous anastomoses can be assessed with the O'Brien test (O'Brien et al. 1987).

a The vessel distal to the anastomosis is occluded with forceps. A second set of forceps is placed next to the first.

b Blood is milked distally with the second forceps, which are tightened to create an empty vascular segment.

c The proximal forceps are released. If the empty segment quickly refills, the anastomosis is patent.

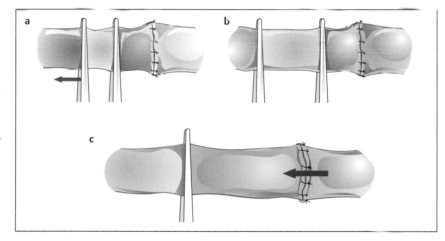

15 Harvesting Bone Graft from the Iliac Crest

Autogenous bone is needed for the reconstruction of defects or to correct cosmetic deformities. Along with the tibia, fibula, scapula, and ribs, the iliac crest is among the most common donor sites for autogenous bone. It can furnish extremely large grafts, which are usually taken in the form of compound or composite flaps that include soft-tissue elements (see **Fig. 14.2**).

Indications:

Cancellous bone chips are used as filling material for mandibular reconstructions and bone cysts, and composite corticocancellous grafts of various sizes are used to correct facial contour deformities, augment the nasal skeleton, and replace portions of the mandible (see **Fig. 15.3**).

Position:

The patient is placed in the supine position, with the hip (generally the right one) elevated on a cushion.

Approach:

The somewhat thicker portions of the iliac crest (~1.3–1.7 cm in diameter) are located in the anterior third between the anterior superior iliac spine (**Fig. 15.1a**, 3) and the iliac tubercle (**Fig. 15.1a**, Tub). The iliac spine is preserved anteriorly. An assistant presses down on the skin medial to the iliac crest, so that the incision, and later the scar, will be lateral to the site where the bone graft is harvested. The incision should not be carried anteriorly past the iliac spine, to avoid injury of the lateral femoral cutaneous nerve, as this would cause anesthesia or hypesthesia on the anterolateral thigh (**Fig. 15.1b**). The incision over the anterior iliac crest extends through

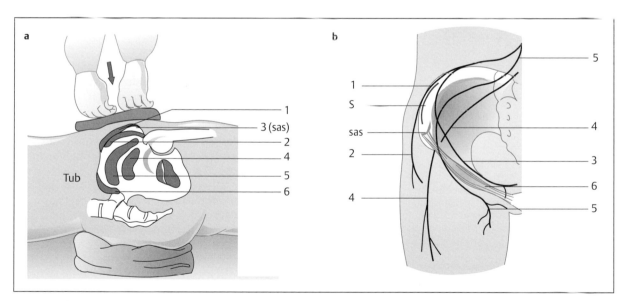

Fig. 15.1a, b Iliac crest bone graft.
a Position of the patient. Pressing down on the abdominal wall draws the skin medially across the iliac crest, positioning the incision and scar lateral to the crest. The diagram shows the inserting muscles, which are partially detached along with the periosteum.
1 Internal and external oblique muscles.
2 Tensor muscle.
3 Sartorius muscle; sas = anterior superior iliac spine.
4 Gluteus minimus muscle.
5 Gluteus medius muscle.
6 Gluteus maximus muscle.
(Tub = iliac tubercle)

b Sensory nerve supply of the leg (in the standing patient).
1 Iliohypogastric nerve.
2 Lateral cutaneous branch.
3 Anterior cutaneous branch.
4 Lateral femoral cutaneous nerve.
5 Ilioinguinal nerve.
6 Inguinal ligament.
(sas = anterior superior iliac spine; S = incision)

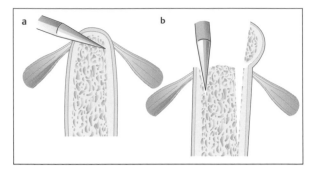

Fig. 15.2a, b
a The periosteum is incised laterally, and the iliac crest is raised with an osteotome, leaving it hinged medially on periosteum and muscle.
b With the cortical cap opened, a straight osteotome is driven along the inner and outer tables of the iliac crest, and a transverse osteotomy is added to free the cancellous bone block.

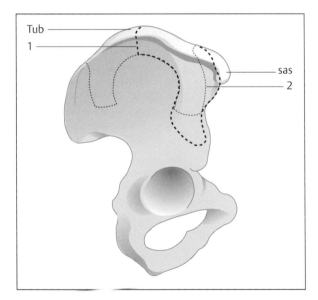

Fig. 15.3   Harvesting of **large two-layer and three-layer grafts**.
1 Graft for hemimandibular reconstruction.
2 Graft for anterior mandibular reconstruction
sas = anterior superior iliac spine; Tub = iliac tubercle; today this graft has been superseded by the fibular graft or pedicled iliac crest graft, see **Fig. 14.2**).

the skin and subcutaneous tissue down to the periosteum. The length of the incision depends on the length of bone graft that will be removed.

Harvesting cancellous bone (**Fig. 15.2**):
The periosteum is first incised along the lateral edge of the iliac crest. Then it is incised transversely behind the iliac spine and anterior to the tubercle, and the bone is divided transversely with an osteotome, to a depth of ~0.5 cm (**Fig. 15.2a**). On the lateral side, the upper portion of the iliac crest is divided with a straight osteotome and fractured on the medial side. This forms a cortical cap that is hinged medially on the periosteum and attached muscles,

and can be opened like a trapdoor to expose cancellous bone (**Fig. 15.2b**).

The straight osteotome is advanced down along the inner surface of the inner and outer tables of the iliac crest, and a transverse osteotomy is made behind the spine and in front of the tubercle. An osteotome curved on the flat is then used to cut through the base of the cancellous block (**Fig. 15.2b**). Harvesting of the cancellous bone is followed by meticulous hemostasis, in which bleeding sites in the bone are first cauterized and then occluded with fibrin glue or bone wax. The outer and inner tables may be fractured toward each other slightly, to reduce the size of the donor cavity. The cavity is packed with blood-soaked fibrin foam or collagen sponge, for example. The cortical cap is returned to its original position, the periosteum is reapproximated with sutures, and the wound is closed in layers. Suction drainage is essential to prevent hematoma formation. Two continuous-suction drains should be used. One is placed at the bone graft donor site, maintaining suction for only ~30 minutes, to prevent excessive blood loss; the other is placed in the soft-tissue mantle, where suction is maintained for 2 to 3 days. The cancellous bone can also be harvested with sharp curettes.

Harvesting corticocancellous bone (**Figs. 15.3 and 15.4**):
Corticocancellous bone can be obtained from various regions of the iliac crest, depending on the necessary graft size (**Fig. 15.3**).

1. **Small grafts** (**Fig. 15.3**): the border of the iliac crest is an excellent donor site for small grafts used to reconstruct the nose, orbital ring, or facial contours. The periosteum is incised along the center and dissected from the inner and outer tables, according to the necessary graft size. The graft is harvested with a straight osteotome or saw (**Fig. 15.4a**). After meticulous hemostasis, the periosteum is closed with absorbable sutures, and the wound is closed in layers over a suction drain.

2. **Larger corticocancellous grafts** (**Figs. 15.3 and 15.4**): the desired graft size will determine whether it is necessary to strip the medial periosteum with the iliac muscles, the lateral periosteum with the attached gluteal muscles, or the periosteum on both sides. The inner table is easier to expose, and larger corticocancellous grafts should be taken from the inner table whenever possible (**Fig. 15.4b**). This leaves the outer table with the gluteal muscle attachments intact. The anterior superior iliac spine with the tensor fasciae latae attachment should also be preserved. The grafts can be harvested with straight and curved osteotomes, or with a motorized saw. After the desired grafts have been obtained, the bone edges are rounded off with burs, rasps, or

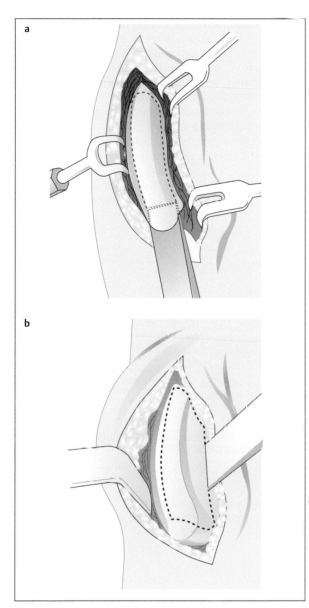

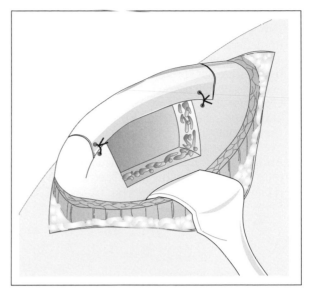

Fig. 15.5 A **three-layer corticocancellous graft** has been removed with preservation of the iliac crest, which is reattached after graft harvest. The iliac crest segment should be slightly larger than the graft.

◄ **Fig. 15.4a, b**
    a A small **cortical bone graft** is obtained from the iliac crest after stripping of the periosteum. The anterior surface of the iliac spine should be preserved (tensor fasciae latae).
    b A **two-layer graft** (dotted line) is taken from the inner table after periosteal stripping. The anterior surface of the iliac spine should be preserved.

ronguers. A three-layer (full-thickness) cortico-cancellous graft can also be harvested, and again it is recommended that the superior border of the iliac crest be preserved (**Fig. 15.5**). In selected cases, bone from the posterior iliac wing can also be used.

Hemostasis:
Heavy bleeding, especially from the cancellous bone, requires meticulous hemostasis. This can be accomplished with bone wax and suction drainage (see above). Donor cavities are packed with blood-soaked fibrin foam or similar material. Blood loss in excess of 500 mL is not unusual.

Wound closure:
The wound should be closed in layers. When large bone grafts have been obtained, the iliac muscles can be sutured to the gluteal muscles over the iliac wing, and the medial and lateral periosteum are sewn together with heavy sutures.

Complications:
1. Hypesthesia or anesthesia on the medial surface of the thigh can occur if the surgeon did not keep strictly below the periosteum while working on the inner table (**Fig. 15.1b**; cutaneous branch of iliohypogastric nerve, ilioinguinal nerve), or if the lateral femoral nerve has been injured (**Fig. 15.1b**).
2. Grating of the fascia lata over the trochanter can cause friction sounds during walking because the surgeon neglected to reattach the tensor fasciae latae to the lateral aspect of the iliac spine (**Fig. 15.1b**).

3. Perforation of the abdominal cavity during removal of graft from the inner table requires immediate closure in layers.
4. A hernia may develop if the medial and lateral muscles are not sutured together after a large graft has been harvested from the iliac wing. Crockford and Converse (1972) suggested that graft harvest be limited to the outer table behind the anterior superior iliac spine in children aged over 2 to 3 years.
5. Atrophy of the gluteal muscles (medius and minimus) can develop if the lateral periosteum is not repaired after graft harvest (**Fig. 15.1a**).
6. The technique of preserving the pelvic brim (**Fig. 15.5**) should be practiced, to avoid contour changes in the iliac wing (Laurie et al. 1984).
7. Scars directly over the iliac crest can lead to problems when wearing belts, girdles, or the like. Also, the scars may be cosmetically objectionable in women, and hypertrophic scars may require later revision.
8. Pain generally lasts from 4 to 6 weeks but may persist longer in some cases.

16 Harvesting Split Calvarian Bone Graft

Calvarian bone graft is usually parietal and harvested above the end of the temporal muscle (see **Fig. 10.93**). It can be used for reconstruction of the facial structures (see **Figs. 8.8** and **14.1**). The incision is made above the temporal muscle (**Fig. 16.1a**) and the pericranium is elevated. The bone is outlined using a pattern made from aluminum foil (suture material wrapper) or glove paper as a guide (**Fig. 16.1b**). A

trough groove several millimeters in size is drilled with a cutting bur (**Fig. 16.1c**), until the diploid space is reached. The bone is freed with an angled chisel or oscillating angled saw (**Fig. 16.1d**). The first graft should only be 1.0 to 1.5 cm wide. Subsequent grafts are easier to harvest because of the larger trough left by the removal of the first graft (Sherris and Larrabee 2009, p. 301).

Fig. 16.1a–d Calvarian bone graft.
a, b The bone graft is taken above the end of the temporalis muscle. The incision, skin and pericranium are elevated.
c A groove 5 to 10 mm wide is drilled with a cutting bur, up to the diploid space.
d The bone graft is taken with an angled chisel or angled oscillating saw. Subsequent grafts can be taken.

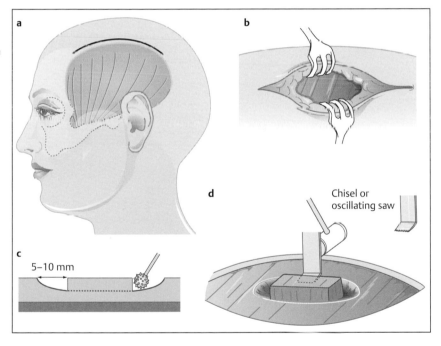

17 Dermabrasion

Dermabrasion is surgical scraping performed with a high-speed motorized handpiece (e.g., Aesculap) that delivers speeds of 15,000 to 25,000 rpm or higher. A large carborundum or diamond abrasive wheel is used.

Indications:
Dermabrasion is done to remove scars above skin level (**Fig. 17.1a, b**) that are due to burns or trauma, to lessen the visibility of traumatic tattooing, and to treat acne scars.

Procedure:
Local anesthesia is the rule, but general anesthesia may be used when large areas are abraded. While the skin is held tense and irrigated with clear, cool saline solution, the skin is uniformly abraded to a level no deeper than the boundary of the epidermis and dermis (Petres and Rompel 1996).

Complications:
Persistent erythema, hyperpigmentation, or hypertrophic scarring.

Postoperative care:
Cold compresses are used on the first postoperative day. Postoperative care also includes emollient skin ointments and protection from sun exposure.

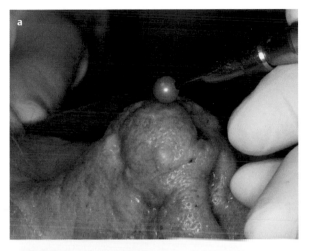

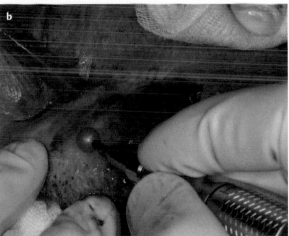

Fig. 17.1a, b   Dermabrasion.
a Situation after reconstruction of the nasal flap. The flap will be thinned by dermabrasion.
b Situation at the end of the operation.

References

Abbé R. A new plastic operation for the relief of deformity due to double harelip. Plast Reconstr Surg 1968;42(5):481–483

Abbé R. A new plastic operation for the relief of deformity due to double harelip. Med Rec 1898;53:477

Abul-Hassan HS, von Drasek Ascher G, Acland RD. Surgical anatomy and blood supply of the fascial layers of the temporal region. Plast Reconstr Surg 1986;77(1):17–28

Antia NH, Buch VI. Chondrocutaneous advancement flap for the marginal defect of the ear. Plast Reconstr Surg 1967;39(5):472–477

Antia N. Repair of segmental defects of the auricle in mechanical trauma. In: Tanzer R, Edgerton M. Symposium on Reconstruction of the Auricle. Vol. 10. St. Louis, MO: Mosby; 1974:218

Argamaso RV, Lewin ML. Repair of partial ear loss with local composite flap. Plast Reconstr Surg 1968;42(5):437–441

Argamaso RV. V-Y S-plasty for closure of a round defect. Plast Reconstr Surg 1974;53(1):99–101

Argamaso RV. Ear reduction with or without setback otoplasty. Plast Reconstr Surg 1989;83(6):967–975

Bakamjian VY. A two-stage method of pharyngoesophageal reconstruction with a primary pectoral skin flap. Plast Reconstr Surg 1965;36:173–184

Barron JN, Emmett AJ. Subcutaneous pedicle flaps. Br J Plast Surg 1965;18:51–78

Baudet J. Reimplantation of the mutilated external ear. New method. [Article in French] Nouv Presse Med 1972;1(5):344–346

Bernard C. Cancer de la lèvre inférieure; restauration à l'aide de lambeaux quadrataires-latéreaux. Scalpel (Brux) 1852;5:162–165

Berson IM. Atlas of Plastic Surgery. New York: Grune & Stratton; 1948

Bethmann W, Zoltan J. Operationen an der Ohrmuschel. In: Bethmann W, ed. Methoden der plastischen Chirurgie. Jena: Fischer; 1968:267–282

Beyer-Machule Ch, Riedel K. Plastische Chirurgie der Lider. 2nd ed. Stuttgart: Enke; 1993

Blasius. Handbuch der Chirurgie. Halle: Anton-Verlag; 1840

Bootz F, Müller H. Mikrovaskuläre Gewebetransplantation im Kopf- und Halsbereich. Stuttgart: Thieme; 1992

Borges AF. Elective Incisions and Scar Revision. Boston, MA: Little, Brown & Co.; 1973

Brent B. Reconstruction of ear, eyebrow, and sideburn in the burned patient. Plast Reconstr Surg 1975;55(3):312–317

Brent B. Earlobe construction with an auriculo-mastoid flap. Plast Reconstr Surg 1976;57(3):389–391

Brent B. Auricular repair with autogenous rib cartilage grafts: two decades of experience with 600 cases. Plast Reconstr Surg 1992;90(3):355–374, discussion 375–376

Brown JB. Switching of vermilion-bordered lip flaps. Surg Gynecol Obstet 1928;46:701–704

Bruns Vv. Handbuch Praktische Chirurgie. Tübingen: Laupp; 1859

Brusati R. Reconstruction of labial commissure by a sliding U-shaped cheek flap. J Maxillofac Surg 1979;7(1):11–14

Burget GC, Menick FJ. The subunit principle in nasal reconstruction. Plast Reconstr Surg 1985;76(2):239–247

Burget GC, Menick FJ. Nasal support and lining: the marriage of beauty and blood supply. Plast Reconstr Surg 1989;84(2):189–202

Burget GC, Menick FJ. Aesthetic Reconstruction of the Nose. St. Louis, MO: Mosby; 1994:315–323

Burow AV. Beschreibung einer neuen Transplantationsmethode (Methode der seitlichen Dreiecke) zum Wiederersatz verlorengegangener Teile des Gesichts. Berlin: Nauck; 1855

Cameron RR. Nasal reconstruction with nasolabial cheek flaps. In: Grabb WC, Myers MB, eds. Skin Flaps. Boston, MA: Little, Brown & Co.; 1975:353

Celsus 25 AD Converse JM. Reconstruction of the auricle. I and II. Plast Reconstr Surg Transplant Bull 1958;22:150–163 and 230–249

Converse 1959, cit. after Converse 1977

Converse JM. Reconstructive Plastic Surgery. 2nd ed. Phildelphia, PA: Saunders; 1977

Converse JM, Brent B. Acquired deformities. In: Converse JM, ed. Reconstructive Plastic Surgery. Vol. 3. 2nd ed. Philadelphia, PA: Saunders; 1977

Cosman B, Crikelair GF. The composed tube pedicle in ear helix reconstruction. Plast Reconstr Surg 1966;37(6):517–522

Crikelair GF. A method of partial ear reconstruction for avulsion of the upper portion of the ear. Plast Reconstr Surg (1946) 1956;17(6):438–443

Crockford DA, Converse JM. The ilium as a source of bone grafts in children. Plast Reconstr Surg 1972;50(3):270–274

Cronin TD. One-stage reconstruction of the helix: two improved methods. Plast Reconstr Surg (1946) 1952;9(6):547–556

Cummings Ch, Fredickson J, Harker C, Krause Ch, Schuller D, eds. Otolaryngology–Head and Neck Surgery. St. Louis: Mosby; 1986

Day HF. Reconstruction of ears. Boston Med Surg J 1921;185:146–147

Dean RK, Kelleher J, Sullivan J, Baibak G. Bi-lobed flaps. In: Grabb WC, Myers MB, eds. Skin Flaps. Boston, MA: Little, Brown & Co.; 1975:289

Denecke HJ, Meyer R. Plastische Operationen an Kopf und Hals, Vol. 1. Nasenplastik. Berlin: Springer; 1964

Di Martino G. Anomalie de pavillon d'oreille. Bull Acad Natl Med 1856/1857;22:17

Dieffenbach JF. In: Fritze HE, Reich OF, eds. Die Plastische Chirurgie in ihrem weitesten Umfange dargestellt und durch Abbildungen erläutert. Berlin: Hirschwald; 1845

Dufourmentel G. Le fermetur des pertes de substance cutanée limitées. Ann Chir Plast 1962;7:61

Dujon DG, Bowditch M. The thin tube pedicle: a valuable technique in auricular reconstruction after trauma. Br J Plast Surg 1995;48(1):35–38

Elliott RA Jr. Rotation flaps of the nose. Plast Reconstr Surg 1969;44(2):147–149

Esser J. Gestielte apikale Nasenplastik mit zweizipfligem Lappen. Deckung des sekundären Defektes vom ersten Zipfel durch den zweiten. Dtsch Z Chir 1918;143:385

Estlander A. Eine Methode aus der einen Lippe Substanzverluste der anderen zu ersetzen. Arch Klin Chir 1872;14:622

Farrior RT. Korrigierende und rekonstruktive plastische Chirurgie an der äußeren Nase. In: Naumann HH, ed. Kopf- und Hals-Chirurgie. VolII/1. Stuttgart: Thieme; 1974

Fries R. Vorzug der Bernardschen Operation als Universalverfahren zur Rekonstruktion der Unterlippe nach Karzinomresektion. Chir Plast 1971;1:45–52

Gersuny R. Über einige kosmetische Operationen. Vienna med Wschr. 1903;53:2253

Gibson T, Davis W. The distortion of autogenous cartilage grafts: its cause and prevention. Br J Plast Surg 1958;10:257

Gillies, et al. 1957, zit. n. Gillies, H., D. Millard 1976

Gillies H, Millard D. The Principles and Art of Plastic Surgery. Vol. II. 4th ed. Boston, MA: Little, Brown & Co.; 1976

Ginestet G, Frézières H, Dupuis A, Pons J. Chirurgie Plastique et Reconstructive de la Face. Paris: Editions Médicales Flammarion; 1967

Gingrass RP, Pickrell KL. Techniques for closure of conchal and external auditory canal defects. Plast Reconstr Surg 1968;41(6):568–571

Goedecke CH. Geschichte der plastisch-rekonstruktiven Chirurgie von erworbenen Ohrmuscheldefekten [Dissertation]. Medizinische Universität zu Lübeck; 1995

Goldstein MA. The cosmetic and plastic surgery of the ear. Laryngoscope 1908;18:826–851

Goldstein MH. The elastic flap: an expanding vermilion myocutaneous flap for lip repairs. Facial Plast Surg 1990a;7(2):119–125

Grimm G. New method of flap plastic surgery for the substitution of total lower lip defects caused by tumors. [Article in German] Zentralbl Chir 1966;91(44):1621–1625

Haas E, Meyer R. Konstruktive und rekonstruktive Chirurgie der Nase. In: Gohrbrand E, Gabka J, Berndorfer A, eds. Handbuch der Plastischen Chirurgie, Vol II/2. Berlin: De Gruyter; 1973

Haas E. Plastische Gesichtschirurgie. Stuttgart: Thieme; 1991

Hamblen-Thomas C. Repair for partial loss of the auricle. J Laryngol Otol 1938;53:259–260

Härle F. Atlas der Hauttumoren im Gesicht. Munich: Hanser; 1993

Imre J. Lidplastik und plastische Operationen anderer Weichteile des Gesichts, Budapest: Studium-Verlag; 1928

Jackson IT. Local Flaps in Head and Neck Reconstruction. St. Louis, MO: Mosby; 1985a

Jackson IT. Lip Reconstruction. In: Jackson IT. Local Flaps in Head and Neck Reconstruction. St. Louis: Mosby; 1985b:327–412

Joseph J. Demonstration operierter Eselsohren. Verl Berl Med Ges; 1896:I:206

Joseph J. Nasenplastik und andere Gesichtsplastiken. Lipezig: Kabitzsch; 1931

Jost G, Danon J, Hadjean E, Mahe E, Vertut J, eds. Reparations plastiques des pertes de substances cutanées de la face. Vol. I Atlas. Vol. II Text. Paris: Librairie Arnette; 1977

Karapandzic M. Reconstruction of lip defects by local arterial flaps. Br J Plast Surg 1974;27(1):93–97

Kastenbauer ER. Special methods of reconstructive surgery in the facial region. [Article in German] Arch Otorhinolaryngol 1977;216(1):123–250

Kazanjian VH. Surgical treatment of congenital deformities of the ears. Am J Surg 1958;95(2):185–188

Kazanjian V, Converse J. The Surgical Treatment of Facial Injuries. Baltimore, MD: Williams & Wilkins; 1974

Koopmann CF Jr, Coulthard SW. "How I do it"—otology and neurotology. A specific issue and its solution. A postauricular muscle-skin flap for conchal defects. Laryngoscope 1982;92(5):596–598

Körte W. Fall von Ohrenplastik. Sitzung am 13.11.1905. Verh Fr Vrgg Chir Berlins 1905;18:91–92

Krespi YP, Ries WR, Shugar JMA, Sisson GA. Auricular reconstruction with postauricular myocutaneous flap. Otolaryngol Head Neck Surg 1983;91(2):193–196

Laurie SW, Kaban LB, Mulliken JB, Murray JE. Donor-site morbidity after harvesting rib and iliac bone. Plast Reconstr Surg 1984;73(6):933–938

Lejour M. One-stage reconstruction of nasal skin defects with local flaps. Chir plastica Berl 1972;1:254–259

Lejour M. The cheek island flap. In: Bohmert H, ed. Plastische Chirurgie des Kopf- und Halsbereichs und der weiblichen Brust. Stuttgart: Thieme; 1975

Lexer E. Wangenplastik. Dtsch Z Chir 1909;100:206

Lexer E. Die gesamte Wiederherstellungschirurgie. Vol I. Leipzig: Barth; 1933:441

Limberg A. Planimetrie und Stereometrie der Hautplastik. Jena: Fischer; 1967

Masson JK. A simple island flap for reconstruction of concha-helix defects. Br J Plast Surg 1972;25(4):399–403

McNichol JW. Total helix reconstruction with tubed pedicles following loss by burns. Plast Reconstr Surg (1946) 1950;6(5):373–386

Mellette JR Jr. Ear reconstruction with local flaps. J Dermatol Surg Oncol 1991;17(2):176–182

Meyer R, Sieber H. Konstruktive und rekonstruktive Chirurgie des Ohres. In: Gohrbrandt, Gabka, Berndorfer, eds. Handbuch der Plastischen Chirurgie. Bd. II/3. Berlin: De Gruyter; 1973:1–62

Meyer R. Secondary and Functional Rhinoplasty. Orlando, NY: Grune & Stratton; 1988

Millard DR Jr. The chondrocutaneous flap in partial auricular repair. Plast Reconstr Surg 1966;37(6):523–530

Mladick RA, Horton CE, Adamson JE, Cohen BI. The pocket principle: a new technique for the reattachment of a severed ear part. Plast Reconstr Surg 1971;48(3):219–223

Mündnich K. Die wiederherstellende Ohrmuschelplastik. In: Sercer A, Mündnich K, eds. Plastische Operationen an der Nase und an der Ohrmuschel. Stuttgart: Thieme; 1962a;325–382, 411–451

Musgrave RH, Garrett WS Jr. Management of avulsion injuries of the external ear. Plast Reconstr Surg 1967;40(6):534–539

Mustardé JCl. Repair and Reconstruction in the Orbital Region. Edinburgh: Churchill Livingstone; 1969

Nagata S. Modification of the stages in total reconstruction of the auricle: Part I. Grafting the three-dimensional costal cartilage framework for lobule-type microtia. Plast Reconstr Surg 1994a, 93(2):221–230

Nagata S. Modification of the stages in total reconstruction of the auricle: Part II. Grafting the three-dimensional costal cartilage framework for concha-type microtia. Plast Reconstr Surg 1994b;93(2):231–242, discussion 267–268

Nagata S. Modification of the stages in total reconstruction of the auricle: Part III. Grafting the three-dimensional costal cartilage framework for small concha-type microtia. Plast Reconstr Surg 1994c;93(2):243–253, discussion 267–268

Nagata S. Modification of the stages in total reconstruction of the auricle: Part IV. Ear elevation for the constructed auricle. Plast Reconstr Surg 1994d;93(2):254–266, discussion 267–268

Nagel F. Reconstruction of a partial auricular loss. Case report. Plast Reconstr Surg 1972;49(3):340–342

Navabi A. One-stage reconstruction of partial defect of the auricle. Plast Reconstr Surg 1964;33:77–79

Nelaton C, Ombredanne L. Troisième partie otoplastie. In: Nelaton C, Ombredanne L, eds. Les Autoplasties. Paris: Steinheil; 1907:125–198

O'Brien B, McCraw W, Morrison A. Reconstructive Microsurgery. Edinburgh: Churchill Livingstone; 1987

Ombredanne L. Reconstruction autoplastique de la moitié du pavillon de l'oreille. Presse Med 1931;53:982–983

Pardue AM. Repair of torn earlobe with preservation of the perforation for an earring. Plast Reconstr Surg 1973;51(4):472–473

Park Ch, Shin KS, Kang HS, Lee YH, Lew JD. A new arterial flap from the postauricular surface: its anatomic basis and clinical application. Plast Reconstr Surg 1988;82(3):498–505

Park C, Chung S. Reverse-flow postauricular arterial flap for auricular reconstruction. Ann Plast Surg 1989;23(4):369–374

Park C, Suk Roh T. Total ear reconstruction in the devascularized temporoparietal region: I. Use of the contralateral temporoparietal fascial free flap. Plast Reconstr Surg 2001;108(5):1145–1153

Pate J, Wilkinson J. Z-advancement rotation flap reconstruction of full-thickness cutaneous defects of the nose. In: Stucker F, ed. Plastic and Reconstructive Surgery of Head and Neck. Philadelphia, PA: Decker; 1991

Peer LA, Walker JC Jr. Total reconstruction of the ear. J Int Coll Surg 1957;27(3):290–304

Peers M. Cheek flaps in partial rhinoplasty. A new variation: the in-and-out flap. Scand J Plast Surg 1967;1:37

Pegram M, Peterson R. Repair of partial defects of the ear. Plast Reconstr Surg (1946) 1956;18(4):305–308

Pennington DG, Lai MF, Pelly AD. Successful replantation of a completely avulsed ear by microvascular anastomosis. Plast Reconstr Surg 1980;65(6):820–823

Pennisi VR, Klabunde EH, Pierce GW. The preauricular flap. Plast Reconstr Surg 1965;35:552–556

Petres J, Rompel R. Operative Dermatologie. Berlin: Springer; 1996

Quetz J. Totalrekonstruktion der Nase: Erfahrungen mit der Septumrekonstruktion durch die Septumrotationstechnik nach Burget. DGPW-Mitteilungen 2009;39:27–32

Quetz J, Ambrosch P. Total nasal reconstruction: a 6-year experience with the three-stage forehead flap combined with the septal pivot flap. Facial Plast Surg 2011;27(3):266–275

Remmert S, Sommer K. More reliable assessment of hand blood circulation by the modified Allen test in removal of a pedicled radialis flap. [Article in German] Laryngorhinootologie 1993;72(5):268–269

Remmert S, Majocco A, Sommer K, Ahrens K-H, Weerda H. A new method of tongue reconstruction with neurovascular infrahyoid muscle-fascia flaps. [Article in German] Laryngorhinootologie 1994;73(4):198–201

Remmert S. Mikrovaskuläre Anastomosen in der rekonstruktiven Kopf- und Halschirurgie. Laryngorhinootologie 1995;73:233–237

Remmert S, Majocco A, Gehrking E. Neurovascular infrahyoid myofascial flap. Anatomic-topographic study of innervation and vascular supply. [Article in German] HNO 1995;43(3):182–187

Remmert S, Kunikowski C, Meyer S, Sommer K. Topographic anatomic study of cells transplanted from the groin region. [Article in German] Ann Anat 1998;180(1):59–68

Renard A. Postauricular flap based on a dermal pedicle for ear reconstruction. Plast Reconstr Surg 1981;68(2):159–165

Rettinger G. Plastisch-rekonstruktive Gesichtschirurgie. In: Theissing J, ed. HNO-Operationslehre. 3rd ed. Stuttgart: Thieme; 1996a

Rettinger G. Plastisch-rekonstruktive Kopf- und Halschirurgie. In: Berghaus H, Rettinger G, Böhme H, eds. Hals-, Nasen-, Ohrenheilkunde. Stuttgart: Hippokrates; 1996b:622–643

Rieger (1957): cited after Kastenbauer 1977

Schmid E, Meyer R. cited after Denecke, H. J., R. Meyer 1964

Scott MJ, Klaassen MF. Immediate reconstruction of the helical rim after bite injury using the posterior auricular flap. Injury 1992;23(5):333–335

Sercer A, Mündnich K. Plastische Operationen an der Nase und an der Ohrmuschel. Stuttgart: Thieme; 1962

Siegert R, Weerda H, Hoffmann S, Mohadjer C. Clinical and experimental evaluation of intermittent intraoperative short-term expansion. Eur Arch Otorhinolaryngol 1992;249:119

Siegert R, Weerda H. Die Hautexpansion, Teil 1 und II. HNO 1994;42:124–137, 182–194

Smith H. Plastic operation for restauration of the auricle, following injury from an explosion. Ann Otol Rhinol Laryngol 1917;26:831–833

Steffanoff DN. Auriculo-mastoid tube pedicle for otoplasty. Plast Reconstr Surg (1946) 1948;3(3):352–360

Streit R. Einige plastische Operationen an der Ohrmuschel. Arch Ohrenheilk 1914;95:300–303

Tagliacozzi T. De curtorum chirurgia per insitionem. Libri duo, Venice: Apud Gasparem Bindonum Iuniorem 1597

Tanzer RC. Correction of the microtia with autogenous costal cartilage. In: Tanzer RC, Edgerton MT, eds. Symposium on Reconstruction of the Auricle. St Louis, MO: CV Mosby & Co; 1974;X:46–57

Tanzer R, Bellucci R, Converse J, Brent B. Deformities of the Auricle. In: Converse J, ed. Reconstructive Plastic Surgery. Vol. 3. 2nd ed. Philadelphia, PA: Saunders; 1977

Tebbetts JB. Auricular reconstruction: selected single-stage techniques. J Dermatol Surg Oncol 1982;8(7):557–566

Templer J, Davis WE, Thomas JR. A rotation flap for low posterior auricular defects. Laryngoscope 1981;91(5):826–828

Tenta LT, Keyes GR. Reconstructive surgery of the external ear. Otolaryngol Clin North Am 1981;14(4):917–938

Tipton JB. Flaps for closure of nasal septal perforations. In: Grabb WC, Myers MB, eds. Skin Flaps. Boston, MA: Little, Brown & Co.; 1975

Toplak FH. Die Totalrekonstruktion der Ohrmuschel (the total reconstruction of the auricle, in German) [Dissertation]. Berlin: Universitätsklinikum Steglitz; 1986

Trendelenburg 1886, cit. after Joseph 1931

Troha FV, Baibak GJ, Kelleher JC. Auriculomastoid tube pedicle for partial ear reconstruction. Plast Reconstr Surg 1990;86(5):1037–1038

von Langenbeck B. Neue Verfahren zur Cheiloplastic durch Ablösung und Verziehung des Lippensaumes. Dtsch Klinik 1855;7:1–3

von Szymanowski J. Ohrbildung. Otoplastik. In: von Szymanowski J. Handbuch der operativen Chirurgie. Braunschweig: F Vieweg & Sohn; 1870:303–306

Wachsberger A. Successful auricular autotransplantation. Arch Otolaryngol 1947;46(4):549–551

Walter C. Plastisch-chirurgische Eingriffe im Kopf-Hals-Bereich. Stuttgart: Thieme; 1997

Webster RC. Cosmetic concepts in scar camouflaging–serial excisional and broken line techniques. Trans Am Acad Ophthalmol Otolaryngol 1969;73(2):256–265

Weerda H. One stage reconstruction of the trachea with an island flap (author's translation). [Article in German] Arch Otorhinolaryngol 1978a;221(3):211–214

Weerda H. Covering defects after extirpation of tumours in the ear region. [Article in German] Laryngol Rhinol Otol (Stuttg) 1978b;57(2):93–98

Weerda H. Der "bi-lobed flap" in der Kopf- und Halschirurgie. Arch Otorhinolaryngol 1978c;219:181–190

Weerda H. The principles of the "bi-lobed flap" and its use for the construction of "multiple flaps". [Article in German] Arch Otorhinolaryngol 1978d;220(1–2):133–139

Weerda H. Remarks about otoplasty and avulsion of the auricle. [Article in German] Laryngol Rhinol Otol (Stuttg) 1979;58(3):242–251

Weerda H. Myocutaneous island flap for one-stage reconstruction of stenoses of the cervical esophagus. [Article in German] HNO 1980a;28(8):271–272

Weerda H. The trauma of the auricle. [Article in German] HNO 1980b;28(7):209–217

Weerda H. Special techniques in one-stage reconstruction of defects of the cheek using rotation or multiple flaps. [Article in German] HNO 1980c;28(12):416–424

Weerda H Special techniques in the reconstruction of cheek and lip defects. [Article in German] Laryngol Rhinol Otol (Stuttg) 1980d;59(10):630–640

Weerda H Special techniques in the reconstruction of cheek and lip defects (author's transl). [Article in German] Otorhinolaryngol 1980e;227:402

Weerda H, Härle F. Special flaps for reconstruction of the lips. [Article in German] HNO 1981;29(1):27–33

Weerda H, Münker G. Der "Bi-lobed flap" in der Rekonstruktion von Defekten der Ohrmuschel. In: Scheunemann H, Schmidseder R, eds. Sonderband der Deutschen Gesellschaft für Plastische Chirurgie. Heidelberg; 1982

Weerda H, Münker G. The "transposition-rotation flap" in the one stage reconstruction of auricle defects. [Article in German] Laryngol Rhinol Otol (Stuttg) 1981;60(6):312–317

Weerda H. Reconstruction of the lower lip. [Article in German] Laryngol Rhinol Otol (Stuttg) 1983a;62(1):23–28

Weerda H. "Bi-lobed and tri-lobed flaps" in head and neck defect repair. Fac Plast Surg 1983c;1:51–60

Weerda H. Die Chirurgie kleiner und mittelgroßer Nasendefekte. Arch Otorhinolaryngol 1983d;(suppl II):65–68

Weerda H. Die Chirurgie der Ohrmuschel nach Unfallverletzungen. In: Jungbluth K, Mommsen U, eds. Plastische und wiederherstellende Massnahmen bei Unfallverletzungen. Berlin: Springer; 1984

Weerda H, Walter C. Surgery of the pinna and the surrounding area. In: Ward PH, ed. Plastic and Reconstructive Surgery of the Head and Neck. St. Louis, MO: Mosby; 1984;827–846

Weerda H. Errors and dangers in rib cartilage removal. [Article in German] Laryngol Rhinol Otol (Stuttg) 1985a;64(4):221–222

Weerda H. Myomucosal flaps of the tongue for covering defects in the mouth area. [Article in German] HNO 1985b;33(7):303–306

Weerda H, Grüner R, Cannive B. Die Einheilungsrate frei transplantierter composite grafts. Arch Otorhinolaryngol 1986;(suppl II):129

Weerda H, Zöllner C. Chirurgie der Tumoren an der alternden Haut der Ohrregion. In: Neubauer H, ed. Plastische und Wiederherstellungschirurgie. Berlin: Springer, 1986

Weerda H. Plastic Surgery of the Ear. In: Kerr AG, ed. Scott Brown's Diseases of the Ear, Nose and Throat. 5th ed. London: Butterworth; 1987

Weerda H. Surgery of lower lip defects. Facial Plast Surg 1990;7(2):84–96

Weerda H, Siegert R. Reconstruction of the upper lip. Facial Plast Surg 1990;7(2):72–83

Weerda H. Das Ohrmuscheltrauma. In: Ganz H, Schätzle W, eds. HNO-Praxis Heute. Berlin: Springer; 1991:11

Weerda H. The auricle. In: Soutar D, Tiwari R, eds. Excision and Reconstruction in Head and Neck Cancer. Edinburgh: Churchill Livingstone; 1994a

Weerda H. Reconstructive surgery of the auricle. Facial Plast Surg 1994b;5:399–410

Weerda H, Siegert R. Complications of otoplasty and their treatment. [Article in German] Laryngorhinootologie 1994;73(7):394–399

Weerda H. Plastic surgery of the ear. In: Booth JB, ed. Scott-Brown Otolaryngology. Vol. 3. 6th ed. Oxford and Boston, MA: Butterworth-Heinemann; 1997

Weerda H, Siegert R, eds. Auricular and Middle Ear Malformations, Ear Defects and their Reconstruction. The Hague: Kugler Publications; 1998

Weerda H. Plastisch-rekonstruktive Chirurgie im Gesichtsbereich. Stuttgart and New York, NY: Thieme; 1999

Weerda H, Siegert R. Otoplastic Procedures and the Treatment of Complications. In: Bull HG, ed. Aesthetic Facial Surgery. Reinbek: Einhorn-Presse Verlag; 1999a

Weerda H, Siegert R. Rekonstruktion der Ohrmuschel In: Kastenbauer E, Tardy ME Jr., eds. Ästhetische und Plastische Chirurgie an Nase, Gesicht und Ohrmuschel. Stuttgart and New York, NY: Thieme; 1999b

Weerda H. Reconstructive Facial Plastic Surgery. A Problem-Solving Manual. Stuttgart: Thieme; 2001

Weerda H. Chirurgie der Ohrmuschel. Verletzungen, Defekte und Anomalien. Stuttgart: Thieme; 2004

Weerda H. Surgery of the Auricle Tumors-Trauma-Defects Anomalies. Stuttgart and NY: Thieme; 2007

Zimany A. The bi-lobed flap. Plast Reconstr Surg (1946) 1953;11(6):424–434

Zisser (1970) zit. u. Köle, H., G. Zisser (1973)

Further Reading

Alanis (1970) zit. u. Converse, J.M., B. Brent (1977)

Argenta LC. The nose. In: Soutar D, Tiwari R, eds. Excision and Reconstruction in Head and Neck Cancer. Edinburgh: Churchill Livingstone; 1994:139

Ariyan S. The pectoralis major myocutaneous flap. A versatile flap for reconstruction in the head and neck. Plast Reconstr Surg 1979;63(1):73–81

Baek SM, Biller HF, Krespi YP, Lawson W. The pectoralis major myocutaneous island flap for reconstruction of the head and neck. Head Neck Surg 1979;1(4):293–300

Baker SR, Krause CJ. Carcinoma of the lip. Laryngoscope 1980;90(1):19–27

Baker PR, Swanson NA. Local Flaps in Facial Reconstruction. St. Louis, MO: Mosby; 1995

Bardach J. Local Flaps and Free Skin Grafts in Head and Neck Reconstruction. St. Louis, MO: Mosby; 1992

Bardach J. Lip reconstruction using local flaps. In: Bardach J. Local Flaps and Free Skin Grafts in Head and Neck Reconstruction. St. Louis, MO: Mosby; 1992:322

Borges AF, Alexander JE. Relaxed skin tension lines, Z-plasties on scars, and fusiform excision of lesions. Br J Plast Surg 1962;15:242–254

Brent B, Byrd HS. Secondary ear reconstruction with cartilage grafts covered by axial, random, and free flaps of temporoparietal fascia. Plast Reconstr Surg 1983;72(2):141–152

Bruns VV. Chirurgischer Atlas. Tübingen: Laupp; 1857

Burg G, Konz B. Mikroskopisch kontrollierte Basaliombehandlung im Gesichtsbereich. In: Bohmert H, ed. Plastische Chirurgie des Kopf- und Halsbereiches und der weiblichen Brust. Stuttgart: Thieme; 1975

Cannon B. The use of vermilion bordered flaps in surgery about the mouth. Surg Gynecol Obstet 1942;74:458–462

Conley J. Concepts in Head and Neck Surgery. Stuttgart: Thieme; 1977

Conley J, Patow C. Flaps in Head and Neck Surgery. 2nd ed. Stuttgart: Thieme; 1989

Converse JM, Wood-Smith D. Techniques for the repair of defects of the lip and cheeks. In: Converse JM, ed. Reconstructive Plastic Surgery. Vol. 3. 2nd ed. Philadelphia, PA: Saunders; 1977:1544–1594

Cook T. Reconstruction of facial defects. In: Cumming Ch, Fredrickson J, Harker L, Krause Ch, Schuller D, eds. Otolaryngology–Head and Neck Surgery. Vol. 1. St. Louis, MO: Mosby; 1986

Cormack GC, Lamberty BG. The Arterial Anatomy of Skin Flaps. 2nd ed. Edinburgh: Churchill Livingstone; 1994

Davidson TM. Lacerations and scar revision. In: Cummings Ch, Fredrickson J, Harker L, Krause Ch, Schuller D, eds. Otolaryngology–Head and Neck Surgery. Vol. 1. St. Louis: Mosby; 1986

Denecke HJ. Besonderheiten bei Schnittführungen, Wundversorgung und Narbenkorrekturen im Bereich des Gesichtes und des Halses. In: Gohrbrandt E, Gabka J, Berndorfer A, eds. Handbuch der Plastischen Chirurgie, Vol. I. Berlin: De Gruyter; 1972

Denecke HJ, Ey W. Die Operationen an der Nase und im Nasopharynx. In: Zenker R, Heberer G, Pichlmayr R, eds. Allgemeine und spezielle Operationslehre, Vol. V., Teil 1. Berlin: Springer; 1984

Denonvillier: cited after Denecke, H. J., R. Meyer 1964

Draf W. Die einzeitige Lippenrekonstruktion nach Tumorentfernung (Meyer-Plastik). In: Düben W, Kley W, Pfeifer G, Schmid E, eds. Fehler und Gefahren in der Plastischen Chirurgie. Stuttgart: Thieme; 1976

Fries R. Advantages of a basic concept in lip reconstruction after tumour resection. J Maxillofac Surg 1973;1(1):13–18

Gersuny R. In: Sercer A, Mündnich K, eds. Plastische Operationen an der Nase und Ohrmuschel. Stuttgart: Thieme; 1962:364

Gohrbrandt E, Gabka J, Berndorfer A. Handbuch der Plastischen Chirurgie. Berlin: De Gruyter, Berlin 1972

Goldstein MH. The elastic flap for lip repair. Plast Reconstr Surg 1990b;85(3):446–452

Grabb W, Myers M. Skin Flaps. Boston, MA: Little, Brown & Co.; 1975

Haas E. Basic techniques of plastic surgical repair in defects of the skull and face (author's transl). [Article in German] Arch Otorhinolaryngol 1977;216(1):1–121

Haas E. Oncological principles of the treatment of facial skin cancer. [Article in German] Laryngol Rhinol Otol (Stuttg) 1982;61(11):611–617

Kastenbauer E, Jahnke V. Zur Problematik maligner Lippentumoren und deren operative Behandlung. In: Bohmert H, ed. Plastische Chirurgie des Kopf- und Halsbereiches und der weiblichen Brust. Stuttgart: Thieme; 1975

Kastenbauer ER. Pedicle transplants in rhinoplasty. [Article in German] Laryngorhinootologie 1983;62(1):19–22

Kastenbauer ER, Tardy ME Jr. Gesicht, Nase und Gesichtsschädel, Band 1, Teil 1. In: Naumann HH, ed. Kopf- und Hals-Chirurgie. Stuttgart: Thieme; 1996

Köle H, Zisser G. Rekonstruktive Chirurgie des Gesichtes, Teil II. In: Gohrbrandt E, Gabka J, Berndorfer A, eds. Handbuch der Plastischen Chirurgie, Vol II/1. Berlin: De Gruyter; 1973

Kunert P. A simple classification system for all skin flaps. [Article in German] Handchir Mikrochir Plast Chir 1995;27(3):124–131

Lentrodt J. Lip reconstruction following neoplasm surgery. [Article in German] Dtsch Zahnarztl Z 1970;25(6):670–677

Longacre J, Converse JM, Knize M. Transplantation of bone. In: Converse JM, ed. Reconstructive Plastic Surgery. Vol. I. 2nd ed. Philadelphia, PA: Saunders; 1977

McCarthy JG. Plastic Surgery. 5 Vol. Philadelphia, PA: Saunders; 1990

McCraw JB, Arnold PG. McCraw and Arnold Atlas of Muscle and Musculocutaneous Flaps. Norfolk, VA: Hampton Press; 1986

McGregor IA. Reconstruction of the lower lip. Br J Plast Surg 1983;36(1):40–47

Menick F. Reconstruction of the nose. In: Baker SH, Swanson N, eds. Local Flaps in Facial Reconstruction. St. Louis, MO: Mosby; 1995

Meyer R. Injuries to the external ear. [Article in German] Arch Klin Exp Ohren Nasen Kehlkopfheilkd 1968;191(2):450–479

Mladick RA, Carraway JH. Ear reattachment by the modified pocket principle. Case report. Plast Reconstr Surg 1973;51(5):584–587

Müller G. Mikrochirurgische Grundtechniken. Aesculap, Wissenschaftliche Informationen, H. 21. Tuttlingen 1989

Naumann HH, Helms J, Herberhold C, et al. Kopf- und Hals-Chirurgie. 3 Vols. Stuttgart: Thieme; 1995–1998

Neukam D. Operative Dermatologie in der Praxis. Stuttgart: Kohlhammer; 1989

Neuner O. Operationen bei Spaltträgern im Erwachsenenalter. In: Gohrbrandt E, Gabka J, Berndorfer A, eds. Handbuch der Plastischen Chirurgie, Vol II/1. Berlin: De Gruyter; 1973

Pfeifer G, Schmitz R, Ehmann G. Freie Transplantation in der Mund-, Kiefer- und Gesichtschirurgie. Fortschr Kiefer- u Gesichts-Chir Vol XX. Stuttgart: Thieme; 1976

Quatela V, Cheney ML. Reconstruction of the auricle. In: Baker PR, Swanson NA, eds. Local Flaps in Facial Reconstruction. St. Louis, MO: Mosby; 1995

Remmert S, Sommer K. Kompendium des mikrovaskulären Gewebetransfers. Hamburg-Norderstedt: Ethicon; 1995

Rosenthal W. Rekonstruktive Chirurgie des Gesichtes. In: Gohrbrandt E, Gabka J, Berndorfer A, eds. Handbuch der Plastischen Chirurgie, Vol II/3. Berlin: De Gruyter; 1973

Schultz-Coulon HJ. The bridge flap concept in closure of large defects of the nasal septum. [Article in German] HNO 1989;37(4):123–127

Sénéchal G, Cachin M, Pech A, Cannoni M, Demard F. La chirurgie Reparatrice en Cancérologie Cervico-faciale. Paris: Atlas and Text. Librairie Arnette; 1977

Song R, Gao Y, Song Y, Yu Y, Song Y. The forearm flap. Clin Plast Surg 1982;9(1):21–26

Soutar DS, Scheker LR, Tanner NS, McGregor IA. The radial forearm flap: a versatile method for intra-oral reconstruction. Br J Plast Surg 1983;36(1):1–8

Spira M. Early care of deformities of the auricle resulting from mechanical trauma. In: Tanzer R, Edgerton M, eds. Symposium on Reconstruction of the Auricle. Vol. X. St. Louis, MO: Mosby; 1974

Staindl O. Defektversorgung im Bereich des Nasenrückens und des Nasen-Augen-Winkels. Laryngol Rhinol Otol (Stuttg) 1983;62:6–18

Staindl O, Chmelizek-Feurstein C. Scars and scar revision. [Article in German] HNO 1983;31(6):183–192

Tanzer R, Edgerton M, eds. Symposium on Reconstruction of the Auricle. Vol. X. St. Louis, MO: Mosby; 1974:312

Taylor GI. Reconstruction of the mandible with free composite iliac bone grafts. Ann Plast Surg 1982;9(5):361–376

Timmons MJ. The vascular basis of the radial forearm flap. Plast Reconstr Surg 1986;77(1):80–92

Walsek E. Plastische Chirurgie der Orbita. In: Gohrbrandt E, Gabka J, Berndorfer A, eds. Handbuch der Plastischen Chirurgie, Vol II/3. Berlin: De Gruyter; 1973

Walter C. Aesthetic surgery of the nose (author's translation). [Article in German] Arch Otorhinolaryngol 1977;216(1):251–350

Webster RC, Coffey RJ, Kelleher RE. Total and partial reconstruction of the lower lip with innervated musclebearing flaps. Plast Reconstr Surg Transplant Bull 1960;25:360–371

Webster R, White M. Flaps for lip reconstruction. In: Grabb W, Myers M, eds. Skin Flaps. Boston, MA: Little, Brown & Co.; 1975

Webster MH, Soutar DP. Practical Guide to Free Tissue Transfer. London: Butterworth; 1986

Weerda H. Removal of the iliac crest bone. [Article in German] Laryngol Rhinol Otol (Stuttg) 1986;65(2):96–98

Weerda H. Reconstructive surgery of the auricle. Facial Plast Surg 1988;5(5):399–410

Weerda H. Kompendium plastisch-rekonstruktiver Eingriffe im Gesichtsbereich. 4th ed. Hamburg-Norderstedt: Ethicon; 1992

Weerda H. Classification and treatment of acquired deformities of the auricle. Face 1998;6:79–82

Yang GF, Chen PJ, Gao YZ, et al. Forearm free skin flap transplantation. A report of 56 cases. 1981. Br J Plast Surg 1997;50(3):162–165

Zhong-ji C, Chao C. Earlobe reconstruction using island flap with postauricular blood vessels. Facial Plast Surg 1990;5:426–430

Index

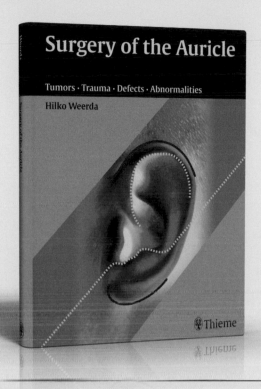 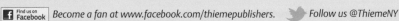
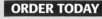
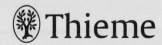